What You Need to Know
To Live a Spiritual Life

Compiled and Edited by
Joan S. Peck

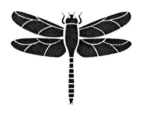

What You Need to Know to Live a Spiritual Life

Authors

Bautista, Precious

Botch, Barbara

Brandon, Magdalena

Carrillo, Cattel

Clark, Mary Jo

Covington, Angi

Dougas, Garry

Dove, Danielle

Garcia, Danielle

Goecke, Susan

Grissett, Carole

Hagen, Beatrice

Hannon, CJ Dr.

Hosmer, Maria

Johnson, Cheryl

Johnson, Dianne

Kaufman, Christian

Moreo, Judi

Murphy, Regina

Pasqui, Barbara

Peck, Joan

Ping, Doreen

Rahim, Elta

Robinson, Leeza

Sterling, Sheila

Strauss, Alice

Vicchiullo, Donna

Wilson, Janice Marie

Bejeweled Press
Henderson, Nevada

What You Need to Know to Live a Spiritual Life
Compiled and Edited By Joan S. Peck

The intent of this material is to provide general information to help your quest for emotional and spiritual growth. The authors and publisher of this book do not dispense medical advice or prescribe any technique as a form of treatment for physical or emotional problems and, therefore, assume no responsibility for your actions.

ISBN: 978-0-9824607-2-6
First Edition: October 2011

Published by:

Bejeweled Press
Phone: 702-423-4342
www.bejeweledpress.com

Cover Art by Mia Heintzelman
Printed in the United States of America

This book is dedicated to each reader

May your life journey be filled with love, joy, and peace.

FOREWARD

One of the most profound results from living a spiritual life is a sense of ease in your daily living, even if surrounded by chaos. This effortless flow of life is easier than your mind may, in the beginning, allow you to believe. It takes only one step, a little peek in the door, a toe dip in the acknowledgment of an ocean of messages, to guide you each and every day. Then you do it, you take that first step...you pick up this book or one similar that calls you. You can almost hear the angels and your guides singing with happiness that you are awakening, as you consume the messages that are meant for you within the lines that you read. Congratulations, you are in for an amazing ride!

There are many wonderful characteristics that immediately drew me to Joan Peck when I first met her in 2009. Her natural, authentic nature is one of my most favorite qualities about her. When you are in Joan's presence you are wrapped in love. It may sound trite to some, maybe even a bit airy-fairy, but the truth of the matter is that feeling that I receive from Joan is what our souls are striving for, that kind of acceptance, love and authenticity. This is part of the path that you will walk when you live a spiritual life. Can you imagine it? Many are living it right now....why not you?

Joan's ability to simplify a subject that countless make so challenging to understand is invaluable to me in my practice of running a center focused on vibrational healing. She has a great gift in bringing spiritual and personal growth material to life clearly, which takes a lot of the mystery out of certain subjects and makes them accessible as with her previous works on the chakras.

One such clarification is that there are many names for the same Source with which you are making a higher connection. Some such names are Higher Power, God, Source, Divine, Universe, Internal Navigation, Creator and so many more. Whatever name feels right to the individual is the perfect name. It is important to understand that this is a personal journey – your name – your connection. Each person has their own inner guidance that will help them on this spiritual path of a renewed way of living. Through the inner voice, your path will be lit up like runway lights guiding you in the right direction and choices to make.

Each author who participated in this book, many whom I know personally from working with them at the center, are incredible souls on their own paths. There is no guru or master per se that has all the answers for you, but their experiences of their spiritual journey will touch you, will assist you to recognize and to encourage your direction. The beauty of this type of book is that you will receive a taste of so many modalities, in so many different voices, collated in one place for you to explore in the comfort of your choosing.

And there again, lies the magnificence of this composition. There are many therapies, viewpoints and personalizations, it is important to remember to take what resonates for you and to discard the rest. To paraphrase what the Historical Buddha once said about the technique of meditation – "So you are eating a fruit salad, you don't like bananas, discard the bananas. It is still a fruit salad."

What resonates with you about these stories will stand out, what may not seem relevant now may prove to be extremely helpful later. As you journey along this course, remind yourself that you are a Divine being, just as you are. Right now, at this moment, the Universe is shining on you, so in love with who you, exactly as you are. Always Divine, and always perfect.

Once you open the door to your own healing, raising your vibration by just the very act of reading this book, changes will occur. There will be a shifting of internal and external forces that will align you to your new vibration. This could look like releasing old habits that no longer serve you, distaste for propaganda news and violent types of movies, a moving away from certain friends or learned negative thought patterns. There will be a thinning of the illusionary veil that shielded you from the very knowing of your Divinity, the very part of you that is the energy that makes up all creation.

You are awakening to your true self. It is quite the difficult path to turn back on. It reminds me of the 1989 movie, "Field of Dreams" with Kevin Costner. His character and his family could clearly see the baseball players from "the other side" playing on this field that he was guided to build; his brother-in-law could not see them until he changed his vibration, opening his heart. It is hard to stop seeing once you have seen. Experiencing living with ease, authenticity and compassion, as well as the joy and love that you feel for all life and humankind could well mean you having to cancel your "bug-man," as you will come to experience all life as being precious and part of you.

There is mention of Extraterrestrials relating to spirituality, which some may find a bit strange or even off-putting. I encourage you to keep an open mind. Explore the subject of Galactic guidance when you are ready - maybe this is the time to do so. Use your internal "feeling" monitor to know when the subject is of interest. From my experience, their loving, non-physical assistance has been extraordinary but, as with all people and energies, there are high vibrational entities and low ones. Use your discerning guidance to know the difference. You can access this knowing, if you will quiet yourself, listen, and allow it.

Everyone's journey to awakening and leading a spiritual life is as diverse as we are individual beings. There is no "right" way. As this book will introduce, there is an array of subjects within the umbrella of spirituality, let your inner knowing guide you to the areas that are meant for you. This combined effort is a beautiful introduction to the God-spark that is truly you and your higher vibrational energy that will transform your life as you know it. Welcome aboard!

Lee Papa

Founder, Ganesha Center, Sanctuary for the Spirit – Las Vegas, NV

Contents

Preface

Today, we all seem to be searching for ways to heal ourselves whether it is for our body, mind or spirit. When you consider what is going on in today's living, there are many reasons to seek out a spiritual side. These reasons usually come from deep within our soul when we can't seem to make sense from everyday happenings. When we look around and see what is going on in the world, we are inspired to turn inward. I know that I'm not the only one who turns on the news to end up wondering why I had bothered to do so. Most of the news is upsetting and negative with no positive outcomes...only conflicts. Once I immerse myself into the political scenarios presented in the news and some of the "educational" talk shows, I literally become ill with either an upset stomach or headache. I feel powerless...I hear things I don't want to hear and see things going on that is painful. What I see happening goes against what I believe in my heart. I then seek to find comfort in what I know is true for me. It is that knowing that led me to write this book with others to give direction and information to those seeking a spiritual life where they can find understanding, peace and joy.

There are many of us in today's world who want to expand our exposure and beliefs beyond what we already know. We are not going to be satisfied until we reach out to discover all the different ways that we can live "to our highest good." We are aware that in today's world, the way most of our societies function is not working on the highest vibrational level. There is too much anger, hatred, violence and greed. Through the media, we are reminded on a daily basis of many people who are or have been in positions of power, who have abused their power in numerous ways that have had disastrous effects on others. We are reminded of sexual abuse by the catholic priests, the financial abuse by Wall Street and the banks and many other examples affecting all aspects of our living. The result of this is that those in power have not only lost their credibility, but have laid an unconscionable lack of trust in those in power at the feet of those less empowered. This is happening on every level, whether it is local, state-wide, nationally or internationally. This abusive power covers all levels of destruction whether it is within a position of intimacy, perhaps within a family, or within a position that is more exposed in a larger, more public way. The reaction that this is causing is our increasing awareness that although we may *feel* helpless with decisions made by others who have power over us, each of us *has* the power and responsibility to get our own life in order. It is only then that we can become strong enough to create an environment that is productive, healthy and lucrative, ultimately benefiting all.

Another reason for us to look into the spiritual way of living may be the idea of extraterrestrials. This is not a new idea and for many of us, it is easily accepted that there has to be something beyond ourselves and our universe...that we cannot be the only ones. Recently, there have been reports where abductees have come forward with their experiences with extraterrestrials, some of whom have had micro-chips removed from them that none of our scientists are able to reproduce. We are shown other examples from both the past and present that demonstrate that it is more than likely we have had visitations from other planets...from drawings in caves and tombs to modern day crop circles. Even the History Channel on our television sets proclaims the existence of alien bodies stored at one of our mid-west Air Force Bases. Our kids are growing up with this knowledge and it does not seem to scare them. Instead, they want to know more and this has opened the doorway for many of us to seek to understand what is beyond our current experience.

However, at the same time, it is important to look realistically at the unknown as presented by the media. There are many movies, books, and TV programs that provide us insights into fantasy sub-cultures that lean toward the more bizarre and unlikely. They feed the human appetite for horror and have de-sensitized us toward violence and created the notion that everyone or everything, real or otherwise, is "out to get us." This theme carries the idea that we are helpless and highlights the "dark side." But when we think about this in an objective way, we recognize that where there is dark, there has to be light. We know the law of the universe means that everything is in balance. And this gives us power. For those of us who believe in Spirituality, the more we become aware of the negative things in our life, we are inspired to find ways to balance them with good. I believe that is why so many of us are turning to Spirituality. We are no longer willing to settle for less than the best it can be. And we accept that each one of us is accountable to learn and understand the different spiritual modalities that can help us reach the goals of love, joy and peace so that we may share our knowledge with others. And these modalities lead us to love, appreciate and connect to our higher power, whether it is God, Allah, Jesus, and any of the others that represent the creator.

We can't ignore that we have war in our lives and how it affects those involved, their families and loved ones. Again, through the media, we at home have even participated in and played an off-stage part in the wars in the near east by watching our soldiers in action in real time on television. Although, for many, this may have resulted in de-sensitizing us toward war itself, in general, the concept of war has provided an ever-increasing conflict within our being because spirituality does not approve of war. This conflict increases when we see "first hand" via television the destruction that it causes. Some say that as long as we have men, we will have wars...that this is part of life. Historically, for the most part, all war has gotten us is dead bodies and an interlude because force is not lasting. We have numerous physical and emotional problems with the returning veterans, "agent orange" and drug addiction, for example, from the Viet Nam war. And now we have veterans from wars in the Middle East returning home not only with addictions and emotional problems, but with a greater sense that war is wrong. And I believe that is happening because our spiritual vibration is higher and the higher vibrations don't accept war as part of living to our highest good. And these confused and unhappy soldiers are seeking spiritual healing for atoning for their past actions; and yet they only did what was asked of them by our country.

In our world today, most of us live so out of balance that it is no wonder that children are coming into this world with little or no addiction and are becoming addicted. We have created an atmosphere where escaping from any struggle through drugs is encouraged and allowed. We keep piling on stress in our daily lives and lay unrealistic expectations on our children without a thought as to enjoying in a healthy way the joy of being who we are as individuals. Even our thoughts are in terms of black and white (not skin color) with no allowance for thoughts to be individual. We came into human form to journey toward our wholeness with the divine. Yet, it has become increasingly easy for us to forget that as we lose our way through our greed, and judgments of others. We need to get our lives in balance before we lose our ability to do so. So where do we go from here?

Our universal consciousness is vibrating at higher levels than ever before and with that comes the knowledge that we are all one...that what we do to one affects us all. There is an innate knowing in our soul that things aren't right on earth at this time and that we must do things differently. That realization alone has made a number of us forego the old staid ways of thinking or just going along with what others dictate to us. Spirituality has led the way for this change.

Even scientists are becoming more accepting to that which is beyond their learning and knowledge. Many of them are endorsing healing practices that work with energy fields and are seeing positive results without being able to explain how it happens. They also are recognizing that our body has the ability to heal without ingesting many of the man-made concoctions that may ultimately poison our bodies. This does not mean that western medicine is bad for us. In fact, western medicine has come a long way in stamping out some of the diseases, like polio and measles, which have provided heartache in the past. What I am saying is that by combining both western and eastern healing methods, we have expanded the opportunity to honor and respect all ways to heal to bring the greatest success.

There are other indicators that times are changing and that people are ready to broaden their beliefs, feelings and emotions beyond their experience. If you have picked up this book, you are already on your way to growing spiritually.

Spirituality is not something to be feared. It is living with the belief that everything is energy, including ourselves, and because of this, when we die, we simply lose our human form, but continue to exist in energy form and can communicate with the living. Although loved ones have died and are on the "other side," it is still possible for us here on earth to work with them to help not only their spiritual growth, but our own spiritual growth and that of our planet, which will provide all of us joy and peace - an unbelievable peace after a frenzied existence of continued stress that we ourselves have created and exists on earth today.

This book is designed to empower you to expand your ideas and beliefs so that you can live a spiritual life to your highest good and the highest good of others. Each author in this book who has shared information with you feels blessed to do so. Each is an extraordinary person in many ways that is unique to them and all are making themselves available to you should you want to seek them out.

I consider the making of the book like the very old story of Stone Soup, which goes something like this. During war time in France, a group of French soldiers were looking for food to satisfy their hunger. Most in the village would not even come to the door when the soldiers knocked and no one would share any food with them. The soldiers built a fire in the center of the village and placed a pot of water with stones in the bottom over the blaze. They stood around the pot and one of the soldiers began to stir round and round. Out of curiosity, one by one the villagers approached the soldiers to ask what they were doing. The soldiers answered, "We're making Stone Soup and we will share it with you." And one by one the villagers would respond by saying that they had a carrot or potato or piece of meat that they would be willing to add to the Stone Soup. As you can now envision, instead of Stone Soup, they ended up with a beautiful, heavy, delicious soup that fed everyone. And that is how I feel about this book. As each author added her or his chapter to this book, it became richer and more beautiful with delicious knowledge that will assist you in understanding Spiritual ways that can help heal you and open a new way of living for you. A kinder, gentler way of living that will give you a sense of joy that you may not have felt before.

All the authors are gifted healers who have much to share with you. We send you blessings and love as you make your way along your own life's path to discover an inner peace and tranquil knowing within your soul that we each are the other...we are all one. Once this is realized, you will be able to accept and love yourself that, in turn, will lead to accepting and loving others in your life. And love is what it is all about; to love is our purpose for living.

Part I

Facts of Dragonflies

Dragonflies have been on earth for 300 million years. A fossilized dragonfly had the wing span of 2 ½ feet. The largest dragonfly today is found in Costa Rica and has a wing span of 7 ½ inches.

There are 5,000 different species of dragonflies in the world; 450 species can be found in the United States. They look much like they did in "dinosaur times" but have gradually gotten smaller.

Dragonflies are fantastic flyers, darting like light, twisting, turning, changing direction, even going backwards as the need arises. They are inhabitants of two realms – beginning in water and moving to the air with maturity, yet staying close to water. After leaving water and becoming flying insects, they only live for about a month.

Dragonflies have two pairs of wings. The wings are mostly transparent and move very fast, so it often appears that they have more than two pairs. They don't have to beat their wings in unison like other insects do. Their front wings can be going up while their back ones are going down. They only flap their wings at approximately 30 beats per second compared to a bee's 300.

The adult dragonfly can see nearly 360 degrees around it at all times. The eyes of the dragonfly contain thousands of tiny lenses while we humans have only one.

Dragonflies are one of the fastest flying insects. Some of the faster species can fly upward of 30 miles an hour and are well suited to eat other insects right out of the air.

Although many people fear them, dragonflies cause no harm to humans whatsoever. They are often curious toward humans and will fly around you for that reason, but they do not sting or bite.

1

Spiritualism Spirituality

When you first choose to live a life of spirituality, there is always confusion on other people's part when they ask you what you mean by that. Does this mean that you denounce organized religion of any kind? Does this mean that you don't believe in God? Does this mean that you sit around holding séances or having tarot cards read? Does this mean you meditate all day? What does it mean?

There is a distinct difference between Spiritualism and Spirituality although by looking at the words, they appear to be much the same. This book is about Spirituality. However, it is important to learn about Spiritualism so that you can understand the differences between the two. If you are a Spiritualist, it does not mean that you can't live a life of Spirituality or vice versa. For many who practice a spiritual life, they adhere to what Spiritualism encompasses. Let's examine both so that the differences, though sometimes subtle, become clear.

Spiritualism

Spiritualism is the belief system or religion that has a belief in God, but with the distinctive belief that spirits of the dead reside in the spirit world and can be contacted by "mediums," who then relay to others messages given to them about the afterlife.

Spiritualism developed and reached its peak from the 1840s to the 1920s, with most of the followers being from the middle and upper classes, both in the United States and Europe. It is interesting to note that when it began, it was not formally organized. Many of the followers were women, who supported causes such as abolition of slavery and women's suffrage and that alone was an incentive for many others to join in the Spiritualist movement. Spiritualism gave power to the mediums (mainly women) and provided women one of the first forums in the U.S. where they could address mixed public audiences. By the late 19th century, spiritualism suffered credibility because of fraud among those who misrepresented themselves as mediums. Eventually, this gave the followers incentive to formalize Spiritualism as an organization by creating Spiritualist churches in the United States and the United Kingdom.

"Spiritualists believe in communicating with the spirits of the dead through mediums. They believe that spirits are capable of growth and perfection, progressing through higher spheres or planes; that the afterlife is not a static place, but one in which spirits evolve. The two beliefs – that contact with spirits is possible, and that spirits may lie on a higher plane – lead to a third belief, that spirits can provide knowledge about moral and ethical issues, as well as about God and the afterlife. Thus many members speak of spirit guides – specific spirits, often contacted, relied upon for worldly and spiritual guidance." [Wikipedia]

Spiritualism has features in common with Christianity, such as the essentially Christian moral system. However, Spiritualists do not believe that a person's level of faith or what he does during his lifetime determines whether a person upon death goes to heaven or hell for eternity. They see the afterlife as different hierarchical planes where a spirit can progress. "Spiritualists differ from Protestant Christians in that the Judeo-Christian bible is not the primary source from which they derive knowledge of God and the afterlife; for them, their personal contacts with spirits provide that." [Wikipedia]

The great majority of Spiritualists do not accept that the death of Jesus Christ on the cross was to pay for all of mankind's sins; they believe that each person is responsible for and has to answer to his own thoughts, words and deeds after death upon his return to the spiritual realms.

They also believe that there is not a single heaven or hell, but a series of higher and lower heavens and hells.

Spirituality

Spirituality is the inner pathway that enables a person to discover the essence of their being. Spiritual practices include meditation, prayer, contemplation and other modalities for healing a person's emotions and allowing for a connectedness with the divine realm. Spirituality is a soul journey to understanding your role in life, the universe and beyond, connecting with your higher self and higher power.

Although many equate spirituality with religion, most consider spirituality to be more personalized, less structured and more open to new ideas and influences than doctrinal faiths of organized religions. Even some atheists are spiritual, believing that in some way the entire universe is connected.

Spirituality is often seen as a spiritual pathway or ascension, along which one advances to a higher state of awareness or communication with God. Plato wrote about this in his "Allegory of the Cave." The spiritual journey is a path that is individual and subjective to the one travelling it. A spiritual path may be of short duration with a specific goal in mind or it may be life-long with every event of living a part of it. Spirituality is also described as a process in two phases: the first on inner growth, and the second on the manifestation of its result in daily living.

"For a Christian, to refer to him or herself as "more spiritual than religious" may (but not always) imply relative deprecation of rules, rituals, and tradition, while preferring an intimate relationship with God. The basis for this belief is that Jesus Christ came to free humankind from those rules, rituals, and traditions, giving humankind the ability to "walk with spirit" thus maintaining a "Christian" lifestyle through that one-to-one relationship with God." [Wikipedia]

Those who define themselves as spiritual but not religious believe that there are many different spiritual paths and that it is important to find one's own individual path. They believe that religion is an outward search while spirituality is a search within oneself.

5

Spirituality plays a large role in self-help movements, such as Alcoholics Anonymous, because it involves a search for inner peace, which is accomplished by spiritual practices. This is where discovering and using the different modalities in this book become so helpful. By using these practices, you can find purpose and meaning in life.

When anyone grows spiritually, it tends to upset those around them because it can force those around them to change, as well. The dynamics are no longer the same, and not everyone is willing to change. Once you involve yourself in the spiritual modalities, your friends may not understand or accept what you are doing, and you may even lose a friendship over it…hard to believe, though it happens.

When you are clear about what spirituality is and stands for in your mind, it is much easier for those around you to accept your choice of exploring your own spirituality and taking part in the different modalities. It is also to your benefit to understand some of the entities and terminology used in spiritual gatherings. And it is for that reason, that the next chapters cover the wonderful, seven Archangels and what they represent, the knowing Ascended Masters and who they are, and often-used references and terms.

Finding your place in the world of spirituality is wondrous. It is personal and quiet. You don't need to convince anyone else of its value because for each person it is something different. Your spirituality is your own relationship with your higher power; you don't need someone to speak for you, although you are grateful for positive blessings from others. Everything becomes clear deep within your soul and you have an understanding of how to live your life to your highest good and the highest good of others. You are provided the strength to make any positive changes in your life that you need to make knowing that you are blessed and loved by your higher power and the universe.

2

The Seven Archangels

When I first joined various spiritual groups when I was much younger, I would hear them talk about the Archangels and the Ascended Masters and I had no idea who they were talking about. I was too shy to ask and didn't want to bring attention to myself. I listened enough to the others to figure out that chances were slim that I would be inducted into the Ascended Masters organization anytime soon, if ever. And I had gleaned that there were seven Archangels, but I didn't know their names or what they stood for although Michael's name came up repeatedly.

As I talked about putting this book together on the spiritual modalities, I realized that it would be beneficial for all of us, myself included, if the book contained information that I wish I had had at my fingertips when I first began my spiritual journey in this lifetime. It would have made more sense than gathering bits and pieces along the way. Here and in the following chapters is additional information that will give you a greater understanding of what and who is involved in the spirituality realm and the importance of the spiritual modalities. So we begin with the seven archangels.

"Angels transcend every religion, every philosophy, and every creed. In fact, angels have no religion as we know it ...their existence precedes every religious system that has ever existed on earth."

St. Thomas Aquinas

Angels are the spirits of God. According to many, angels are spirits without bodies, who possess superior intelligence, gigantic strength, and surpassing holiness. They enjoy an intimate relationship with God as His special adopted children, contemplating, loving, and praising Him in heaven. Each one of us has our own special angel. They were created to serve and minister to us, and to answer our prayers, and is their special reason for being. Angels never leave or ignore you and will listen to you whatever the time of day or night.

Angels can help bring success to your work, finances and relationships. They help to heal you, your family and friends and bring you closer to your higher self. Angels protect against all forms of danger and help to end war and bring peace and promote brotherhood and understanding.

Archangels

"Archangel is a term meaning an angel of high rank. Archangels are found in a number of religious traditions, including Judaism, Christianity and Islam. Michael and Gabriel are the Archangels named in the Bible as recognized by both Jew and many Christians. The book of Tobit mentions Raphael, who is also considered by some to be an archangel. Tobit is included in the Catholic Canon of the Bible, as well as in the Orthodox Septuagint; however, this book is considered apocryphal (mystical) by others outside of those faiths. The Archangels Michael, Gabriel and Raphael are venerated in the Roman Catholic Church with a feast on September 29, formerly March 24 for Gabriel. The named Archangels in Islam are Gabriel, Michael, Raphael and Azrael. Other traditions have identified a group of Seven Archangels, the names of which vary, depending on the source. The fallen archangel Lucifer (also known as Satan) was an archangel until he rebelled against God and was cast out of heaven by the other angels." [Wikipedia]

The Seven Archangels

Michael – the archangel of Protection and Defender of Faith

"Before you begin your day, call upon me, Michael, to equip you with armor of light and I will imbue it with my love and power. I, Michael, assure you, if you remember this, you will be protected from any imperfection of the outer world. However, you must maintain the consciousness that you are protected in this armour!

...I cut you free from all negative memories and burdens of the ages. If you do not bring them back to life through your thoughts and words, you will remain free from them.

...My great desire for earth's humanity is to help them strengthen their faith. Countless angels work for this just as I do, and always new helpers join them." [Wikipedia]

Michaels' name is said to be "He who is like God." Michael is referred to as the greatest of all angels and was the first angel that God created. In Revelations 12:7-12, it's Archangel Michael who leads his army of angels in the fight against Satan and his angels at the end of the world. Michael protects you with his mighty sword, cutting the cords that bind us to people, places and things. Call on Archangel Michael when you are in need of courage, strength and protection. He was put in charge of nature, including weather, and his purpose is to guard and protect all of God's creations. He is the patron saint of policemen. Michael loves to help anyone who reaches out to him and helps people overcome their hopelessness and easily manifest their sacred dreams.

Archangel Michael is associated with the ROOT CHAKRA invoking safety and trust for your journey in life.

Gabriel – the archangel of Resurrection

"The term resurrection is mainly known to Christians in relation to the feats of Jesus Christ, the resurrection out of the tomb and the ascension.

...but resurrection is constantly taking place in each person as well as in nature. Resurrection is magical when, after a long winter's sleep, growth starts again and renews all life. Each person who knows, can use the power of Resurrection flame for his own life stream, for his perfection and his future victory.

...may your hearts assimilate the Resurrection Energies, so that they can contribute to the renewal and to the resurrection of the Christ-consciousness in the lower self." [Wikipedia]

Gabriel's name means "God is my strength" and he is said to rule the spirit of mankind. He is said to be the angel that connects the astral and heavenly worlds. He gives guidance and helps with prophecy and vision. If your goals seem unobtainable, call on Archangel Gabriel and ask for his guidance. Famous for announcing to the Virgin Mary that she was to bear the "Son of God," Gabriel is often linked as the angel of childbirth. His symbol is the trumpet. He brings mercy, forgiveness, change and transformation. Call on Gabriel when you need clarity, vision and discipline to follow your path. Call on Gabriel when times are tough and you need direction or an important decision is to be made.

Archangel Gabriel is associated with the THIRD EYE CHAKRA, bringing emphasis to your prophetic side of life.

Raphael – the archangel of Healing and Consecration

"Illuminating streams of light connect you with the Divine World, and they will be strong and powerful, especially when your consciousness is open and uplifted. By way of this connection, the current of power flows into you as needed, and serves you and your work or being filled with your energy, is sent on by you to bless life.

...your Divine Self is the leader of these powers and you are part of Him. Never see yourself separated from your Divine Source, whose light flows constantly into you.

...we are thankful for every helper, who is willing to be a focal point for the healing powers – call on me, Raphael, if you want to bring about a blessing for the earth.

Sanctify yourself daily when you focus your attention on imperfections and ask forgiveness for the misuse of energy. Only that life current is in danger who no longer raises himself up, or fails to keep trying." [Wikipedia]

Raphael's name means "God heals," and is the last of the well-known angels who is mentioned in the bible. Raphael is the angel who helped Tobias cure his dad's blindness in the book of Tobit. Raphael gives healing, both physically and emotionally through giving and receiving love. He encourages you to communicate and share your inner wisdom to heal with thoughts, words, and creativity – a sage, seer, a healer. Archangel Raphael is also the angel of abundance. He will help eradicate any negative blocks, disease, and help you create everything you want, through visualization and focus. Raphael is associated with spring and the evening wind and can be called upon to assist in the healing of the Earth. He is charged with guiding the sun as it travels on its heavenly journey.

Raphael is associated with the CROWN CHAKRA connecting body, mind and spirit with God.

Uriel – the archangel of Service

"I, Uriel, come in your presence to strengthen the light in your hearts with my breath, to activate love and devotion, which will put you in a state to further carry on your service.

…your helpers from the angelic realm are not only delicate, charming beings, but also powerful servants of the light, with which they work and put at your disposal. Work even more with the angels who love you with devotion, who see your efforts and want to help to realize the great goal which the whole spiritual world pursues.

…your friends cover you in powerful, protective mantle as often as you ask for this, so your protection will be strong when you descend into the lower spheres to purify them." [Wikipedia]

Archangel Uriel's name means "Fire of God." He is the angel of Peace and can help you release your fears and anger, letting go of the past, bringing inner peace, transformation and harmony into your life while helping you to achieve your goals in life. Call on Uriel when you need his assistance in developing inner peace with yourself and God, and bringing peace to social and emotional relationships. Uriel is said to be the most powerful and formidable angel and his presence is said to reflect the unimaginable brightness of the throne of God, for Uriel is the keeper of the gates of Zion. Uriel's purpose is to teach truth, wholeness and Unity. He was the angel sent to Noah to warn him of impending floods. Call on Uriel to save you if you find yourself in a crisis and it's the twelfth hour.

Archangel Uriel is associated with the SACRAL CHAKRA, allowing us to create using both our feminine and masculine balance.

Chamuel – the archangel of Worship

"Holy Elixir of Life in the hearts of man, we call You forth, out of the sleep of the ages, to be kindled again to a flaming fire.

…This fire has again become active in you, yet, it needs to shine still more beautifully and radiantly and permeate your whole being. Only then will you become Christ in Action! You should direct your attention even more to this…Nothing else is so important for you, for your progress and for the awakening of all humanity. Everything external is, in comparison, of little consequence.

We answer your call to kindle this inner fire with our breath and to bring it to a brilliant shine so that you can be better assistants and helpers for me, Chamuel and the Others – on the physical plane. Standing in this Divine Fire, you should rule as lord over the lower realms when events occur that require your full engagement." [Wikipedia]

Archangel Chamuel's name means "He who seeks God." He is often described as "pure love in a winged form." Chamuel is the angel of unconditional love that lifts you from your sorrow, helping you to love yourself and others, to express your inner feelings and to release your negative emotions, mending your bruised and battered heart. There are many that claim that Archangel Chamuel was the angel who helped Jesus in Gethsemane (Luke 22:43). Call upon Chamuel when you need assistance in the matters of the heart, particularly personal relationships or when additional nurturing is required for the caring of a sick loved one or the comforting of a friend. Chamuel is there to help you release judgmental attitudes, even if you are unaware of them. He will help you use your shortcomings as an opportunity to connect with your spirit, rather than as a burden.

Archangel Chamuel is connected to the HEART CHAKRA, bringing solace of heart to your journey.

12

Jophiel – the archangel of Protection and Defender of Faith

"Through many opportunities, you have become conscious of your inner strength. Always when the situation has called for it you have had more than the usual amount of strength.

This strength grows out of our Divine Self, which takes over in exceptional situations. When your outer self becomes quiet, this power will flow into your world as enlightenment, strength and especially as inspiration.

…you, yourself, are the ones who limit this flow. Accustom yourselves to let your inner light express itself by putting your outward behavior, your intellect and emotions into the background. You can learn to always keep this light in motion, by often using a quiet moment to direct your attention to it. You will feel how your strength multiplies. Remain concentrated on the connection with me, Jophiel or the other Archangels, which is always present but needs acknowledgement in order to become active. Call upon me and I will help you." [Wikipedia]

Archangel Jophiel's name means "beauty of God," and is the archangel of wisdom and illumination. Jophiel is believed to be the first angel mentioned in the Bible. He guards the Tree of Life and drove Adam and Eve from the Garden of Eden, freeing them so that they could experience life more fully. His sword cuts through illusion. His divine purpose is to provide us with wisdom with sudden flashes of wonderful inspiration and answers to problems. Jophiel brings joy, laughter and light, helping with exams, studying and concentration, as well as developing intuition, inner wisdom and insight. Call upon Jophiel to fill your mind, body and spirit with light, enlightenment, wisdom, joy and laughter along your spiritual pathway.

Archangel Jophiel is associated with the SOLAR PLEXUS CHAKRA, discerning how to react to the feelings of others.

Zadkiel – the archangel of Invocation and Transformation

"The forgiving, purifying power of the Violet Flame is a holy ray of grace from Divine Love. The karma one earth life alone would often be too much for a person to bear. He would be crushed to death from the load, had not the greatness of Divine Grace provided for this purifying and redeeming ray.

13

...even without mankind being aware of it, this stream of grace has flowed through the atmosphere throughout the ages, being guided and watched over by the Divine Messengers, who have devoted themselves to this service of love. One cannot measure with human understanding the amount of energy needed to remove, time and again, at least the greatest of imperfections.

...thanks be to the efforts of the Great Hierachy – Brothers of Light – for having allowed the knowledge of the powerful Flame of Purification to be given to the unascended for some time.

...the success, seen through the work of humankind justifies the energy spent, and if every human would only redeem his own disharmonious creations, much would be accomplished." [Wikipedia]

Archangel Zadkiel's name means "righteousness of God." He is the angel of Forgiveness and brings comfort, gentleness, freedom and grace into the lives of anyone who asks for his help. Call on Zadkiel to purify your body, mind and soul, to heal your emotions, relationships and negative beliefs, to help you move on with your life, bringing forgiveness for yourself and others for true happiness and joy. Zadkiel is a very giving angel who presides over matters such as prosperity, speculation and money. Call on Archangel Zadkiel when you are having troubles forgiving a friend or loved one for their actions, or when you need to be forgiven by others. Zadkiel works with cellular memory to deepen your connection with your divine nature.

Archangel Zadkiel is associated with the THROAT CHAKRA as we learn to speak to our truths.

Michael, Gabriel, Raphael and Uriel are considered to be the main archangels. Some believe that these four display spiritual activity over the seasons: Spring (Raphael); Summer (Uriel); Autumn (Michael) and Winter (Gabriel).

A Catholic variation lists the archangels according to the days of the week: St. Michael (Sunday); St. Gabriel (Monday); St. Raphael (Tuesday); St. Uriel (Wednesday); St. Selaphiel (Thursday); St. Jhudiel (Friday) and St. Barachiel (Saturday).

The Seven Archangels

Michael – The Archangel of Protection and Defender of Faith (Protection)

Gabriel - The Archangel of Resurrection (Guidance)

Raphael – The Archangel of Healing and Consecration (Healing)

Uriel -   The Archangel of Service (Peace)

Chamuel – The Archangel of Worship (Love)

Jophiel –   The Archangel of Protection and Defender of Faith (Wisdom)

Zadkiel -   The Archangel of Invocation and Transformation (Forgiveness)

In Islam, there are two angels, Rakeeb and Atheed, who are believed to record the Good deeds and the mis-deeds of a person in his entire life time. Rakeeb is believed to be on the Right Shoulder of a person only recording the Good deeds and Atheed is believed to be on the Left Shoulder recording the mis-deeds. [Wikipedia]

Isn't it nice to know that you are surrounded by spiritual entities that are there to help and protect you? Isn't it comforting to realize that at different times in your life when you may have felt all alone, there were always angels, spirits and guides with you wanting the best for you? In the past, if things didn't turn out the way that you wanted them to, it might have been because they weren't supposed to according to the contract you made before you were born or simply because you made other choices using your free will that interfered with a successful outcome.

Although the angels, spirits and guides are always around you, it is important for you to ask for their help when you need help. Oftentimes, we humans, particularly we women, think that the universe knows or should know what we want or need. But it doesn't work that way. You need to be clear in what you are asking. Otherwise, your spirits won't step in unless it is an emergency or part of your plan. Talk to them and get to know them. They get so excited with each spiritual success in your life and are a terrific cheering section for you. So acknowledge them. At night, thank them for being with you and see how you become filled with love. It is amazing!

3

Ascended Masters

An Ascended Master is a being who has become Self-Realized and serves humanity; a being who has raised his or her vibration to a sustained frequency of light. He or she can come and go at will from the earth plane without the Birth/Death cycle.

There have been many Ascended Masters, both male and female, who have assisted mankind along the way. One of them was Sanat Kumara, also known in the Bible as the "Ancient of Days," or by others known as the "Lord of the World." Sanat Kumara came long ago to give assistance to the Earth when it would have been dissolved otherwise. He offered His own free will to supply the Light required to sustain the Earth and keep the Earth in the system until mankind could be raised to a point where we could carry the responsibility of emitting sufficient Light.

There are many stories about all of our Ascended Masters who have played a role in our lives from past life times. It is further claimed by various groups and teachers that the Ascended Masters serve as the teachers of mankind from the realms of spirit, and that all people will eventually attain their Ascension and move forward in spiritual evolution beyond this planet. According to these teachings, they remain attentive to the spiritual needs of humanity, and act to inspire and motivate its spiritual growth.

The Ascended Masters can seem somewhat confusing as the hierarchy can appear complicated and very broad. For simplicity's sake, I quote the information of the Ascended Masters from the spiritualhealing-now.com website:

"The Ascended Masters are a spiritual organization that consists of the highest initiates of our cosmic system. Only one who has mastered and is able to practice the first three leaves of the Book of Wisdom has access to the Brothers of Light. Since the beginning of human spiritual evolution, those who have achieved the highest state of magical perfection and have not yet consciously dissolved their individuality are to be found in the Brothers of Light.

Ascended Masters assume responsibility for the well-being and development of humankind. Though the task of the Brotherhood of Light is maintaining that development, it may not always require physical incarnation.

The Ascended Masters, Brothers of Light, are structured in accordance with a hierarchy which corresponds to the initiated members' degree of perfection. Their superior is the so-called Prime Initiator who has a rank equal to a Mahatma, the Deputy of Divine Order and the Custodian of All Secrets.

In the hierarchy he is call Urgaya, the Wise Man of the Mountain or the Old Master. He has been the Prime Initiator since the beginning of the world, but rarely manifests himself. He customarily takes on a form only for very short periods of time when he chooses to stand by and give advice to a Brother of Light regarding his task.

In the hierarchy, the Old Master has twelve subordinate adepts who have reached the highest spiritual perfection. These adepts take over the most difficult tasks, but they too are very seldom incarnate; therefore, they usually do their work through the zone which girdles the earth. Some of these adepts are only incarnated once in a hundred or a thousand years.

The Old Master and the twelve adepts form the Council of Elders and meet regularly or have special meetings to make important decisions concerning the fate of the peoples of the earth.

The Ascended Masters who guide and help with the expansion of light on this planet are God-Free Beings, not bound by time and space. Having come into embodiment, as you and I through the portals of birth, they walked the earth fulfilling the inner calling of their God Presence day by day, lifetime after lifetime. They mastered all the lesser things of this world, learning the lessons of life, balancing karma, fulfilling their earthly mission and manifesting and becoming God in action. At the completion of their mission, they achieved the ultimate Victory through the Ascension, the permanent integration with the Light of their own true reality, their mighty I AM Presence. They continue to stand ready to assist mankind of earth to accomplishing this same goal and will continue to extend the fires of their hearts till all are received into the Brotherhood of Light.

The hosts of Ascended Masters are tangible beings of Great Light! They are real, visible, glorious, living and caring friends of old who have such love, wisdom and power that the human mind gasps at its immensity. They work everywhere in the universe with complete freedom and limitless power, to do naturally all that the average individual would consider supernatural.

An Ascended Master is an individual who by self-conscious effort has generated enough love and power within himself to snap the chains of all human limitation, and so stands free and worthy to be entrusted with the use of forces beyond those of human experience. He realizes himself to be the Oneness of Omnipresent God - "Life." Hence, all forces and things obey his command because he is a self-conscious being of free will, controlling all by the manipulation of the Light within himself.

These glorious beings, who guard and help the evolving human race, are called the Ascended Masters of Love, Light, and Perfection. They are all the word Master implies because by bringing forth the love, wisdom and power of the God Self within, they manifest their mastery over all that is human. Hence, they have "Ascended" into the next expression above the human - which is Superhuman Divinity, Pure, Eternal, All-Powerful Perfection.

It is through the radiation or outpouring of his own pure and luminous essence of Divine Love that an Ascended Master is able to help those who come under his care and direction. This luminous essence has within it the highest force in the universe, for it dissolves all discord and establishes perfect balance in all manifestations. The Ascended Master's body is constantly pouring out rays of his light essence upon the discords of earth, dissolving them like the rays of force which we call light and heat from our physical sun dissolves a fog. The radiation which they pour out to humanity on earth is consciously drawn energy to which they give quality, and again send it out to accomplish a definite result. In this way, they give protection thousands and thousands of times to persons, places, conditions, and things of which mankind are totally oblivious.

The Ascended Master has the All-Knowing Mind and the All-Seeing Eye of God. From Him nothing can be hidden. Each Master knows and sees all concerning the student, for he reads clearly the record which the student has made. This reveals the state of the disciple's development, his strengths, as well as his weaknesses.

They are the wielders of such power and manipulators of such concentrated force as to stagger the imagination of the person in the outer world. The Ascended Masters are really great batteries of tremendous power and energy, and whatever touches their radiance becomes highly charged with their light essence through the same activity that makes a needle kept in contact with a magnet take on its qualities, and become a magnet also. All their help and radiation is forever a free gift of love. For this reason they never use any of their force to compel.

The Ascended Masters are the guardians of the race of men, and as in the world of physical education, various grades of teachers are provided to guide the development of the individual's growth from childhood to maturity, so do the Ascended Masters of Perfection exist to educate and help the individual that he too may expand his consciousness beyond ordinary, human, expression. Thus, he develops his superhuman attributes, until like the student graduating from college, the one, under the care and instruction of an Ascended Master, graduates out of his humanity into the full, continuous expression of his divinity.

Personal association with one or more Ascended Masters produces an intense feeling of love and gratitude that can never be put into words. Following such contact with their living presence, there can be but one overwhelming desire displacing all other desires and that is to BE ALL THAT THEY ARE! Once a student has truly, even for a fraction of a second, experienced the ecstatic bliss radiating from an Ascended

Being, there is nothing in human experience that one would not endure or sacrifice in order to reach their height of attainment and express the selfsame dominion and love.

Since 1880, the Ascended Masters have carefully released to the mankind of earth the understanding of how each individual might cooperate in winning their final freedom, and attaining the original purposes of incarnation. Precept upon precept, they have built a magnificent, cohesive understanding of true identity. Further, they have clearly outlined The Path, which has been delineated, but which has yet to be put to the test by men and women who have scarcely ventured into the mildest forms of the teaching." [www.spiritualhealing-now.com]

I recommend reading about Saint Germain, an ascended master, who has worked for 12,000 years to bring about a nation of Ascended Masters. What a fascinating entity! He has chosen to be embodied for many lifetimes from living in Atlantis to being in our lives today. It is said that he was Joseph, the father of Jesus, and held powerful positions during most of his lifetimes and assisted many others in positions of power to bring forth Light and Love. He assisted many highly recognized artists and musicians and powerful people in politics. It is said that he even helped with the construction of our own American constitution through Thomas Jefferson. It is also said that his most recent work with mankind was in the 1930's when he worked with Mr. and Mrs. Ballard to establish the focus on the "I AM" Presence.

Ascended Master Saint Germain's Cosmic Name is "Freedom." He is the Cosmic Father of the people of America. Saint Germain's work for the freedom of mankind began in that civilization seventy thousand years ago when a whole civilization could have been raised into the Ascension had they continued to give obedience instead of becoming rebellious.

An unascended Master has, according to later teachings, overcome the limitations of the physical, emotional, mental, but has chosen to postpone the final Initiation of the Ascension to remain in time and space to externalize and focus the Consciousness of God for the evolutions of the Earth.

Many of us here on the earth plane are Masters having lived many lifetimes and ascended upward on our individual journeys. This also explains the difference between an Ancient Soul and an Old Soul.

Ancient Souls are usually Masters while an Old Soul may have lived many times, but has not been able to ascend that far. It becomes clear then that an Ascended Master is one who has travelled up the spiritual ladder to completion.

Get to know the Ascended Masters and know that you can call on them at any time that you need some support. They are generous with their attention to our needs and come to our aid with much love and caring. We are so blessed to have them at our call.

4

Terminology

A

Affirmation
In personal development, an affirmation is a form of autosuggestion in which a statement of a desirable intention or condition of the world or the mind is deliberately meditated on and/or repeated in order to implant it in the mind.

Afterlife (or life after death)
A generic term referring to a continuation of existence, typically spiritual and experiential, beyond this world, or after death.

Ahimsa
A religious concept which advocates non-violence and a respect for all life. *Ahimsa* is Sanskrit for avoidance of injury. It is interpreted most often as meaning peace and reverence toward all sentient beings. Ahimsa is the core of Hinduism, Jainism and Buddhism. It's first mentioned in Indian philosophy and is found in the Hindu scriptures called the Upanishads, the oldest dating about 800 BC. Those who practice Ahimsa are often vegetarians or vegans.

Agnosticism
Denies that man can know whether or not God exists. Therefore, it also denies the validity of the Bible. The only certainties are those that can be "proved" by science.

Aikido
Literally means "harmony energy way", or with some poetic license, "way of the harmonious spirit." It is a modern Japanese martial art. It was developed by Morihei Ueshiba over the period of the 1930s to the 1960s.

Technically, the major parts of aikido are a form of jujutsu with many joint techniques, and Japanese sword technique. Aikido is also considered to contain a significant spiritual component.

Akashic Records
Akasha is a Sanskrit word meaning "sky" or "space," and is said to be a collection of mystical knowledge that is stored on a non-physical plane of existence. The concept is common in some New Age religious groups. The Akashi Records are said to have existed since the beginning of the planet. Just as we have various specialty libraries, there are said to exist various Akashic Records with most writings referring to the Akashi Records in the area of human experience.

Alpha and Omega
Appellation of God in the book of Revelation (verses 1:8, 21:6, and 22:13). Its meaning is found in the fact that Alpha and Omega are respectively the first and last letters of the Greek alphabet. This would be similar to referring to someone in English as "the A to Z".

Altered States of Consciousness
Any state which is significantly different from a normative waking beta wave state. The expression was coined by Charles Tart and describes induced changes in one's mental state, almost always temporary. A synonymous phrase is "altered states of awareness".

Altruism
Selfless concern for the welfare of others. It is a traditional virtue in many cultures, and central to many religious traditions. In English, this idea was often described as the Golden rule of ethics. In Buddhism it is considered a fundamental property of human nature.

Angels
An angel is a supernatural being found in many religions. In scripture, they typically act as messengers, as held by the three prominent monotheistic faiths, Christianity, Judaism and Islam.

Ancestor worship
A religious practice based on the belief that one's ancestors possess supernatural powers.

Animism
Refers to belief systems that, unlike Christianity, attribute personalized souls to animals, plants, and other material objects, governing, to some degree, their existence.

Anomalous Phenomenon
An observed phenomenon for which there is no suitable explanation in the context of a specific body of scientific knowledge (e.g. astronomy or biology).

Archetype
The concept of psychological archetypes was advanced by the Swiss psychiatrist Carl Jung, c. 1919, and generally adopted in the social sciences. In Jung's psychological framework archetypes are innate, universal prototypes for ideas and may be used to interpret observations.

24

A group of memories and interpretations associated with an archetype is a complex, e.g. a mother complex associated with the mother archetype.

Aromatherapy
Commonly associated with complementary and alternative medicine (CAM), is the use of volatile liquid plant materials, known as essential oils (EOs), and other scented compounds from plants for the purpose of affecting a person's mood or health.

Ascended Master
In various descendants and offshoots of theosophy, are held to be a group of spiritually-enlightened beings, who in past incarnations were ordinary humans, but who have undergone a process of spiritual transformation.

Asceticism
Describes a life characterized by abstinence from worldly pleasures (austerity). Those who practice ascetic lifestyles often perceive their practices as virtuous and pursue them to achieve greater spirituality.

Ashram
An Ashram in ancient India was a Hindu hermitage where sages lived in peace and tranquility amidst nature. Today, the term ashram is used to refer to an intentional community formed primarily for spiritual upliftment of its members, often headed by a religious leader or mystic.

Astral
Relating to a subtle body and plane of existence that coexist with and survive the death of the human physical body.

Astral body
The astral body refers to the concept of a subtle body which exists alongside the physical body, as a vehicle of the soul or consciousness. It is usually understood as being of an emotional nature and, as such, it is equated to the desire body or emotional body.

Astral plane
The astral plane, also called the astral world or desire world, is a plane of existence according to esoteric philosophies, some religious teachings and New Age thought.

Astral Projection
Out-of-body experiences (OBEs) achieved either awake or via lucid dreaming, deep meditation, or use of psycho tropics. The consciousness or soul has transferred into an astral body which moves in the astral plane.

Astrological Age (Cycles of the ages)
An astrological age is a time period in astrology which is believed by some to cause major changes in the Earth's inhabitants' development. It roughly corresponds to the time taken for the vernal equinox to move through one of the twelve constellations of the zodiac.

Astrological Age of Aquarius
Thought to bring with it an era of universal brotherhood rooted in reason where it will be possible to solve social problems in a manner equitable

to all and with greater opportunity for intellectual and spiritual improvement. It is generally described by astrologers that in the Age of Aquarius there will be a blending of religion and science to such a degree that a religious science and a scientific religion will be formed.

Atheism

Denies the existence of any God, though it is traditionally focused on the rejection of the Biblical God.

Aura

Energy field emanating from the surface of a person or object. This emanation is visualized as an outline of cascading color and may be held to represent soul vibrations, chakric emergence, or a reflection of surrounding energy fields.

Autosuggestion

Process by which an individual trains the subconscious mind to believe something, or systematically schematizes the person's own mental associations, usually for a given purpose. This is accomplished through self-hypnosis methods or repetitive, constant self-affirmations.

Avatar

In Hindu philosophy, most commonly refers to the incarnation (bodily manifestation) of a higher being (diva), or the Supreme Being (God) onto planet Earth. The Sanskrit word avatar a- literally means "descent" and usually implies a deliberate descent into lower realms of existence for special purposes.

B

Bagua (concept)

literally means "eight trigrams," and is a fundamental philosophical concept in ancient China. It is an octagonal diagram with eight trigrams on each side. The concept of *bagua* is applied not only to Chinese Taoist thought and the I Ching, but is also used in other domains of Chinese culture, such as Feng Shui, and Martial arts.

Baha'i Faith

The Baha'i Faith is the religion founded by Baha'u'llah in 19th century Persia. According to Baha'i teachings, religious history is seen as an evolving educational process for mankind, through God's messengers, which are termed Manifestations of God.

Bhagavad Gita

The Bhagavad Gita is a Sanskrit text from the Bhishma Parva of the Mahabharata epic. Krishna, as the speaker of the Bhagavad Gita is referred to within as Bhagavan (the divine one), and the verses themselves are written in a poetic form that is traditionally chanted; The Bhagavad Gita is revered as sacred by the majority of Hindu traditions, and especially so by followers of Krishna.

Bhakti Yoga

Term within Hinduism which denotes the spiritual practice of fostering of loving devotion to God, called bhakti. Bhakti yoga is generally considered the easiest of the four general paths to liberation, or moksha (the others being Karma, Raja and Jnana Yoga), and especially so within the current age of Kali yuga (according to the Hindu cycle of time).

Biofeedback

Biofeedback is a form of complementary and alternative medicine (CAM) which involves measuring a subject's bodily processes such as blood pressure, heart rate, skin temperature, galvanic skin response (sweating), and muscle tension and conveying such information to him or her in real-time in order to raise his or her awareness and conscious control of the related physiological activities.

Blessing

Old English that originally meant "sprinkling with blood" during the pagan sacrifices. A blessing, (also used as a bestowing of such) is the infusion of something with holiness, divine will, or one's hopes. Within Roman Catholicism, Eastern Orthodoxy, and similar traditions, formal blessings of the church are performed by bishops, priests, and sometimes deacons, but as in many other religions, anyone may formally bless another.

Bodhi

Bodhi is the Pali and Sanskrit word for (spiritual) "awakening".

Bodhisattva

In Buddhist thought, a bodhisattva (Sanskrit) or bodhisatta (Pali) is a being who is dedicated to attaining Nirvana. Bodhisattva literally means "enlightenment ('bodhi') being ('sattva')" in Sanskrit; it also refers to the Buddha himself in his previous lives. In Mahayana philosophy, Bodhisattvas take an extra vow of not attaining Enlightenment (Nirvana) before all sentient beings have achieved complete Buddhahood.

Brahman

Brahman is the concept of the supreme spirit found in Hinduism. Brahman is the unchanging, infinite, immanent, and transcendent reality which is the Divine Ground of all matter, energy, time, space, being, and everything beyond in this universe. The nature of Brahman is described as transpersonal, personal and impersonal by different philosophical schools.

Buddha

In Buddhism, a buddha is any being who has become fully awakened (enlightened), and has experienced Nirvana. Buddhists do not consider Siddhartha Gautama to have been the only Buddha.

Buddhism

Buddhism is a dharmic, non-theistic religion and a philosophy. Buddhism is also known as Buddha Dharma or Dhamma, which means the "teachings of the Awakened One" in Sanskrit and Pali, languages of ancient Buddhist texts. Buddhism was founded around the fifth century BCE by Siddhartha Gautama, hereafter referred to as "the Buddha".

Bushido
Meaning "Way of the Warrior", is a Japanese code of conduct and a way of life, loosely analogous to the European concept of chivalry. According to the Japanese dictionary Shogakukan Kokugo Daijiten, "Bushido is defined as a unique philosophy (ronri) that spread through the warrior class from the Muromachi (chusei) period."

C

Causal body
The Causal body - originally Karana-Sarira - is a Yogic and Vedantic concept that was adopted and modified by Theosophy and Neo-Theosophy. It generally refers to the highest or innermost subtle body that veils the true soul.

Chakra
In Hinduism and its spiritual systems of yoga and in some related eastern cultures, as well as in some segments of the New Age movement—and to some degree the distinctly different New Thought movement—a chakra is thought to be an energy node in the human body. Nexus of biophysical energy residing in the human body, aligned in an ascending column from the base of the spine to the top of the head. In various traditions chakras are associated with multiple physiological functions, an aspect of consciousness, a classical element, and other distinguishing characteristics.

Chant
The rhythmic speaking or singing of words or sounds, either on a single pitch or with a simple melody involving a limited set of notes and often including a great deal of repetition or status. Chant may be considered speech, music, or a heightened form of speech which is more effective in conveying emotion or expressing ones spiritual side.

Channelling
The act of having spirits enter or possess one's body in order to speak and act through one as practiced in many cultures and religions. Process of receiving messages or inspiration from invisible beings or spirits.

Chi (Ch'i, Qi, Ki)
Fundamental concept of traditional Chinese culture, Qi is believed to be part of every living thing that exists, as a kind of "life force" or "spiritual energy." It is frequently translated as "energy flow," or literally as "air" or "breath."

Christ
The word is often misunderstood to be the surname of Jesus due to the numerous mentions of Jesus Christ in the Christian Bible. The word is in fact a title, hence its common reciprocal use Christ Jesus, meaning The Anointed One, Jesus. Followers of Jesus became known as Christians

because they believed that Jesus was the Christ, or Messiah, prophesied about in the Tanakh (which Christians term the Old Testament).

Christianity
Christianity is a monotheistic religion centered on the life and teachings of Jesus of Nazareth as presented in the New Testament. Christians believe Jesus to be the Son of God and the Messiah prophesied in the Old Testament. Refers to the exercise of faith in the atoning and saving work of Jesus Christ through His sacrificial death and victorious resurrection as revealed through God's holy Word. But today, as in previous centuries, it's being twisted into whatever form of faith/salvation/works combination fits today's emerging "Christian" communities.

Chromotherapy
Chromotherapy, sometimes called color therapy or colorology, is an alternative medicine method. It is claimed that a therapist trained in chromotherapy can use colour and light to balance energy wherever our bodies are lacking, be it physical, emotional, spiritual, or mental.

Clairaudience
Ability to hear things not audible within normal hearing ranges. It includes the audible perceptions of ghosts, spirits and those who are in the astral realm.

Clairsentience
A clairsentient person is able to perceive energy fields (through physical sensations), including a person's aura and vibrations (such as voice and how words are strung together). This may also explain the ability to "sense" the presence of non-corporeal entities, such as ghosts.

Clairvoyance
Extra-sensory perception whereas a person perceives distant objects, persons, or events, including perceiving an image hidden behind opaque objects and the detection of types of energy not normally perceptible to humans. Typically, such perception is reported in visual terms, but may also include auditory impressions (sometimes called clairaudience) or kinesthetic impressions.

Cognition
Refer to the mental functions, mental processes and states of intelligent entities (humans, human organizations, highly autonomous robots), with a particular focus toward the study of such mental processes as comprehension, inferencing, decision-making, planning and learning.

Consciousness
A quality of the mind generally regarded to comprise qualities such as subjectivity, self-awareness, sentience, sapience and the ability to perceive the relationship between oneself and one's environment. Many philosophers divide consciousness into phenomenal consciousness which is experience itself and access consciousness which is the processing of the things in experience.

Many cultures and religious traditions place the seat of consciousness in a soul separate from the body. Conversely, many scientists and philosophers consider consciousness to be intimately linked to the neural functioning of the brain dictating the way in which the world is experienced. This aspect of consciousness is the subject of much debate and research in philosophy of mind, psychology, brain biology, neurology and cognitive science.

Contemplation
A type of prayer or meditation in the Christian, especially Catholic tradition. It is an attempt to experience God directly. It is connected to Christian mysticism, and authors such as Teresa of Avila, Margery Kempe, Augustine Baker and Thomas Merton have written about it extensively. It is briefly described in the Catechism of the Catholic Church, paragraphs 2709 onwards, where the Song of Songs is quoted.

Cosmogony
The coming into existence and the creation and origination of the universe. It is also the *study* of these aspects. So *a cosmogony* describes how the universe came to be; hence, the creation myth in the Book of Genesis is one such cosmogony, and there are many others, both scientific and mythological. This contrasts with cosmology, which studies the Universe at large, throughout its existence.

Cosmic consciousness
Cosmic consciousness is the concept that the universe is a living superorganism with which animals, including humans, interconnect, and forming a collective consciousness which spans the cosmos.

Creation myth
The term creation myth refers to myths that describe the beginnings of humanity, earth, life and the universe). Creation myths may explain that the beginnings of the universe were a deliberate act of "creation" by a supreme being. As with any set of beliefs, opinions regarding the validity of particular creation myths differ—points of view on these subjects vary widely.

Cult
In religion and sociology, a cult is a term designating a cohesive group of people (generally, but not exclusively a relatively small and recently founded religious movement) devoted to beliefs or practices that the surrounding culture or society considers to be outside the mainstream.

D

Deism
Historical and modern deism is defined by the view that reason, rather than revelation or tradition should be the basis of belief in God. Deists reject organized religion and promote reason as the essential element in making moral decisions. This "rational" basis was usually founded upon the cosmological argument (first cause argument), the teleological

argument (argument from design), and other aspects of what was called natural religion. Deism has become identified with the classical belief that God created but does not intervene in the world, though this is not a necessary component of deism.

Deity(or a god)

A postulated preternatural being, usually, but not always, of significant power, worshiped, thought holy, divine or sacred, held in high regard, or respected by human beings. They assume a variety of forms, but are frequently depicted as having human or animal form. Sometimes it is considered blasphemous to imagine the deity as having any concrete form. They are usually immortal. They are commonly assumed to have personalities and to possess consciousness, intellects, desires, and emotions much like humans. Such natural phenomena as lightning, floods, storms, other "acts of God", and miracles are attributed to them, and they may be thought to be the authorities or controllers of every aspect of human life (such as birth or the afterlife). Some deities are asserted to be the directors of time and fate itself, to be the givers of human law and morality, to be the ultimate judges of human worth and behavior, and to be the designers and creators of the Earth or the universe. Some of these "gods" have no power at all-they are simply worshipped.

Demon

In religion, folklore, and mythology a demon (or daemon) is a supernatural being that has generally been described as a malevolent spirit, and in Christian terms it generally understood as an angel not following God.

Demonology

Demonology is the systematic study of demons or beliefs about demons. Insofar as it involves exegesis, demonology is an orthodox branch of theology.

Devil

The Devil is a title given to the supernatural entity, who, in Christianity, Islam, and other religions, is a powerful, evil entity and the tempter of humankind. The Devil commands a force of lesser evil spirits, commonly known as demons.

Dharma

Dharma is the underlying order in nature and human life and behaviour considered to be in accord with that order. Ethically, it means 'right way of living' or 'proper conduct,' especially in a religious sense. With respect to spirituality, dharma might be considered the Way of the Higher Truths. Dharma is a central concept in religions and philosophies originating in India. These religions and philosophies are called Dharmic religions. The principal ones are Hinduism, Buddhism, Jainism and Sikhism.

A Sanskrit word meaning roughly *law* or *way* - the way of the higher Truths. Beings that live in harmony with Dharma proceed quicker towards nirvana or personal liberation, a concept first taught in Indian religions (Hinduism, Buddhism, Jainism and Sikhism).

Dhikr Arabic. ("invocation" or "remembrance")

Also spelled *zikr* based on its pronunciation in Turkish and Persian. Dhikr is the remembrance of God commanded in the Qur'an for all Muslims. To engage in dhikr is to have awareness of God according to Islam. Dhikr as a devotional act includes the repetition of divine names, supplications and aphorisms from hadith literature, and sections of the Qur'an. More generally, any activity in which the Muslim maintains awareness of God is considered dhikr.

Dogma

Dogma is the established belief or doctrine held by a religion, ideology or any kind of organization, thought to be authoritative and not to be disputed or doubted.

Druid

In Celtic polytheism the word druid denotes the priestly class in ancient Celtic societies, which existed through much of Western Europe north of the Alps and in the British Isles until they were supplanted by Roman government and, later, Christianity.

Dualism

Dualism is the view that two fundamental concepts exist, which often oppose each other, such as good and evil, light and dark, or male and female. The word's origin is the Latin dualis, meaning "two" (as an adjective).

E

Enlightenment

As a concept is related to the Buddhist Bodhi, but is a cornerstone of religious and spiritual understanding in practically all religions. It literally means being illuminated by acquiring new wisdom or understanding.

Epiphany "miraculous phenomenon"

A Christian feast intended to celebrate the 'shining forth' or revelation of God to mankind in human form, in the person of Jesus. The observance had its origins in the eastern Christian churches, and included the birth of Jesus; the visit of the three Magi (Caspar, Melchior and Balthasar) who arrived in Bethlehem; and all of Jesus' childhood events up to his baptism in the Jordan by John the Baptist. The feast was initially based on, and viewed as a fulfillment of, the Jewish Feast of Lights. This was fixed on January 6.

Eckankar

Eckankar, Path of the Light and Sound of God is a teaching founded by Paul Twitchell in 1965. The teaching emphasizes the value of personal spiritual and physical experiences as the most natural way back to God and does not advocate reliance on external authority, books or dogmatic beliefs.

Ego

In spirituality, and especially nondual, mystical and eastern meditative traditions, the human being is often conceived as being in the illusion of individual existence, and separateness from other aspects of creation. This "sense of doership" or sense of individual existence is that part which believes it is the human being, and believes it must fight for itself in the world, is ultimately unaware and unconscious of its own true nature.

Empath

Possesses the ability to sense the emotions of other sentient life forms.

Energy

Energy in spirituality refers to a widespread belief in an inter- or intra-personal forces. Believers assume spiritual energy to be of a different type than those known to science, and therapies involved are often classed as alternative medicine.

Enlightenment

In religious use, enlightenment is most closely associated with South and East Asian religious experience, being used to translate words such as (in Buddhism) Bodhi or satori, or (in Hinduism) moksha.

Entity

An entity is something that has a distinct, separate existence.

Eschatology

A part of theology concerned with the final events in the history of the world or the ultimate fate of human kind, commonly phrased as the end of the world. In many religions, the end of the world is a future event prophesied in sacred texts or folklore.

ESP (Extra Sensory Perception)

Perception that involves awareness of information about something (such as a person or event) not gained through the senses and not deducible from previous experience. Classic forms of ESP include telepathy, clairvoyance, and precognition.

Esoteric (Esotericism)

The term Esotericism refers to the doctrines or practices of esoteric knowledge, or otherwise the quality or state of being described as esoteric, or obscure. Esoteric knowledge is that which is specialized or advanced in nature, available only to a narrow circle of "enlightened", "initiated", or highly educated people. In contrast, exoteric knowledge is knowledge that is well-known or public.

Esotericism

Refers to knowledge suitable only for the advanced, privileged, or initiated, as opposed to exoteric knowledge, which is public. It is used especially for mystical, occule and spiritual viewpoints.

Eternity

While in the popular mind, eternity often simply means existing for an infinite or limitless amount of time, many have used it to refer to a timeless existence altogether outside of time. There are a number of arguments for eternity, by which proponents of the concept, principally, Aristotle, purported to prove that matter, motion, and time must have existed eternally.

Etheric plane

In Theosophy, the etheric plane is related to the Prana principle and is understood as the vital, life-sustaining force of living beings and the vital energy in all natural processes of the universe.

Etheric body

The etheric body, or vital body is one of the subtle bodies in esoteric philosophies, in some religious teachings and in New Age thought. It is understood as a sort of life force body or aura that constitutes the "blueprint" of the physical body, and which sustains the physical body.

Ethics

Ethics, a major branch of philosophy, is the study of values and customs of a person or group. It covers the analysis and employment of concepts such as right and wrong, good and evil, and responsibility.

Evil

In religion and ethics, evil refers to the morally or ethically objectionable behaviour or thought; behavior or thought which is hateful, cruel, excessively sexual, or violent, devoid of conscience.

Evolution (Spiritual)

Spiritual evolution is the philosophical, theological, esoteric or spiritual idea that nature and human beings and/or human culture evolve along a predetermined cosmological pattern or ascent, or in accordance with certain pre-determined potentials. The term higher evolution is used in Theosophy and in Buddhism to indicate the development of consciousness in human beings, as distinct from, although continuous with, the 'lower' or biological evolution within the animal kingdom up to the human level.

Existentialism

Existentialism is a philosophical movement which claims that individual human beings have full responsibility for creating the meanings of their own lives.

Exorcism

The practice of evicting demons or other evil spiritual entities which are supposed to have possessed (taken control of) a person or object. The practice, though ancient in roots, is still part of the belief system of many religions. The word "exorcism" means "I cause [someone] to swear," referring to the exorcist forcing the spirit to obey a higher power.

F

Faith healing

The use of solely spiritual means in treating disease, sometimes accompanied with the refusal of modern medical techniques. Another term for this is spiritual healing. Faith healing is a form of alternative medicine.

FastingThe act of willingly abstaining from all food and in some cases drink, for a period of time. Depending on the tradition, fasting practices may forbid sexual intercourse, as well as refraining from eating certain types or groups of food, such as meat. Fasting for religious and spiritual reasons has been a part of human custom since pre-history.

Feng Shui

Feng shui (fengshui) is the ancient Chinese practice of placement and arrangement of space to achieve harmony with the environment. The literal translation is "wind-water". Feng shui involves the use of geographical, psychological, philosophical, mathematical, aesthetic and astrological concepts in relation to space and energy flow.

Flotation Tank (Isolation Tank)

An isolation tank is a lightless, soundproof tank in which subjects float in salty water at skin temperature. They were first used by John C. Lilly in 1954 in order to test the effects of sensory deprivation. Such tanks are now also used for meditation, relaxation, and in alternative medicine.

Four Noble Truths

The Four Noble Truths are one of the most fundamental Buddhist teachings. They are among the truths Gautama Buddha realized during his experience of enlightenment. The Four Noble Truths are a formulation of his understanding of the nature of "suffering", the fundamental cause of all suffering, the escape from suffering, and what effort a person can go to so that they themselves can "attain happiness."

Freemasonry

Freemasonry is a fraternal organization with millions of members. It exists in various forms worldwide, with shared moral and metaphysical ideals and in most of its branches requires a constitutional declaration of belief in a Supreme Being.

G

Gaia

The Gaia hypothesis is an ecological hypothesis that proposes that living and nonliving parts of the earth are viewed as a complex interacting system that can be thought of as a single organism. Named after the Greek earth goddess.

Gestalt Therapy

Gestalt Therapy is a psychotherapy that focuses on experience in the now, the therapist-client relationship, and personal responsibility. It was co-founded by Fritz Perls, Laura Perls and Paul Goodman in the 1940s-1950s.

Ghost

A ghost is a non-corporeal manifestation of the spirit or soul of a dead person which has remained on Earth after death.

Glossolalia

Comprises the utterance of what appears to the casual listener either as an unknown foreign language, simple nonsense syllables, or utterance of an unknown mystical language; the utterances sometimes occur as part of religious worship.

Certain Christians regard the act of speaking in tongues as a gift of God through the Holy Spirit; one of the Gifts of the Spirit. Other religions also use glossolalia as a component of worship.

Gnosticism

Gnosticism (from Greek gnosis, knowledge) is a term created by modern scholars to describe a diverse, syncretistic religious movement, especially in the first centuries C.E. Gnostics believed in gnosis, the knowledge of God enabled by secret teachings. A blanket term for various mystical initiatory religions, sects and knowledge schools, which were most prominent in the first few centuries AD. It is also applied to modern revivals of these groups and, sometimes, by analogy to all religious movements based on secret knowledge gnosis, can lead to confusion.

God

The name God refers to the deity held by monotheists to be the supreme reality. God is generally regarded as the sole creator of the universe. Theologians have ascribed certain attributes to God, including omniscience, omnipotence, omnipresence, perfect goodness, divine simplicity, and eternal and necessary existence.

Great Awakenings

Commonly said to be periods of religious revival in Anglo-American religious history. They have also been described as periodic revolutions in American religious thought. The Great Awakenings appear to form a cycle, with a period of roughly 80 years. There are three generally accepted Great Awakenings in American history: The First Great Awakening (1730s - 1740s); The Second Great Awakening (1820s - 1830s); The Third Great Awakening (1880s - 1900s).

The importance of discerning between a true guru and a false one is explored in scriptures and teachings of religions in which a guru plays a role, and by skeptics both in the West and in India.

Guardian Spirit (Guardian Angel)

A guardian angel is a spirit who protects and guides a particular person.

Guru

A teacher in Hinduism, Buddhism or Sikhism. Based on a long line of philosophical understanding as to the importance of knowledge, the guru is seen in these religions as a sacred conduit, or a way to self-realization.

In India and among people of Hindu, Buddhist or Sikh belief, the title retains a hallowed meaning.

In Western usage, the original meaning of guru has been extended to cover anyone who acquires followers, and not necessarily in an established school of philosophy or religion. In a further metaphorical extension, guru is used of a person who has authority because of his or her perceived knowledge or skills in a domain of expertise.

H

Hatha Yoga
Is a particular system of Yoga introduced by Yogi Swatmarama, a sage of 15th century India, and compiler of the Hatha Yoga Pradipika. In this treatise Swatmarama introduces Hatha Yoga as 'a stairway to the heights of Raja Yoga', hence a preparatory stage of physical purification that renders the body fit for the practise of higher meditation. Hatha Yoga is what most people in the West associate with the word "Yoga".

Heaven
Heaven is a plane of existence in religions and spiritual philosophies, typically described as the holiest possible place, accessible by people according to various standards of divinity (goodness, piety, etc.) Christians generally hold that it is the afterlife destination of those who have accepted Jesus Christ as their savior.

Hell
Hell, according to many religious beliefs, is an afterlife of suffering where the wicked or unrighteous dead are punished. Hells are almost always depicted as underground. Christianity and Islam traditionally depict hell as fiery, Hells from other traditions, however, are sometimes cold and gloomy. Alternatively, Hell would not be a place or locality but a state of being, where one is seperated of God - thought to be held back by unrepented sin and/or corruption of spirit.

Herbalism
Herbalism, also known as medicinal Botany (a neologism by Dr. K. Seshagirirao, University of Hyderabad, India), medical herbalism, herbal medicine, herbology, botanical medicine and phytotherapy, is a traditional medicinal or folk medicine practice based on the use of plants and plant extracts.

Heresy
Heresy is a "theological or religious opinion or doctrine maintained in opposition, or held to be contrary, to the Roman Catholic or Orthodox doctrine of the Christian Church, or, by extension, to that of any church, creed, or religious system, considered as orthodox.

Higher consciousness (Christ consciousness, super consciousness, Buddhic consciousness, God-consciousness)
Expressions used in various traditions of spiritual science and psychology to denote the consciousness of a human being who has

reached a higher level of evolutionary development and who has come to know reality as it is.

Higher Self

Higher Self is a term associated with multiple belief systems and is sometimes associated with the eternal, conscious, and intelligent being. The term has been popularized by those involved in new age and new religious movements (Neopaganism).

Hinduism

Hinduism is a religion that originated on the Indian subcontinent. With its origins in the Vedic civilization and, to a minor degree, in the Indus Valley Civilization it has no known founder, being itself a conglomerate of diverse beliefs and traditions. Hinduism contains a vast body of scriptures. Divided as revealed and remembered and developed over millennia, these scriptures expound on a broad of range of theology, philosophy and mythology, providing spiritual insights and guidance on the practice of dharma (religious living). Among such texts, Hindus consider the Vedas and the Upanishads as being among the foremost in authority, importance and antiquity.

Holism (Holistic)

Holism is the idea that all the properties of a given system cannot be determined or explained by the sum of its component parts alone. Instead, the system as a whole determines in an important way how the parts behave.

Holiness

The state of being holy or sacred, that is, set apart for the worship or service of God or gods. It is most usually ascribed to people, but can be and often is ascribed to objects, times, or places. The word holy is related to the word whole.

Homeopathy

Homeopathy is a system of alternative medicine that aims to treat "like with like." Homeopathic formulas are based on the theory that even when a remedy is diluted with water to the point where no starting material remains, the water will retain a "memory" of what it was once in contact with.

Horoscope

In astrology, a horoscope is a chart or diagram representing the positions of the Sun, Moon, and planets, the astrological aspects, and sensitive angles at the time of an event, such as the moment of a person's birth.

Hymn

A song specifically written as a song of praise, adoration or prayer, typically addressed to a god.

A writer of hymns is known as a hymnist or hymnodist, and the process of singing a hymn is called *hymnody*; the same word is used for the collectivity of hymns belonging to a particular denomination or period (e.g. "nineteenth century Methodist hymnody" would mean the body of hymns written and/or used by Methodists in the nineteenth century).

Books called hymnals are collections of hymns, which may or may not include music.

Hypnagogia (Hypnogogic)

Hypnagogia are the experiences a person can go through in the hypnagogic (or hypnogogic) state, the period of falling asleep. Hypnagogic sensations collectively describe the vivid dream-like auditory, visual, or tactile sensations that can be experienced in a hypnagogic or hypnopompic state.

Hypnosis

Psychological condition of altered state of consciousness in which some people may be induced to show various differences in behaviour and thinking, like heightened suggestibility and receptivity to direction.

Hypnotherapy

Hypnotherapy is therapy that is undertaken with a subject in hypnosis. A person who is hypnotized displays certain unusual characteristics and propensities, compared with a non-hypnotized subject, most notably hyper-suggestibility, which some authorities have considered a sine qua non of hypnosis.

I

I Ching

The oldest of the Chinese classic texts. It describes an ancient system of cosmology and philosophy which is at the heart of Chinese cultural beliefs. The philosophy centers on the ideas of *the dynamic balance of opposites, the evolution of events as a process,* and *acceptance of the inevitability of change.* In Western cultures, the *I Ching* is regarded by some as simply a system of divination; others believe it expresses the wisdom and philosophy of ancient China.

Iconolatry

Icon in Greek simply denotes a picture but has now come to be closely associated with religious art used by the Orthodox and the Roman Catholic Churches. Icons are used by Orthodox Churches to assist in prayer and worship of God. Icon (image) is the same word used in the Bible in Genesis 1:27, Colossians 1:15.

Incarnation

Incarnation, which literally means enfleshment, refers to the conception, and live birth of a sentient creature (generally human being) who is the material manifestation of an entity or force whose original nature is immaterial.

Incorporeal

Incorporeal, from Latin, means without the nature of a body or substance. The idea of the incorporeal refers to the notion that there is an incorporeal realm or place, that is distinct from the corporeal or material world.

Infinity

The word infinity comes from the Latin infinitas or "unboundedness." It refers to several distinct concepts which arise in philosophy, mathematics, and theology.

InitiationInitiation is a rite of passage ceremony marking entrance or acceptance into a group or society. It could also be a formal admission to adulthood in a community. It can also signify a transformation in which the initiate is reborn into a new role.

Inner peace (or peace of mind)

A colloquialism that refers to a state of being mentally or spiritually at peace, with enough knowledge and understanding to keep oneself strong in the face of discord or stress. Being "at peace" is considered by many to be healthy and the opposite of being stressed or anxious. Peace of mind is generally associated with bliss and happiness. Most religious people believe that it is only truly possible to achieve inner peace with divine intervention of some form or another.

Peace of mind, serenity, and calmness are descriptions of a disposition free from the effects of stress. In some cultures, inner peace is considered a state of consciousness or enlightenment that may be cultivated by various forms of training, such as prayer, meditation, T'ai Chi Ch'uan or yoga, for example. Many spiritual practices refer to this peace as an experience of knowing oneself.

Integrity

Comprises the personal inner sense of "wholeness" deriving from honesty and consistent uprightness of character. Evaluators, of course, usually assess integrity from some point of view, such as that of a given ethical tradition or in the context of an ethical relationship.

Interconnectedness

Interconnectedness is part of the terminology of a worldview which sees a oneness in all things. A similar term, interdependence, is sometimes used instead, although there are slightly different connotations. Both terms tend to refer to the idea that all things are of a single underlying substance and reality, and that there is no true separation deeper than appearances.

Intuition

Intuition is an immediate form of knowledge in which the knower is directly acquainted with the object of knowledge. Intuition differs from all forms of mediated knowledge, which generally involve conceptualizing the object of knowledge by means of rational/analytical thought processes.

Intuitive

A person sensitive to the feelings of other life forms, as well as signals of nature.

Involution

In integral theory, the process by which the Divine manifests the cosmos is called involution. The process by which the creation rises to higher states and states of consciousness is the evolution. Involution prepares the universe for the Big Bang; evolution continues from that point forward. The term *involution* comes from the idea that the divine *involves* itself in creation.

Islam

Islam is a monotheistic religion originating with the teachings of Muhammad, a 7th century Arab religious and political figure. The word Islam means "submission", or the total surrender of one's self to God, and the word Muslim means "one who submits (to God)". Muslims believe that God revealed the Qur'an to Muhammad, God's final prophet, and regard the Qur'an and the Sunnah (the words and deeds of Muhammad) as the fundamental sources of Islam.

J

Jainism

Jainism is a dharmic religion and philosophy originating in Ancient India. The Jains follow the teachings of Tirthankaras. The 24th Tirthankara Lord Mahavira lived in ca. 6th century BC.

Japa: (or Japam)

A spiritual discipline in which a devotee repeats a mantra or the name of the God. The repetition can be aloud or just the movement of lips or in the mind. This spiritual practice is present in the major religions of world. This is considered as one of the most effective spiritual practices.

Jihad

An Islamic term, from the Arabic root *jhd* ("to exert utmost effort, to strive, struggle"), which connotes a wide range of meanings: anything from an inward spiritual struggle to attain perfect faith to a political or military struggle to further the Islamic cause. The meaning of "Islamic cause" is of course open to interpretation. The term is frequently mistranslated into English as "holy war," although jihad can apply to warfare. Mainstream Muslims consider jihad to be the most misunderstood aspect of their religion by non-Muslims. The Islamic religious legitimacy of the goals or methods of various Islamist movements who adopt the terminology of jihad is often brought into question, usually by moderate and liberal Muslims.

Jnana Yoga

Jnana yoga is one of the four basic paths in yoga (jnana, bhakti, raja and karma.), according to Yoga and Vedanta philosophies. Jnana in Sanskrit means "knowledge" and is often interpreted to mean "knowledge of the true self".

Judaism

Judaism is the religion of the Jewish people, based on principles and ethics embodied in the Bible (Tanakh) and the Talmud. According to Jewish tradition, the history of Judaism begins with the Covenant between God and Abraham (ca. 2000 BCE), the patriarch and progenitor of the Jewish people. Judaism is one of the first recorded monotheistic faiths and among the oldest religious traditions still in practice today.

K

Kabbalah

Kabbalah literally means "receiving", and is sometimes transliterated as Cabala, Kabbala, Qabalah, or other permutations. According to its adherents, intimate understanding and mastery of the Kabbalah brings man spiritually closer to God and as a result man can be empowered with higher insight into the inner-workings of God's creation effectively enabling prophecy and even control over nature.

Karma

A term in several Indian religions that comprises the entire cycle of cause and effect. Karma is a sum of all that an individual has done and is currently doing. The effects of those deeds actively create present and future experiences, thus making one responsible for one's own life. In religions that incorporate reincarnation, karma extends through one's present life and all past and future lives as well.

Karma is the concept of "action" or "deed" in Dharmic religions understood as denoting the entire cycle of cause and effect described in Hindu, Jain, Sikh and Buddhist philosophies. Karma is believed to be a sum of all that an individual has done, is currently doing and will do. The effects of all deeds actively create past, present and future experiences, thus making one responsible for one's own life, and the pain and joy it brings to others.

Karma Yoga

Karma yoga or the "discipline of action" is based on the teachings of the Bhagavad Gita, a sacred Sanskrit scripture of Hinduism. One of the four pillars of yoga, Karma yoga focuses on the adherence to duty (dharma) while remaining detached from the reward. It states that one can attain Moksha (salvation) or love of God (bhakti) by performing their duties in an unselfish manner for the pleasure of the Supreme.

Koan

A story, dialog, question, or statement in the history and lore of Chan (Zen) Buddhism, generally containing aspects that are inaccessible to rational understanding, yet that may be accessible to intuition. Koans are often used by Zen practitioners as objects of meditation to induce an experience of enlightenment or realization, and by Zen teachers as *testing questions* when a student wishes to validate their experience of enlightenment.

Kundalini

Kundalini according to various teachings is believed to be a type of "corporeal energy". Kundalini is envisioned as a serpent coiled at the base of the spine. According to Hindu tradition, through specific meditative exercises, Kundalini rises from the root chakra up through the spinal channel, called sushumna, and it is believed to activate each chakra it goes through.

Kundalini Yoga

Kundalini Yoga is a system of meditative techniques and movements within the yogic tradition that focuses on psycho-spiritual growth and the body's potential for maturation.

L

Law of Attraction

The Law of Attraction is commonly associated with New Age and New Thought theories. It states people experience the corresponding manifestations of their predominant thoughts, feelings, words, and actions and that people therefore have direct control over reality and their lives through thought alone.

Love

Has many different meanings in English, from something that gives a little pleasure ("I loved that meal") to something one would die for, such as patriotism. It can describe an intense feeling of affection, an emotion or an emotional state. In ordinary use, it usually refers to interpersonal love. Probably due to its psychological relevance, love is one of the most common themes in art.

Just as there are many types of lovers, there are many kinds of love. Love is inherent in all human cultures. It is precisely these cultural differences that make any universal definition of love difficult to establish. Definitions of love may include the love for a "soul" or mind, the love of laws and organizations, love for a body, love for nature, love of food, love of money, love for learning, love of power, love of fame, love for the respect of others, et cetera. Different people place varying degrees of importance on the kinds of love they receive. Love is essentially an abstract concept, easier to experience than to explain.

M

Magic

Magic and sorcery are the influencing of events, objects, people and physical phenomena by mystical, paranormal or supernatural means. The terms can also refer to the practices employed by a person to wield this influence, and to beliefs that explain various events and phenomena in such terms.

Mandala

Mandala is a term used to refer to various objects. It is of Hindu origin, but is also used in other Dharmic religions, such as Buddhism. In the Tibetan branch of Vajrayana Buddhism, they have been developed into sandpainting. In practice, mandala has become a generic term for any plan, chart or geometric pattern that represents the cosmos metaphysically or symbolically, a microcosm of the universe from the human perspective. A mandala, especially its center, can be used during meditation as an object for focusing attention.

Manifesting

Manifesting is a term often used in New Thought and New Age circles to refer to the belief that one can by force of will, desire, and focused energy, make something come true on the physical level.

Mantra

A religious syllable or poem, typically from the Sanskrit language. Their use varies according to the school and philosophy associated with the mantra. They are primarily used as spiritual conduits, words and vibrations that instill one-pointed concentration in the devotee. Other purposes have included religious ceremonies to accumulate wealth, avoid danger, or eliminate enemies. Mantras originated in India with Vedic Hinduism and were later adopted by Buddhists and Jains, now popular in various modern forms of spiritual practice which are loosely based on practices of these Eastern religions.

Maya (illusion)

Maya, in Hinduism, is a term describing the phenomenal world of separate objects and people, which creates for some the illusion that it is the only reality. For the mystics this manifestation is real, but it is a fleeting reality; it is a mistake, although a natural one, to believe that maya represents a fundamental reality.

Medium

A person who posess the ability to communicate with spirits of deceased people (and sometimes pets). Some mediums claim to be able to channel the spirit, by allowing the deceased to speak or write messages using the medium's body.

Meaning of life

The question "What is the meaning of life?" means different things to different people. The ambiguity of the query is inherent in the word "meaning", which opens the question to many interpretations, such as: *"What is the origin of life?"*, *"What is the nature of life (and of the universe in which we live)?"*, *"What is the significance of life?"*, *"What is valuable in life?"*, and *"What is the purpose of, or in, (one's) life?"*. These questions have resulted in a wide range of competing answers and arguments, from practical scientific theories, to philosophical, theological and spiritual explanations. Similar questions people ask themselves about the origin and purpose of life are "Why am I here?" and "Why are we here?"

Meditation

Refers to any of a wide variety of spiritual practices which emphasize mental activity or stillness. The English word comes from the Latin *meditatio*, which could perhaps be better translated as "contemplation." This usage is found in Christian spirituality, for example, when one "meditates" on the sufferings of Christ; as well as Western philosophy, as in Descartes'Meditations on First Philosophy, a set of six mental exercises which systematically analyze the nature of reality. Meditation describes a state of concentrated attention on some object of thought or awareness. It usually involves turning the attention inward to the mind itself. Meditation is often recognized as a component of Eastern religions.

Meridian

The concept of meridians or acu-tracts arises from the techniques and doctrines of Traditional Chinese Medicine (TCM), including acupuncture, acupressure, and qigong. According to these practices, the body's vital energy, "qi", circulates through the body along specific interconnected channels called meridians.

Metaphysics

A branch of philosophy concerned with the study of "first principles" and "being." Problems that were not originally considered metaphysical have been added to metaphysics. Other problems that were considered metaphysical problems for centuries are now typically relegated to their own separate subheadings in philosophy, such as philosophy of religion, philosophy of mind, philosophy of perception, philosophy of language and philosophy of science. In rare cases subjects of metaphysical research have been found to be entirely physical and natural, thus making them a part of physics. More recently, the term "metaphysics" has also been used more loosely to refer to "subjects that are beyond the physical world".

Mind

Mind refers to the collective aspects of intellect and consciousness which are manifest in some combination of thought, perception, emotion, will and imagination. In popular usage mind is frequently synonymous with thought: It is that private conversation with ourselves that we carry on "inside our heads."

Mindfulness

Mindfulness is a technique in which a person becomes intentionally aware of his or her thoughts and actions in the present moment, non-judgmentally.

Mind's eye (or third eye)

A phrase used to refer to one's ability to "see" things, such as Visions with the mind. This is, essentially, a reference to imagination and memory, although it can have religious or occult connotations. Also, the term "third eye" has been associated with the Pineal gland.

Miracle

According to many religions, a miracle, derived from the Latin word miraculum meaning 'something wonderful', is a striking interposition of divine intervention by God in the universe by which the operations of the ordinary course of Nature are overruled, suspended, or modified. One must keep in mind that in Judaism, Christianity, Islam and in other faiths people have substantially different definitions of the word *miracle*. Even within a specific religion there is often more than one usage of the term. Sometimes the term *miracle* may refer to the action of a supernatural being that is not a god. Then the term divine intervention refers specifically to the direct involvement of a deity.

Moksha

Refers, in general, to liberation from the cycle of death and rebirth. In higher Hindu philosophy, it is seen as a transcendence of phenomenal being, of any sense of consciousness of time, space and causation (karma). It is not seen as a soteriological goal in the same sense as in, say, a Christian context, but signifies dissolution of the sense of self, or ego, and the overall breakdown of *nama-roopa* (name-form).

Muraqaba

The Sufi word for meditation. Literally it means "to watch over", "to take care of' or "to keep an eye". Metaphorically, it implies that with meditation, a person watches over or takes care of his spiritual heart (or soul), and acquires knowledge about it, its surroundings and its creator.

Mysticism

Mysticism is the pursuit of achieving communion or identity with, or conscious awareness of, ultimate reality, the divine, spiritual truth, or God through direct experience, intuition, or insight; and the belief that such experience is one's destiny, purpose, or an important source of knowledge, understanding, and wisdom.

N

Nadi (yoga)

Nadis (Sanskrit: channel or vein) are the channels through which, in traditional Indian medicine and spiritual science, the energies of the subtle body are said to flow. They connect at special points of intensity called chakras. Nadis correspond to the meridians of traditional Chinese medicine.

Nasma

A body made of the purest form of light (called Noor) which is more pure than any visible color. This body is actually controlling the human physical body and these visible lights called Aura are visible only through Kirlian photography.

Near-death experience

A near-death experience (NDE) is an experience reported by a person who nearly died, or who experienced clinical death and then revived. The experience has become more common in recent times, especially since the development of cardiac resuscitation techniques. Popular interest in near-death experiences was sparked by Raymond Moody Jr's 1975 book Life after Life and the founding of the International Association for Near-death Studies (IANDS) in 1978.

Neopaganism (sometimes Neo-Paganism)

describes a heterogeneous group of new religious movements which attempt to revive ancient, mainly pre-Christian and often pre-Judaic Indo-European religions. As the name implies, these religions are Pagan in nature, though their exact relationship to older forms of Paganism is the source of much contention. Neopaganism or Neo-Paganism is an umbrella term used to identify a wide variety of new religious movements, particularly those influenced by ancient and pre-Abrahamic Pagan religions. Many Neopagans practice a spirituality that is entirely modern in origin, while others attempt to reconstruct or revive culturally historic Pagan and indigenous belief systems.

Neuro-linguistic programming

Neuro-linguistic programming (NLP) is a personal development system developed in the early 1970s by Richard Bandler and linguist John Grinder, in association with Gregory Bateson. NLP's core idea is that an individual's thoughts, gestures and words interact to create one's perception of the world. By changing one's outlook, a person can improve his attitudes and actions.

New Age

New Age is the term commonly used to designate the broad movement of late 20th century and contemporary Western culture, characterised by an eclectic and individual approach to spiritual exploration. Self-spirituality, New spirituality, and Mind-body-spirit are other names sometimes used for the movement. Describes a broad movement of late twentieth century and contemporary Western culture characterized by an individual eclectic approach to spiritual exploration. It has some attributes of a new, emerging religion but is currently a loose network of spiritual seekers, teachers, healers and other participants. The name "New Age" also refers to the market segment in which goods and services are sold to people in the movement.

Nirvana

Sanskrit word that means extinguishing of the passions. It is a mode of being that is free from mind-contaminants such as lust, anger or craving; a state of pure consciousness and bliss unobstructed by psychological conditioning (sankhara). All passions and emotions are transformed and pacified such that one is no longer subject to human suffering. The Buddha in the Dhammapada says of Nirvana that it is "the highest happiness". This is not the sense-based happiness of everyday life but rather an enduring, transcendental happiness integral to the calmness attained through enlightenment. In the Indian religions Buddhism,

Jainism and Hinduism, nirvāna literally means "extinction" and/or "extinguishing," and is the culmination of the yogi's pursuit of liberation.

Noble Eightfold Path

The Noble Eightfold Path is, in the teachings of the Buddha, declared to be the way that leads to the end of dukkha, or suffering. Essentially a practical guide of bringing about ethical and meditative discipline, the Noble Eightfold Path forms the fourth part of the Four Noble Truths, which have informed and driven much of the Buddhist tradition.

O

Occult

The word has many uses in the English language, popularly meaning 'knowledge of the paranormal'. For most practicing occultists it is simply the study of a deeper spiritual "reality" that extends beyond pure reason and the physical sciences.

Oneness

A spiritual term referring to the 'experience' of the absence of ego identity boundaries, and, according to some traditions, the realization of the awareness of the absolute interconnectedness of all matter and thought in space and time, or one's ultimate identity with God.

Out-of-body experience

An out-of-body experience (OBE or sometimes OOBE) is an experience that typically involves a sensation of floating outside of one's body and, in some cases, seeing one's physical body from a place outside one's body.

P

Paganism

Paganism is a term which, from a Western perspective, has come to connote a broad set of spiritual or cultic practices or beliefs of any folk religion, and of historical and contemporary polytheism religions in particular.

Pandeism

A term that has been used at various times to describe religious beliefs. This use has been inconsistent over time - some 19th century figures used the term to describe a particular set of religious beliefs; today, the term is generally used to describe broader philosophical systems, often mixing elements of pantheism (all in God, meaning All is God) and Deism (reason). The term of all that is was and shall be is represented or personified in the theological principle of 'God'.

Paradigm

Since the late 1960s, the word paradigm has referred to a thought pattern in any scientific discipline or other epistemological context.

Paranormal

Paranormal is an umbrella term used to describe a wide variety of reported anomalous phenomena. According to the Journal of Parapsychology, the term paranormal describes "any phenomenon that in one or more respects exceeds the limits of what is deemed physically possible according to current scientific assumptions."

Parapsychology

The study of the evidence involving phenomena where a person seems to affect or to gain information about something through a means not currently explainable within the framework of mainstream, conventional science. Proponents of the existence of these phenomena usually consider them to be a product of unexplained mental abilities.

Past life regression (therapy)

Past life regression is a technique used by some hypnotherapists to try to get clients to remember their past lives. Implicit in this procedure is the spiritual belief that souls exist and come back many times, living in different times and places, experiencing different genders, races, social classes and so forth in an attempt to learn.

Pilgrimage

A term primarily used in religion and spirituality of a long journey or search of great moral significance. Sometimes, it is a journey to a sacred place or shrine of importance to a person's beliefs and faith. Members of every religion participate in pilgrimages. A person who makes such a journey is called a pilgrim.

Plane (cosmology)

In metaphysics and esoteric cosmology, a plane of existence (sometimes called simply a plane, dimension, vibrating plane, or an inner, invisible, spiritual, supra physical world) is a theoretical region of space and/or consciousness beyond the known physical universe, or the region containing the universe itself. Many esoteric teachings propound the idea of a whole series of subtle planes or worlds or dimensions which, from a center, interpenetrate themselves and the physical planet in which we live, the solar systems, and all the physical structures of the universe.

Prana

Prana is a Sanskrit word meaning 'breath' and refers to a vital, life-sustaining force of living beings and vital energy in natural processes of the universe.

Prayer

An effort to communicate with God, or to some deity or deities, or another form of spiritual entity, or otherwise, either to offer praise, to make a request, or simply to express one's thoughts and emotions.

Predestination

Predestination is a religious concept which involves the relationship between the beginning of things and its destiny. Predestination concerns God's decision to determine ahead of time what the destiny of groups and/or individuals will be and also includes all of Creation.

Premonition

Premonition refers to a situation when future events are foreknown or forecast. Premonitions are usually treated as a result of paranormal or supernatural feat. However, it is possible that the human mind is capable of forecasting an accurate view of the future.

Prophecy

In a broad sense, is the prediction of future events. The etymology of the word is ultimately Greek, from *pro-* "before" plus the root of *phanai* "speak", i. e. "speaking before" or "foretelling", but prophecy often implies the involvement of supernatural phenomena, whether it is communication with a deity, the reading of magical signs, or astrology. It is also used as a general term for the revelation of divine will.

Throughout history, people have sought knowledge of future events from special individuals or groups who were thought to have the gift of prophecy, such as Oracles at Delphi in ancient Greece. Cultures in which prophecy played an important role include the North American Indians, Mayans, Celts, druids, Chinese, Egyptians, Hindus, Hebrews, Tibetans, Greeks and many in the Christian tradition, among others.

Psychic

Person who possess extra-sensory abilities, including: clairvoyance, psychometry and precognition, who can sometimes communicate with spirits, ghosts or entities.

Q

Qi

Also commonly spelled *ch'i*, *chi* or *ki*, is a fundamental concept of everyday Chinese culture, most often defined as "air" or "breath" (for example, the colloquial Mandarin Chinese term for "weather" is *tiān qi*, or the "breath of heaven") and, by extension, "life force" or "spiritual energy" that is part of everything that exists. References to qi or similar philosophical concepts as a type of metaphysical energy that sustains living beings are used in many belief systems, especially in Asia.

Qigong

An increasingly popular aspect of Chinese medicine involving the coordination of different breathing patterns with various physical postures and motions of the body. Qigong is mostly taught for health maintenance purposes, but there are also some who teach it, especially in China, for therapeutic interventions. Various forms of traditional qigong are also widely taught in conjunction with Chinese martial arts, and are especially prevalent in the advanced training of what are known as the nei chia (internal martial arts).

Quantum mechanics

Fundamental branch of physics with wide applications in experimental physics and theoretical physics that replaces classical mechanics and classical electromagnetism at the atomic and subatomic levels.

R

Raja Yoga
One of the six orthodox schools of Hindu philosophy, outlined by Patanjali in his Yoga Sutras. Raja yoga is concerned principally with the cultivation of the mind using meditation (dhyana) to further one's acquaintance with reality and finally achieve liberation.

Reality
The term reality, in its widest sense, includes everything that is, whether it is observable, comprehensible, or apparently self-contradictory by science, philosophy, or any other system of analysis. Reality in this sense may include both being and nothingness, whereas existence is often restricted to being (compare with nature). In everyday usage means "everything that exists." The term "Reality," in its most liberal sense, includes everything that is, whether or not it is observable, accessible or understandable by science, philosophy, theology or any other system of analysis. Reality in this sense may include both being and nothingness, whereas "existence" is often restricted to being.

Rebirthing-Breathwork
Branch of alternative medicine which postulates that specialized breathing techniques may have therapeutic benefits.

Reflexology
It is the practice of stimulating nerves on the feet, hands and ears, in order to encourage a beneficial effect on some other parts of the body, or to try to improve general health.

Reiki
Mikao Usui developed Reiki in early 20th century Japan, where he said he received the ability of 'healing without energy depletion' after three weeks of fasting and meditating on Mount Kurama. Practitioners use a technique similar to the laying on of hands as well as gestures in the air, which they say will channel healing energy (ki).

Reincarnation
Reincarnation, literally "to be made flesh again", is a doctrine or mystical belief that some essential part of a living being survives death to be reborn in a new body. According to such beliefs, a new personality is developed during each life in the physical world, but some part of the being remains constantly present throughout these successive lives as well. As a doctrine or mystical belief, holds the notion that one's 'Spirit' or 'Soul' depending on interpretation, 'Higher or True Self', 'Divine Spark', 'I' or 'Ego' (not to be confused with the ego as defined by psychology) or critical parts of these returns to the material world after physical death to be reborn in a new body. The natural process is considered integrative of all experiences from each lifetime. A new personality feature, with the associated character, is developed during each life in the physical world, based upon past integrated experience and new acquired experiences.

Some Reincarnation theories express that usually rebirth is made each time in alternated female and male type of bodies. Also that there is interaction between pre-determinism of certain experiences or lessons intended to happen during the physical life, and the free-will action of the individual as they live that life.

Religion

A religion is a set of beliefs and practices generally held by a community, involving adherence to codified beliefs and rituals and study of ancestral or cultural traditions, writings, history, and mythology, as well as personal faith and mystic experience.Sometimes used interchangeably with faith or belief system—is commonly defined as belief concerning the supernatural, sacred, or divine; and the moral codes, practices, values, institutions and rituals associated with such belief. In its broadest sense some have defined it as the sum total of answers given to explain humankind's relationship with the universe. In the course of the development of religion, it has taken many forms in various cultures and individuals. Occasionally, the word "religion" is used to designate what should be more properly described as "organized religion" – that is, an organization of people supporting the exercise of some religion, often taking the form of a legal entity. There are many different religions in the world today.

Religious ecstasy

A trance-like state characterized by expanded mental and spiritual awareness and is frequently accompanied by visions, hallucinations, and physical euphoria. Such an experience usually lasts about a half-hour. However, there are many records of such experiences lasting several days, and some people claim to have experienced ecstasy over a period of over three decades, or to have recurring experiences of ecstasy during their lifetime.

Repentance

The feeling and act in which one recognizes and tries to right a wrong, or gain forgiveness from someone that they wronged. In religious contexts it usually refers to repenting for a sin against God. It always includes an admission of guilt, and also includes at least one of: a solemn promise or resolve not to repeat the offense; an attempt to make restitution for the wrong, or in some way to reverse the harmful effects of the wrong where possible.

Responsibility assumption

A doctrine in the spirituality and personal growth fields holding that each individual has substantial or total responsibility for the events and circumstances that befall them in their life. While there is little notable about the notion that each person has at least some role in shaping their experience, the doctrine of responsibility assumption claims that the individual's mental contribution to his or her own experience is substantially greater than is normally thought. "I must have wanted this" is the type of catchphrase used by adherents of this doctrine when encountering situations, pleasant or unpleasant, to remind them that their own desires and choices led to the present outcome.

The term *responsibility assumption* thus has a specialized meaning beyond the general concept of taking responsibility for something, and is not to be confused with the general notion of making an assumption that a concept such as "responsibility" exists.

Revelation

Refers to an uncovering or disclosure of that which had been previously wholly or partly hidden via communication from the divine. In monotheistic religions, revelation is the process in which God makes himself, his will, and/or other information known to mankind. The recipient of revelation is commonly referred to as a prophet, and sometimes is termed a messenger.

There are a number of ways that religious thinkers have traditionally approached this topic; many widely differing views have been proposed. Generally speaking, one can find all of the following viewpoints in varying segments of Judaism and in varying groups within Christianity.

Revivalism

A revival is the apparent restoration of a living creature from a dead state to a living state. In a New Testament story, Lazarus was revived by divine intervention. In religious terms, Revival is the substitution of religious fervor in life and worship, for an intellectualized, pragmatic approach to everyday conduct (often stigmatized by revivalists as 'pride').

Ritual

A ritual is actually the words of a "rite", which are said as a part of a ceremony which is a set of actions, performed mainly for their symbolic value, which is prescribed by a religion or by the traditions of a community. A formalized, predetermined set of symbolic actions generally performed in a particular environment at a regular, recurring interval. The set of actions that comprise a ritual often include, but are not limited to, such things as recitation, singing, group processions, repetitive dance, manipulation of sacred objects, etc. The general purpose of rituals is to express some fundamental truth or meaning, evoke spiritual, numinous emotional responses from participants, and/or engage a group of people in unified action to strengthen their communal bonds. The word ritual, when used as an adjective, relates to the noun 'rite', as in rite of passage.

Rosicrucian

The Rosicrucian Order is a legendary esoteric order with its roots in the western mystery tradition. This hermetic order is viewed among earlier and many modern Rosicrucianists as a "College of Invisibles" from the inner worlds, composed of great Adepts, aiming to give assistance in humanity's spiritual development.

S

Sacred (Holiness)

Holiness, or sanctity, is the state of being holy or sacred, that is, set apart for the worship or service of God or gods. It is most usually ascribed to people, but can be and often is ascribed to objects, times, or places. The word holy is related to the word whole.

Sacrifice

from a Middle English verb meaning 'to make sacred,' and commonly known as the practice of offering food, or the lives of animals or people to the gods, as an act of propitiation or worship. The term is also used metaphorically to describe selfless good deeds for others.

Saint

Generally refers to someone who is exceptionally virtuous and holy. It can be applied to both the living and the dead and is an acceptable term in most of the world's popular religions. The Saint is held up by the community as an example of how we all should act, and his or her life story is usually recorded for the edification of future generations.

The process of officially recognizing a person as a Saint, practiced by some churches, is called canonization, though many Protestant groups use the less formal, broader usage seen in Scripture to include all who are faithful as saints.

Salvation

Refers to deliverance from undesirable state or condition. In theology, the study of salvation is called soteriology and is a vitally important concept in several religions. Christianity regards salvation as deliverance from the bondage of sin and from condemnation, resulting in eternal life with God.

Samadhi

Samadhi is a Hindu and Buddhist term that describes a non-dualistic state of consciousness in which the consciousness of the experiencing subject becomes one with the experienced object, and in which the mind becomes still (one-pointed or concentrated) though the person remains conscious.

Satan

Satan, from the Hebrew word for "adversary", is a term that originates from the Abrahamic faiths, being traditionally applied to an angel. Religious belief systems other than Judaism relate this term to a demon, a rebellious fallen angel, devil, minor god and idolatry, or as an allegory for evil

Satguru (or Sadguru)

Means true guru or true teacher. The title means that his students have faith that the guru can be trusted and will lead them to moksha, enlightenment, or inner peace, and that the teacher, guru, is the sacred conduit to self-realization.

Satori

Satori is a Japanese Buddhist term for enlightenment. The word literally means "to understand". Satori refers to "deep" or lasting enlightenment.

SBNR

Acronym used by individuals who define themselves as Spiritual But Not Religious.

Self

The Self is a complex and core subject in many forms of spirituality. Two types of self are commonly considered - the self that is the ego, also called the learned, superficial self of mind and body, an egoic creation, and the self which is sometimes called the "True Self", the "I" (or "I AM"), the "Atman", the "Observing Self", or the "Witness".

Self-realization

In yoga, self-realization is knowledge of one's true self. This true self is also referred to as the atma to avoid ambiguity. The term "self-realization" is a translation of the Sanskrit expression atma jnana (knowledge of the self or atma). The reason the term "realization" is used instead of "knowledge" is that it is knowledge based on experience, not mere intellectual knowledge.

Seminar

A seminar is, generally, a form of academic instruction, either at a university or offered by a commercial or professional organization. It has the function of bringing together small groups for recurring meetings, focusing each time on some particular subject, in which everyone present is requested to actively participate.

Seven Virtues

Derived from the Psychomachia, an epic poem written by Prudentius (c. 410). Practicing these virtues is alleged to protect one against temptation toward the Seven Deadly Sins. The *Seven Virtues* considered by the Roman Catholic Church are those of humility, meekness, charity, chastity, moderation, zeal and generosity. These are considered to be the polar opposite of the seven deadly sins, namely pride, wrath, envy, lust, gluttony, sloth and greed.

Shamanism

Shamanism refers to a range of traditional beliefs and practices concerned with communication with the spirit world. Also, refers to the traditional healing and religious practices of Northern Asia and Mongolia. By extension, the concept of shamanism has been extended in common language to a range of traditional beliefs and practices that involve the ability to diagnose, cure, and sometimes cause human suffering by forming a special relationship with, or gaining control over spirits. Shamans have been credited with the ability to control the weather, the interpretation of dreams, astral projection, and traveling to upper and lower worlds. Shamanistic traditions have existed throughout the world since prehistoric times.

Shinto (sometimes called Shintoism)
A native religion of Japan and was once its state religion. It involves the worship of kami, which can be translated to mean gods, spirits of nature, or just spiritual presences. Thus, Shinto means "the way of the gods."

Sin
Sin is a term used mainly in a religious context to describe an act that violates a moral rule, or the state of having committed such a violation.

Soul
The soul, according to many religious and philosophical traditions, is the *ethereal substance* — spirit — particular to a unique living being. Such traditions often consider the soul both immortal and innately aware of its immortal nature, as well as the true basis for the ability to feel and sense in each living being.

The concept of the soul has strong links with notions of an afterlife, but opinions may vary wildly, even within a given religion, as to what happens to the soul after death. Many within these religions and philosophies see the soul as immaterial, while others consider it possibly material.

Spacetime
In physics, space time is any mathematical model that combines space and time into a single construct called the space-time continuum. Spacetime is usually interpreted with space being three-dimensional and time playing the role of the fourth dimension. According to Euclidean space perception, our universe has three dimensions of space, and one dimension of time.

Spirit Guides
Term used by mediums and spirituals to describe an entity that remains a disincarnate spirit in order to act as a spiritual counselor or protector to a living incarnated human being.

Spiritual evolution
The philosophical/theological/esoteric idea that nature and human beings and/or human culture evolve along a predetermined cosmological pattern or ascent, or in accordance with certain pre-determined potentials. Predeterminism of evolution concept is also complemented with the idea of a creative impulse of human beings, known as epigenesis. Within this broad definition, theories of spiritual evolution are very diverse. They may be cosmological (describing existence at large), personal (describing the development of the individual), or both. They can be holistic (holding that higher realities emerge from and are not reducible to the lower), idealist (holding that reality is primarily mental or spiritual) or nondual (holding that there is no ultimate distinction between mental and physical reality). All of them can be considered to be teleological to a greater or lesser degree.

Spiritism
Spiritism is a philosophical doctrine akin to Spiritualism, established in France in the mid 19th Century, which has become a sort of religious

movement. Like Spiritualists, Spiritists believe in the survival of the souls after death and the importance of eventual communications received from them. Spiritism derives most of its principles from works by the French educator Hippolyte Léon Denizard Rivail written under the pseudonym Allan Kardec.

Spiritualism

Spiritualism is a religious movement that began in the United States and was prominent in the 1840s-1920s, especially in English-speaking countries. The movement's distinguishing feature is the belief that the spirits of the dead can be contacted by mediums. These spirits are believed to lie on a higher plane of existence than humans, and are therefore capable of providing guidance in both worldly and spiritual matters. May refer to a variety of modern religious ideologies, primarily active in the United States and Europe. Central tenets of Spiritualist liturgy and dogma are the beliefs and practices of mediumship which purports to be evidence of the continued existence of an individual's spirit or soul after deasth. The origin of Spiritualism is commonly considered to be the Modern Spiritualist movement of the 19th century United States.

Spirituality

Spirituality, in a narrow sense, concerns itself with matters of the spirit. It may include belief in supernatural powers, as in religion, but the emphasis is on personal experience. It may be an expression for life perceived as higher, more complex or more integrated with one's worldview, as contrasted with the merely sensual.

The spiritual, involving (as it may) perceived eternal verities regarding humankind's ultimate nature, often contrasts with the temporal, with the material, or with the worldly. Spirituality often focuses on personal experience. Many spiritual traditions share a common spiritual theme: the "path", "work", practice, or tradition of perceiving and internalizing one's "true" nature and relationship to the rest of existence (God, creation (the universe), or life), and of becoming free of the lesser egoic self (or ego) in favor of being more fully one's "true" "Self".

Spiritual healing

Use of spiritual means in treating disease. Spiritual healing can also refer to the self-empowerment or self-actualization process or steps within those processes that often occurs with individuals seeking enlightenment or meaning in their lives.

Subconscious

In the strict psychological sense, the adjective is defined as "operating or existing outside of consciousness". The term also appears in Sigmund Freud's very early work, to denote the unconscious mind but was soon eliminated due its ambiguity.

Subliminal message

A subliminal message is a signal or message embedded in another object, designed to pass below the normal limits of perception. These messages are indiscernible to the conscious mind, but are alleged to be perceptible to the subconscious or deeper mind.

Sufism

A mystic tradition of Islam, which is based on the pursuit of spiritual truth as a definite goal to attain. In modern language it might also be referred to as Islamic spirituality or Islamic mysticism. While fiqh focuses on the legal aspects of Islam , Sufism focuses on the internal aspects of Islam, such as perfecting the aspect of sincerity of faith and fighting one's ego. Sufi practitioners are organized into a diverse range of brotherhoods and sisterhoods, with a wide diversity of thought.

Sufi whirling

The practice of Sufi whirling (or Sufi spinning), is a twirling meditation that originated among the ancient Indian mystics and Turkish Sufis, which is still practiced by the Dervishes of the Mevlevi order. Following a recommended fast of several hours, Sufi whirlers begin with hands crossed onto shoulders and may return their hands to this position if they feel dizzy. They rotate on their left feet in short twists, using the right foot to drive their bodies around the left foot. The left foot is like an anchor to the ground, so that if the whirler loses his or her balance, he or she can think of their left foot, direct attention towards it and regain balance back.

Supernatural

The supernatural refers to forces and phenomena which are not observed in nature, and therefore beyond verifiable measurement.

Supplication (also known as petitioning)

The most common form of prayer, wherein a person asks a supernatural deity to provide something, either for that person who is praying or for someone else on whose behalf a prayer of supplication is being made. One example of supplication is the Catholic ritual of novena (from *novem*, the Latin word for "nine") wherein one repeatedly asks for the same favor over a period of nine days. This ritual began in France and Spain during the Middle Ages when a nine day period of hymns and prayers led up to a Christmas feast, a period which ended with gift giving.

Swami

Swami is primarily a Hindu honorific title, loosely akin to "master" or "teacher". It is derived from Sanskrit and means "owner of oneself", that is, a complete master over instinctive and lower urges. It is a title added to one's name to emphasize learning and mastery of a specific field of knowledge, most often religious or spiritual.

Sweat lodge

The sweat lodge is a ceremonial sauna used by North American First Nations or Native American peoples.

Synchronicity

Synchronicity is the experience of two or more events which occur in a meaningful manner, but which are causally inexplicable to the person or persons experiencing them.

Synergy

Synergy refers to the phenomenon in which two or more discrete influences or agents acting together create an effect greater than that predicted by knowing only the separate effects of the individual agents.

Synesthesia

Synesthesia is a neurological condition in which two or more bodily senses are coupled.

T

Tai chi chuan

Tai chi chuan is an internal Chinese martial art often practiced with the aim of promoting health and longevity. Tai chi chuan is considered a soft style martial art - an art applied with internal power - to distinguish its theory and application from that of the hard martial art styles.

Tantra

Tantra, tantricism or tantrism is any of several esoteric traditions rooted in the religions of India. Rather than a single coherent system, Tantra is an accumulation of practices and ideas which has among its characteristics the use of ritual, energy work, in some sects transgressional acts, the use of the mundane to access the supramundane and the identification of the microcosm with the macrocosm.

Tao Te Ching

The Tao Te Ching, roughly translatable as The Book of the Way and its Virtue, is a Chinese classic text. According to tradition, it was written around 600 BCE by the Taoist sage Laozi (or Lao Tzu, "Old Master"), a record-keeper at the Zhou Dynasty court.

Taoism

Taoism (Daoism) is the English name referring to a variety of related Chinese philosophical and religious traditions and concepts. These traditions influenced East Asia for over two thousand years and some have spread internationally. Taoist propriety and ethics emphasize the Three Jewels of the Tao; namely, love, moderation, and humility. Taoist thought focuses on wu wei ("non-action"), spontaneity, humanism, and emptiness. The Tao Te Ching is widely considered to be the most influential Taoist text.

Telepathy

Communication of information from one mind to another by means other than the known perceptual senses.

Thanatology

Thanatology is the academic, and often scientific, study of death among human beings. It investigates the circumstances surrounding a person's death, the grief experienced by the deceased's loved ones, and larger social attitudes towards death such as ritual and memorialization.

Theism

The belief in one or more gods or goddesses. More specifically, it may also mean the belief in God, a god, or gods, who is/are actively involved in maintaining the Universe. This secondary meaning is shown in context to other beliefs concerning the divine. The term is attested in English from 1678, and was probably coined to contrast with *atheism* attested from ca. 1587.

Theology

Theology finds its scholars pursuing the understanding of and providing reasoned discourse of religion, spirituality and God or the gods.

Theophysics

Theophysics is a merger between theology and physics. A branch of theology with the aim of proving the existence of a higher supreme of all (God) using physics arguments. The main area of interest for theophysicists is the Big Bang.

Theosophy

Theosophy designates several bodies of ideas in history, but the word was revived in the nineteenth century by Helena Petrovna Blavatsky to designate her religious philosophy which holds that all religions are attempts by humanity to approach the absolute, and that each religion therefore has a portion of the truth.

Theosis

In Eastern Orthodox and Eastern Catholic theology, theosis, meaning *divinization* (or *to become god*), is the call to man to become holy and seek union with God, beginning in this life and later consummated in the resurrection. *Theosis* comprehends salvation from sin, is premised upon apostolic and early Christian understanding of the life of faith, and is conceptually foundational in both the East and the West.

Tibetan Book of the Dead (Bardo Thodol)

The Bardo Thodol is a funerary text that describes the experiences of the consciousness after death during the interval known as bardo between death and rebirth. The Bardo Thodol is recited by lamas over a dying or recently deceased person, or sometimes over an effigy of the deceased.

Tibetan Buddhism

Tibetan Buddhism is the body of religious Buddhist doctrine and institutions characteristic of Tibet. It is a Mahayana Buddhist tradition, meaning that the goal of all practice is to achieve full enlightenment (or Buddhahood) in order to remove all limitation on one's ability to help all other living beings to attain this state.

Tithe (from Old English"tenth")

A one-tenth part of something, paid as a voluntary contribution or as a tax or levy, usually to support a Jewish or Christian religious organization. Today, tithes (or *tithing*) are normally voluntary and paid in cash, checks, or stockks, whereas historically tithes could be paid in kind, such as agricultural products. There are still European countries today that allow some churches to assess a mandatory tithe which is enforced by law.

Torah
A Hebrew word meaning "teaching," "instruction," or "law." It is the central and most important document of Judaism revered by Jews through the ages. It primarily refers to the first section of the Tanakh–the first five books of the Hebrew Bible, but the term is sometimes also used in the general sense to also include both of Judaism's written law and oral law, encompassing the entire spectrum of authoritative Jewish religious teachings throughout history, including the Mishnah, the Talmud, the midrash, and more.

Totem
A totem is any entity which watches over or assists a group of people, such as a family, clan or tribe. Totems support larger groups than the individual person. In kinship and descent, if the apical ancestor of a clan is nonhuman, it is called a totem. Normally this belief is accompanied by a totemic myth.

Trance
An altered state of consciousness is any state which is significantly different from a normative waking beta wave state. A synonymous phrase is "altered states of awareness".

Transcendentalism
The name of a group of new ideas in literature, religion, culture, and philosophy that advocates that there is an ideal spiritual state that 'transcends' the physical and empirical and is only realized through a knowledgeable intuitive awareness that is conditional upon the individual. The concept emerged in New England in the early-to mid-nineteenth century. It is sometimes called "*American Transcendentalism*" to distinguish it from other uses of the word transcendental. It began as a protest against the general state of culture and society at the time, and in particular, the state of intellectualism at Harvard and the doctrine of the Unitarian church which was taught at Harvard Divinity School.

Transpersonal psychology
School of psychology that studies the transpersonal, the transcendent or spiritual aspects of the human mind. Issues considered in transpersonal psychology include spiritual self-development, peak experiences, mystical experiences and other metaphysical experiences of living.

U

Unitarian Universalism (UU)
A theologically liberal, inclusive religion formed by the merger of Unitarian and Universalist organizations in the mid 20th century. UUs generally: cherish creativity, freedom, and compassion; embrace diversity and interconnectedness; and promote personal spiritual growth and justice-making through worship, fellowship, personal experience,

social action, deeds, and education. While one UU may differ from another in personal creed, the term UU is a distinct theological signifier and Unitarianism or Universalism should not be confused or interchanged with Unitarian Universalism.

Upanishad

The Upanishads are part of the Vedas and form the Hindu scriptures which primarily discuss philosophy, meditation, and the nature of God; they form the core spiritual thought of Vedantic Hinduism.

Urantia Book

The Urantia Book is a spiritual and philosophical book that discusses God, science, religion, history, philosophy, and destiny. The exact circumstances of the origin of The Urantia Book are unknown. There is not a human author associated with the book.

V

Vedas

The Vedas are a large corpus of texts originating in Ancient India. They are the oldest scriptural texts of Hinduism.

Vedanta

Vedanta is a school of philosophy within Hinduism dealing with the nature of reality.

Veneration

In traditional Christian churches (for example, Catholicism and Eastern Orthodoxy), veneration or veneration of saints, is a special act of honoring a dead person who has been identified as singular in the traditions of the religion, and through them honoring God who made them and in whose image they are made. Veneration is often shown outwardly by respectfully bowing or making the sign of the cross before a saint's icon, relics or cult image. These items are often also kissed.

Vipassana

The practice of Insight Meditation. While it is often referred to as Buddhist meditation, the practice taught by the Buddha was non-sectarian, and has a universal application. It does not require conversion to Buddhism. While the meditation practices themselves vary from school to school, the underlying principle is the investigation of phenomena (Sanskrit: dharmas) as they manifest in the five aggregates namely, matter or form, sensation or feelings, perception, mental formations & consciousness. This process leads to direct experiential perception, Vipassanā.

W

Wabi-sabi

represents a comprehensive Japanese world view or aesthetic. It is difficult to explain wabi-sabi in Western terms, but the aesthetic is sometimes described as one of beauty that is imperfect, Impermanent, or incomplete.

Wicca

Wicca is a religion found in various countries throughout the world. It was first popularised in 1954 by a retired British civil servant named Gerald Gardner after the British Witchcraft Act was repealed. He claimed that the religion, of which he was an initiate, was a modern survival of an old witchcraft religion, which had existed in secret for hundreds of years, originating in the pre-Christian Paganism of Europe.

Witchcraft

Witchcraft is the use of certain kinds of alleged supernatural or magical powers. A witch is a practitioner of witchcraft. While the term "witchcraft" can have positive or negative connotations depending on cultural context, most contemporary people who self-identify as witches see it as beneficent and morally positive. The term witch is typically feminine, masculine equivalents include wizard, sorcerer, warlock and magician.

Worship

Usually refers to specific acts of religious praise, honor, or devotion, typically directed to a supernatural being such as a god or goddess. It is the informal term in English for what sociologists of religion call cultus, the body of practices and traditions that correspond to theology. Religious worship may be performed individually, in informally organized groups, or as part of an organized service with a designated leader (as in a church, synagogue, temple, or mosque). In its older sense in the English language of *worthiness* or *respect*, *worship* may sometimes refer to actions directed at members of higher social classes (such as lords or monarchs) or to particularly esteemed persons (such as a lover). Typical acts of worship include: prayer; sacrifice (korban in Hebrew; rituals; meditation; holidays; festivals; pilgramages; hymns or psalms; the construction of temples or shrines; the creation of idols of the deity.

Y

Yana (Buddhism)

A Sanskrit word with a range of meanings including nouns such as vehicle, journey, and path; and verbs such as going, moving, riding, and marching. In the Indian religions Buddhism and Hinduism, both *yana* and maraga (road or path) express the metaphor of spiritual practice as a path or journey. Ancient texts in both religions discuss doctrines and practices associated with various *yanas*. In Buddhism, *yana* often augments the metaphor of the spiritual path with the idea of various vehicles that convey a person along that path. The *yana/marga* metaphor is similar to the Chinese image of the Tao (path or way) but Indian and Chinese cultures appear to have evolved such similar metaphors independently.

Yin and yang
The concept of yin and yang originates in ancient Chinese philosophy and metaphysics, which describes two primal opposing but complementary forces found in all things in the universe. Yin, the darker element, is passive, dark, feminine, downward-seeking, and corresponds to the night; yang, the brighter element, is active, light, masculine, upward-seeking and corresponds to the day. The concept is the cornerstone for Taoism and traditional Chinese medicine.

Yoga
A family of spiritual practices that originated in India, where it is seen primarily as a means to enlightenment). Traditionally, Karma Yoga, Bhakti Yoga, Jnana Yoga, and Raja Yoga considered the four main yogas. In the West, yoga has become associated with the postures of Hatha Yoga, which are popular as fitness exercises. Yoga as a means to enlightenment is central to Hinduism, Buddhism, and Jainism. Major branches of Yoga include: Hatha Yoga, Karma Yoga, Jnana Yoga, Bhakti Yoga, and Raja Yoga.

Yogi
A yogi or yogin is a term for one who practices yoga. These designations are mostly reserved for advanced practitioners.

Z

Zazen
A meditative discipline practitioners perform to calm the body and the mind and experience insight into the nature of existence. While the term originally referred to a sitting practice, it is now commonly used to refer to practices in any posture, such as walking.

Zen
Zen is a school of Mahayana Buddhism notable for its emphasis on practice and experiential wisdom -particularly as realized in the form of meditation known as zazen- in the attainment of awakening. As such, it de-emphasizes both theoretical knowledge and the study of religious texts in favor of direct individual experience of one's own true nature. From China, Zen subsequently spread southwards to Vietnam and eastwards to Korea and Japan.

These terms are a collection from Wikipedia, and numerous and varied spiritual websites, books, etc. where usage of the terms is commonplace.

Part II

Symbolisms of Dragonflies

Dragonflies in almost every part of the world symbolize change in the perspective of self-realization, and the kind of change that has its source in mental and emotional maturity and the understanding of the deeper meaning of life.

Dragonflies scurry across water in their flight representing an act of going beyond what's on the surface and looking deeper into the implications and aspects of life.

Dragonflies are reminders that we are light and can reflect the light in powerful ways if we choose to do so. "Let there be light" is the divine prompting to use the creative imagination as a force within your life. They help you to see through your illusions and allow your own light to shine in a new vision.

Some Native American beliefs state that dragonflies are a symbol of renewal after a time of great hardship. Others say that the dragonflies are the souls of the dead and are symbols of happiness, speed and purity (because the dragonfly eats from the wind itself).

Faerie stories say that dragonflies used to be real dragons.

Dragonflies are the most powerful in the summer under the effects of warmth and sunlight. The dragonfly's agile flight and its ability to move in all six directions exude a sense of power and poise – something that comes only with age and maturity. The dragonfly is a reminder that we can accomplish our objectives with simplicity, effectiveness, elegance and grace.

When a dragonfly lands on you, you will hear excellent news from someone far away from home. A dead dragonfly symbolizes sad news. Dragonfly symbolism crosses and combines with that of the butterfly and change. The dragonfly symbolizes going past self-created illusions that limit our growing and changing and are a symbol of the sense of self that comes with maturity.

The dragonfly symbolizes success, victory, happiness, strength and courage to the Japanese, and in China, dragonflies symbolize prosperity, and harmony.

Angels

Danielle Garcia

My life has been blessed and enriched through my communication with the mighty and benevolent spiritual beings of the Angelic Realm. I have developed a partnership with angels, and this relationship assists me in my daily life, as well as in my business practices.

I have a nickname here in Las Vegas, "The Angel Lady," so I am continuously asked questions about angels and the role they play in our lives. In this chapter, I explain more about angels and the fascinating impact they have had upon my spiritual experience, not only as a woman, wife and mother, but also as a healer, teacher and intuitive.

What is an Angel? Angels exist on the other side of the veil. They reside at home with Mother/Father God and are a bridge from the other side to here, on this earth plane. In history, angels have been termed as "divine beings who act as messengers of God" or "spirits that protect and offer guidance." I believe that both these definitions are correct. These loving beings hold the absolute pure vibration of unconditional love and this is the true essence of home. They have never incarnated in physical form, so they do not have the same experiences that we humans have. They have no knowledge of hate, anger, or negativity other than what they witness by watching life here on this plane and on other planes as well.

How Do Angels Appear? Angels may appear in many forms. They have been depicted as beautiful, graceful human forms complete with wings and halos. This is probably the most common way people see them, or visualize them. They appear in this form because it is what is widely accepted here – it is what has been taught to us through religions and through the history of time. Angels may also appear as bright colors, as balls of energy or flashes of light. The way that they are perceived, strictly depends on the level a person is who is perceiving them – meaning, if you are someone who is more spiritual, you may recognize them in a different manner than someone who is not. Or, if you are a visual person, you may see them in complete form, whereas someone who is not as visual may see them only in colors. You may not even "see" an angel, but you may sense them through vibration, energy, and even through sound.

Many years ago, while taking intuitive training, I began a practice of calling in angels before I would go to sleep and asking for guidance and assistance. I put forth the intention for my subconscious to come through to connect with these other realms so that I would be able to receive personal messages. One night, I awoke around two or three o'clock in the morning, and standing next to my bed was an enormous ten foot tall angel. He was completely black from head to toe and had amazingly huge wings covered in black feathers. The angel stared at me with his violet eyes, not speaking a word. You can imagine my fright! I thought the Angel of death was coming to get me and I must be on my way out! As I laid there, this angel continued making deep eye connection, and then basically disintegrated before my very eyes. I had no sense of alarm or panic by this time. I was merely the actively engaged witness watching this visitation unfold before my eyes. Nothing bad happened, and now I truly believe that this experience happened so that I would learn that not everything is as it seems. I had taken my past history of watching movies, reading books and seeing TV shows that associated darkness and black colors as being negative, and applied that reaction to this angel that stood less than a foot away from me. It was a lesson well learned for me that night.

On another evening, weeks later, I awoke to a beautiful light show playing out on the bedroom wall in front of me. This anomaly looked like a giant curtain of radiant sapphire and indigo blue, dancing and twinkling in waves across the wall. I blinked me eyes several times, to make sure nothing was amiss with my eyesight. I sat up and watched the heavenly occurrence continue with the fascination and awe of partaking in a thrilling ballet production. My mind and body were at a complete state of peace and utter happiness. This energy was one of my first conscious connections with the energy of Archangel Michael.

Do We All Have Guardian Angels? Yes, we all have guardian angels. An angel is assigned to you – actually you contract with this angel before you enter into this lifetime. You make the agreement with them that they will assist and guide you throughout your incarnation. They help you work towards your highest good and learn the life lessons you have chosen to learn. This angel matches the vibration of your higher self; of your soul's vibration, and this is why you work so well together. A Guardian Angel is always at hand to assist in any and every situation, no matter how large or how small. The thing to remember is that you need to ASK for their assistance. As we are beings living on a planet of free will, angels will not intervene with our lives unless there is imminent danger present. An angel will intercede with accidents and tragedies if it is not our time to exit the planet, meaning we have more work to do here. They will not interfere with other situations, such as finances, romance, health or the like, without our request for guidance. Remember, unless you ask for assistance, they cannot give it. You have the blessing of free will to make this decision and this is how it is.

Free will means that you have a choice. You get to choose how you act and react every single moment of the day. If an angel were to interfere with your choices, even if they appeared to be for your highest good, you would not necessarily learn the soul lessons you came here to complete. Always remember, you can CHOOSE to ask these amazing beings of light for assistance. Form that connection, and you will find it is like having access to the most incredible set of life coaches and tour guides twenty-four hours a day, seven days a week.

Many people don't realize that because we are blessed with this wonderful gift of free will, angels cannot always intervene. There are instances, however, when divine intervention is allowed. I experienced this myself when I was seven months pregnant with my son. I had gone for a drive by myself in the mountains of Julian in San Diego, California. As I exited the freeway, I came to a complete stop at the head of the line at a stoplight. I was in a rush to get home, and was anxiously thinking about plans for the rest of my day as I waited for the light to turn green. Normally, when the light turns green, I step on the gas because I am always on the go. Especially this day, after drinking a full bottle of water and being seven months pregnant, I needed to get home quickly. The light turned green, and I heard a very distinct, deep male voice exclaim, "Stop!" My foot would not move from the brake pedal to the gas pedal. I used all my might to lift my foot off the brake pedal, rolling forward a few inches, and again the same voice cried out, "Stop!" My foot slammed on the brakes just as I witnessed a pickup truck flying through the intersection doing about fifty-five to sixty-five miles an hour. Had I driven when the light changed to green, this truck would have plowed into my driver side door. I have no doubt my life and the life of my son was saved that afternoon. I will always be grateful for Archangel Michael's protection and for my ability to listen and heed his words of warning. I know that he watched over us that day because we have much work to complete here on this planet. It was not our time to go home.

Our Guardian Angels are always close by. In fact, they may be closer than you think! Many times when I am in session with a client, I will see their Angels behind them or beside them. Sometimes, they will be on the floor on their knees and just staring up at the person that I'm reading. Imagine watching your best friend and observing every moment of their life, good times and bad times, and knowing they do not see or hear you. Picture having this extraordinary, unconditional love for your dearest friend, and yet never able to embrace them, share laughter or offer a shoulder to lean on. This is my interpretation of what many angels experience. It does not make them sad, but when you do make the effort to connect with them, I can most assuredly tell you, they become thrilled and excited beyond measure.

How Does the Angelic Realm Communicate With You? There are many ways angels communicate with us. These communications may be very subtle, and at other times are extremely loud and clear.

Angels facilitate Divine Intervention when they step into our world to prevent accidents, pain or tragedy. They can connect to you through signs that may be a feeling you suddenly have about not taking a certain route home for example, or the voice you hear that says "Don't go through that green light." It could be the hairs that stand up on the back of your neck notifying you to be on guard of danger. Angels even take physical form when they need to intercede in certain situations.

I assist souls during their transition from the physical plane to crossing over to the other side. As I was helping my husband's grandfather, Don, through the deathing work that I do, a most unusual, yet heartwarming incident occurred. We were in the hospital's Intensive Care Unit, and Don had been removed from the machines that had been sustaining his life. I could feel his chakra centers begin to close down, one by one, and I continued the energy practice to help him pass comfortably. It was a few minutes before midnight, and a nurse we had not previously met, entered the hospital room. She spoke to Don as she inspected the monitors, and touched him on the arm as she told the family that it would not be too much longer before his transition. There was the most amazing calm and peaceful energy that filled the room as she spoke these loving and supportive words to the family. Don passed shortly after midnight, and as we left his room, I stopped at the information desk to thank this nurse for her care and reassurance. The nurse was nowhere to be found. As I described her to the supervisor, they did not know who I was talking about, nor did they have anyone working in the unit that fit that description. My heart jumped as I realized this woman was an angel, who had appeared not only for Don's comfort, but also to console and soothe his family.

Many times, angels will come to us through music. This is one of their most favorite ways to convey messages. You may be in the grocery store busy shopping, when suddenly you tune into the music playing in the background and it is a sign for you. Or, you may be sad, and the instant you turn on your radio an uplifting song that reminds you of a happy memory comes on. Many times, angels will come to me through song lyrics that are played in my head. These come through as personal messages for me, and at times, I will hear them when I am giving a session to a client. I have learned not to take all these lyrics literally because I have to remember that angels also have a brilliant sense of humor.

Angels also leave feathers around to remind us of their continued presence here. These feathers can be of any shape or color, it truly matters not. If you continue to see feathers throughout your day, know that angels are close by. Pay close attention to what is going on at the exact moment you notice these heavenly signs. What are the thoughts going on in your mind? Where are you concentrating your energy? Is there a song playing when you see these feathers, or were you thinking about a memory when you found them?

Another way that the angels send signs is through repetitive numbers. Angel numbers act as messages from these celestial beings. Look for number sequences that are repeated throughout the day, or even several times a week.

You can always set forth the intention to receive signs and communications from your angels. Watch to see what happens. When you do, the results can be astonishing.

How Can You Open Yourself Up To The Angelic Realm? This is a very simple process. Setting your intention to communicate is the most important part. Once your intention is set, you put forth the energy out to the universe that this is what you desire, and the message is received. It is then your responsibility to watch for the signs that follow, or to take an active role in bringing these messages through.

Meditation is one way to facilitate communication with the angelic realm. First of all and most importantly, put that positive intention forth of what you want to accomplish – make sure you are specific. This could be anything from "I want to know my Guardian Angel's name" to "I want guidance and assistance from my angels with this situation." Relax yourself and begin the meditation while focusing on your intention. Await the messages that will follow. It is always a good idea to have a notebook close by to take notes on what you have seen, sensed or heard during your time of connection.

An additional method to open up to the angels is by writing a personal letter to your guardian angel or one of the Archangels you feel drawn to. You need not know your guardian angel's name, so do not concern yourself with labels when it comes time to write the letter. Quiet your mind, and let the feelings and questions come forth and be written down. See what messages and signs come through during and after this process.

Singing is a beautiful method to open you to these celestial beings. The angels are so highly attuned to the vibration of music and love to communicate in this fashion. When you open your heart to sing to them, it is a blessing that is well received on the other side. Trust and know that they hear you and accept your vocal melodies as they would a most honored and admired gift.

Speaking aloud to the angels also opens the doors to their world. It may seem silly at first, but you can carry on conversations with them. Try this and see what happens. Ask your questions out loud or simply vent or express your emotions to them and see what comes through when you are finished with your dialogue.

Prayer, as always, is an instant pathway into the angelic realm, be they quiet prayers you recite inside your mind, or those that are chanted or spoken aloud.

What Tools Can Be Used to Assist With Communication? There are many tools that can be used to achieve angelic communication. Again, your intention is the strongest tool of all, and they urge me to continue to reinforce that statement.

Crystals – There are certain crystals that hold the vibration that attract the angelic realm. These crystals include the following: angel aura quartz, spirit quartz, aqua aura quartz and Celestite.

Oracle Cards or Angel Cards are another marvelous tool used to connect to the angelic realm. These cards are different than tarot cards in that the spreads are different, and each card conveys a message from the angel or angelic realm that it represents. I love Angel Cards and use them all the time. This is how I personally started connecting with the higher dimensions and it was a wonderful stepping stone for me. It was not as daunting to me as some of the other tools, and it was fun! That is what this whole spiritual path is supposed to be about anyway – bliss and joy, so you might as well be happy and having fun while you're learning about it. I enjoy the colors and scenes depicted on the Oracle Cards as they hold their own individual messages along with the written ones that appear on the cards.

Automatic Writing is another way to assist in contacting the angels. This is a process of relaxing and letting spirit guide you while you write the messages that come through. It is a form of channeling and what some consider being a wakened state of meditation.

Everyone is Different – Use What Works For You! Remember, we all have our own individual perspectives and ideals. What may work well for one person, may not work for another. Always trust your own instincts when using any type of energy work or divination tools. Use the information that I have provided as a guideline only. I share this information with you showing you what works for me personally, based on my own perception and beliefs – it is in no way, shape or form the ONLY way that works.

Part of the joy is finding out your own techniques that work for you along this blessed journey of life. Have fun while doing this. Enjoy them – go out and explore all that you can and find what truly makes your heart sing. Know that the angels are always there to assist and guide you every step along the way.

About the Author

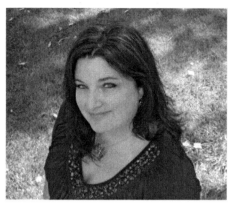

Danielle Garcia is a dedicated Intuitive, Medium, Channel, Spiritual Counselor and Author. She is a licensed Minister and Metaphysician, Reiki and Zenith Master, Crystal Therapist, and Overlight Facilitator in Spiritual Communication, Inverse Wave Therapy, Medulla and Pineal Activation, Sexual Energy, and Spiritual Psychology.

Danielle also has created her own modality, Dimensional Connection, and has written the book, "Angel Blessings – A Collection of Channeled Messages from the Angelic Realm." Her articles have appeared in the magazines: Spectrum, Energy Exchange, and Children of the New Earth.

Danielle's featured segment, "Angel Blessings" has been a part of the Virtual Light Broadcast. She communicates with the Angelic Realm to bring through messages and guidance. By using her gifts of Mediumship, Intuition, Channeling and Counseling, she assists others on their spiritual journey. It is her divine purpose to empower others and through teaching, she instructs others on the purity and power of Intuitive Development.

Danielle Garcia can be contacted at:
www.intuitiveangels.com
Danielle@intuitiveangels.com
(702) 376-2726

Astrology

Carole Grissett

Why have your chart done? Since the horoscope is a report card of where you've been and what you've done in the past and also shows what you intend to experience in this lifetime, it stands to reason that this knowledge gives you power. The power to take advantage of your strengths and those you have just discovered and the power of being forewarned of challenges on the road ahead. Forewarned is forearmed. Doesn't it make sense to get as much understanding as possible about your relationships, career opportunities, financial decisions, and all the other areas of your life? Astrology can give you insights that will allow you to confidently face life secure in the knowledge that you are taking every possible advantage available to you.

One of the most ancient of the predictive sciences, astrology can be traced back to the Bronze Age (circa 1700 BCE) when Chinese astronomers divided the sky into segments roughly equivalent to the Moon's path through the heavens each month. Two hundred years later, the Mayans created their long count calendar, which famously ends on December 21, 2012. In 900 BCE, ancient Indian astrologers developed their own system to track the Moon, followed by Third Century (CE) Babylonians who developed the mathematical schema to list planetary positions by date. One hundred years later, Arab astronomers developed the astrolabe which measured the location of stars. The 1500 CE reformation of the Church caused the decline of astrology in Europe and with the Age of Reason, around 1650, astrology lost favor in Europe.

In the 1800's almanacs grew in popularity, and by 1890, astrology was reborn. Another big shift came with the emergence of modern psychology. Astrology, once the tool of rulers and their astronomers, now was applied to the study of individual lives. In the 1970s, astrology computer programs produced the most dramatic change in the way astrology is practiced. Before that, it took as much as four to eight hours to construct a person's birth chart, and now anyone interested in astrology can purchase software to calculate astrological charts.

Although a belief in reincarnation is not necessary to make use of this science, you will find that most astrologers do believe that we've all lived before and will return again. Following that belief, your birth chart (natal chart, horoscope) is a combination of a report card of the cumulative lessons you've learned, the karmic "credits" you've built up, as well as those areas where more work is needed, and it outlines the major areas of growth you've chosen to address in this lifetime. We all have challenges; we all possess gifts. What is important is how we use our gifts and how we respond to the various experiences this lifetime provides. To quote the late astrologer, Max Heindel, "The stars incline, they do not compel." It is up to us, as individuals, what we make of the debits and credits we bring with us on our balance sheet. Even identical twins that are born three minutes apart can live very different lives because of the influences from previous lives.

In today's world, almost everyone knows their Sun Sign. Every day, millions of us peek at our daily horoscope to see what the day might bring. However, they only give a broad picture of what could happen. If you choose to know only three elements of your chart, they should be the zodiacal signs of your Sun (your Self), your Moon (your emotions), both determined by the date and time you were born and your Ascendant (rising sign).

If you look at your horoscope as a clock face, the Ascendant is the zodiacal sign at the nine o'clock position. This is the sign that is 'rising' on the horizon at the moment you took your first breath. Your Ascendant is the "mask" you wear for this lifetime. It is how people first perceive you. It is also the lens through which your Sun (Self) looks out into the world. The combination of these three influences form the tripod on which the rest of your chart rests.

Astrology is complex and fascinating. Take your time to read on to discover the talent it takes by an Astrologer to unfold your uniqueness and your individual journey this lifetime.

Once the horoscope is drawn, it resembles the face of a clock divided into twelve sections, or "houses". Each house represents an arena of life, and any planets within it describes various energies, personal will, and desires that will be experienced in that area, as well as describing the people who will impact this segment of your life. The positions of these houses are defined by the Earth's 24-hour rotation on its axis. This is why knowing the correct time of birth is so important. The houses are numbered one through twelve. Any planets residing in a house adds emphasis as well as any interaction those planets have with other planets throughout the chart.

Beginning with the Ascendant or rising sign, the 1st house indicates your manner of self-expression, character, abilities and appearance. It describes your early environment. Moving counter-clockwise, the 2nd house shows your financial assets, attitudes toward money, and basic value system. The 3rd house represents how you communicate, siblings, neighbors, and short journeys. The 4th house illustrates your home and family life, your roots, either mother or father (whichever is or was the most influential), and the conditions at the latter fourth of your life. Children, love affairs, creative outlets and entertainment are indicated by the 5th house. Working conditions and environment, your competence and skill and your general health are described by the 6th house, which completes the lower (or northern) half of the horoscope.

Opposite the Ascendant and beginning the upward (southern) climb is the 7th house which describes partnerships in general, marriage and the marriage partner, as well as those with which you have open conflicts. Continuing counter-clock wise, the 8th house indicates transformation of all kinds (including death), regeneration, inheritances, sexuality, and is also one of the so-called 'psychic' houses. The 9th house represents philosophy and religion, foreign travel and interests, higher education and relatives of the marriage partner. Your career status, mother or father (the less influential parent), public life, and people in power over you (your boss) are shown by the 10th house. The 11th house indicates friends, group associations and your hopes and wishes. The final house, the 12th represents your unconscious that you haven't integrated yet into yourself, and is also called the house of self-undoing and limitations.

The "patterns" or concentrations of planet placement are the next thing we look at. A majority of planets in the left-hand (eastern) half of the circle indicates a "sowing" lifetime, showing that you are a person who is self-determined, acting on your choices, and generally blazing your own trail. If you have a majority of planets in the right-hand (western) half of the chart, you are experiencing a "reaping" lifetime and will usually find that your path is strongly influenced by society in general and the significant others in your life. A concentration of planets in the upper half of the horoscope (south), or "above the horizon," describes you as a person who tends to be more outgoing and sociable, wanting to be in the public eye. Planets heavily weighted in the lower half of the circle (north) indicates you as a personality who may be more intellectually and physically introspective and private.

The twelve signs of the zodiac are next divided into your threefold spiritual nature (the triplicates of cardinal, fixed, and mutable signs) and then, again, into the four elements (earth, air, fire and water) which together combine to produce your individuality. Looking at your spiritual nature, if you have planets in the four cardinal signs (Aries, Cancer, Libra, and Capricorn), you have an active temperament. This makes you ambitious, ardent, energetic, and independent. Planets in the four fixed signs (Taurus, Leo, Scorpio, and Aquarius) give a set temperament. If you have planets here you can be unyielding, determined, organized, and dignified. If you have a concentration in these signs you achieve results slowly, but surely. The four mutable signs (Gemini, Virgo, Sagittarius, and Pisces) give you a more versatile, flexible, and diplomatic temperament.

Each of the four elements consists of a cardinal, a fixed, and a mutable sign. The earthy signs (Taurus, Virgo and Capricorn) yield a materialistic temperament. These folks tend to be practical, conservative and lovers of material comfort. The watery signs (Cancer, Scorpio, and Pisces) generally are intuitive, and can be susceptible to moods and impressions. The fiery signs (Aries, Leo, and Sagittarius) give an impulsive temperament and what seems to be inexhaustible energy. Folks who have a concentration of planets in the fire signs can be impulsive, sharp, and magnetic. Intellectual temperament is bestowed by the airy signs (Gemini, Libra, and Aquarius). These signs give a versatile, pleasing personality which enjoys an interchange of ideas and needs companionship. If there are too many planets in air, these folks may be a little superficial and lack stability.

The spiritual triplicates and the four elements are combined to describe you as an individual. For example, Aries is both cardinal and fire. If you have several Aries planets you will be much more impulsive than Leo, who is also fire but fixed. A Taurus would be much more unmovable (earth/fixed) than a Capricorn (earth/cardinal) who, in turn, would be harder to convince than a Virgo (earth/mutable). Mercury is the planet that shows how you think. A Gemini Mercury (air/mutable) is much more changeable than one in Aquarius (air/fixed). Venus shows how you love. A Cancer Venus (water/cardinal) is emotional, but not as intense as Scorpio (water/fixed), yet Pisces (water/mutable) would be the most flexible and considerate of the three.

We next look at how the various planets relate to (or aspect) one another. An aspect is a geometric angle between two points in the heavens, some of which are considered beneficial and others that are considered challenging. Aspects can be either "approaching" (the motion of the planets is bringing them into closer alignment), or "separating" (planetary motion is in the process of increasing the distance between them). Approaching aspects are thought to be lessons from the past that are now being brought into focus for you to work through, whereas separating aspects are considered to be experiences you've addressed in another lifetime and whose influence is now fading.

A natal chart calculated for the time of birth can be progressed (brought forward) to the present, and can be taken to any point in the future. Progressions are based on "a degree of movement per year" since birth, then transits (the current daily planetary positions) are placed as overlays to the natal chart to get a snapshot of what is going on in your life (as reflected by the heavenly patterns).

To this point we've discussed only your natal (birth) chart. There are many other branches of this science that can be extremely valuable in charting your path through life.

In the area of personal relationships, there are two chart types that I believe are very revealing. The first is the comparison of the natal horoscopes of the two people involved. The relationship can be romantic, business-based, parent and child, between siblings, neighbors, or friends. The benefit is that you can get a detailed understanding of areas of compatibility, as well as those challenging aspects of the relationship. The second takes the two natal charts in question and combines them, producing a third chart of the relationship itself. This results in a different, but complementary analysis of the interaction in question. In any relationship, the more the people involved understand where the others are coming from, the greater the communication between them, and the greater success possible for both.

Horary astrology answers specific questions. It is similar to having a Tarot reading and can address virtually anything. Where is my lost pet? How will my job interview go? Will I be offered the job? Am I going to sell my house, when and will I be pleased with the price? What's ahead on my vacation? What's the future of my current relationship? This specialty is not as well-known as some of the other astrological branches, but can provide amazingly detailed information on nearly any question posed. The key here is pinpointing the exact time the question presented itself.

Electional horoscopes are similar to Horary charts, but here you plan the beginning or birth of something ahead of time to take the greatest advantage of heavenly patterns. Examples would be scheduling a wedding, starting a business (opening the doors or signing the incorporation papers), starting a new job, beginning a major process like building a home, leaving on a special vacation, etc. An Electional chart not only allows you to select the best date and time to initiate important activities, but also gives you a forecast of what to expect along the way. This gives you as much control as possible as to the final outcome of the event in question.

Relocation astrology uses your birth date and time, but calculated for the latitude and longitude for the place in question. If the new location isn't far from your birth place, the difference in your chart will be small. But the longer the distance from your birth place, the greater the possibility the house cusps (the horoscope house markers) will change, which may also change the house placement of the planets. The value in looking at this, if you're considering a major move, is to see what areas of your life may be either emphasized or minimized in the new location. It's also helpful to compare your natal chart and the actual birth chart of the city, state or country to which you're thinking of moving. Just like in personal relationship astrology, this comparison will show you how you will get along with folks who live there, how you will fare financially, if your health will be affected or strengthened, etc. In other words, it gives you a preview of what life will be like in the new location.

Mundane astrology involves world events such as wars, political elections, current events, weather patterns, geo-physical conditions, the economy, etc. Mundane astrology is much more popular during election years such as this one and will be again in 2012. This branch also can calculate the horoscope of a city, state, or nation and plot that entity's future as if it were a living being.

Past Life and Karmic astrology are two branches of the science that, using your birth chart, delve into your past experiences and lessons learned, or lessons yet to be mastered. It cannot specify actual place of past lives, but rather concentrates on the general conditions your soul experienced, giving an overview of what was gained or lost in talents, strengths, and weaknesses,
 as a result.

To recap, the advantages of an astrological viewpoint is that you have the opportunity of moving with the natural flow of the life you've chosen, rather than going against it, swimming upstream. Your chart is a map, a forecast. It is not destiny. Your free will and the choices you make determine your life experiences. As the ancient Irish blessing says, "May your journey be one with the road rising with you and the wind always at your back."

About the Author

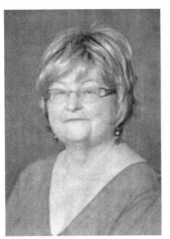

Carole Grissett has utilized Tarot, numerology, and astrology in an intuitive consulting practice serving an international clientele for over 30 years.

In her corporate business career, Carole served in a Human Resources management capacity with several Fortune 500 companies and holds a BA in Journalism, an MBA, and a MA (abt) in Industrial and Organizational Psychology.

She is an ordained minister in both the American Holistic Church and the Universal Church of the Master. Using her practical, positive approach, she continues business and individual consulting practices, as well as continuing to lecture and write.

Carole Grissett can be contacted at:
www.mypsychicpathfinder.com
polestar@netscape.com

Brainwave Optimization with Real-Time Balancing (RTB)™

Angi Covington

What it Brainwave Optimization™? Where did it come from? How does it work? How has it helped others? How might it help you or someone you love?

I am so privileged to be able to share something with you that may change your life. Before we begin, I'd like to share a little of my background and how I met this amazing technology.

While I now know I've been on a spiritual path my whole life, I certainly was not aware of it until I was 41. I'd spent my life working to be successful by traditional standards. I guess I thought I'd made it. I made a 6 figure income, drove luxury cars, purchased a nice home in a golf course community, maintained some healthy relationships with friends and family, traveled for business and treated myself to spa visits regularly. In 2005, I was faced with a lesson in attachment. My outside world took a hit when the company I loved went through a merger, a merger that experts consider to be one of the worst in history. It, however, proved Divine in *my* history!

Luckily for me, I got out pretty early with enough stock options to pay my mortgage for a few years. But, I was completely clueless about what I was going to do with the rest of my life.

My first stop was at a Tony Robbins seminar, where I received a consciousness raising energy known as Deeksha. Seven hours later I met God. I wasn't prepared for this at all! I didn't have a religious background. The most religious I'd felt was when I was in the church choir as a teen. I remember telling Him, "There are 2000 other people in this room, surely you can find one who goes to church. You've got the wrong girl!" He didn't listen...interesting to be 41 and shown for the first time that life doesn't work at all like I'd once believed.

I ended up on a 3 year sabbatical that took me to hundreds of books, seminars, modalities and three visits to India's Oneness University. Since my awareness of this path was coming to me later in life, I felt a sense of urgency to "catch up" with those who'd been aware of their spiritual path for some time. I crammed, just like in college, loading in as much as my brain could handle. The Oneness University's founder believes that if we have too much activity in our parietal lobes, we feel disconnected from others, but if we quiet the activity there, we feel a greater sense of connection to not only others, but to all that is... Oneness. Deeksha, he explained, makes that physiological shift in one's brain activity. After hearing this, I took courses about the brain to learn how its functionality affects our experience of this amazing thing called Life. I had a deep knowing that the brain was somehow going to be a part of my future. While in India, I became a Deeksha Giver and later, a Trainer for the Oneness University. No matter how much I enjoy and continue to support the Oneness Movement, there is not a viable career there for me.

I began sharing what I learned with anyone who'd listen. After a year of resistance, I wrote a book, "7 Course Meal for the Soul," and began sharing Deeksha with prison inmates on a weekly basis, during a class I teach at nearby prisons. I've been blessed to witness the transformation of many men and women over the past two years who have been in my class. Many miracles are happening behind bars, I assure you.

I continued to sample modalities like a Vegas buffet. I was looking for the best. If I found the best, the one that consistently delivered results that lasted, then that could be my life's next chapter, my purpose, my joy and my living. I found many modalities that definitely had some positive results, but usually didn't offer long-term discernable results for me. One of the modalities I tried in 2007 was then called brain training. My interest in the brain gave me high hopes, but initially I was less than impressed. In hindsight, I think I had expectations that may have been a bit unreasonable. I guess I was looking for a lightning bolt, something so amazing and profound that no one could deny it. Everyone would want it and I could offer it to them. I could make lots of money and help everyone improve their lives! Can you hear the birds singing? Anyway, my friend who'd tried the brain training along with me got the lightning bolt. He could focus and his sleep improved dramatically. It obviously did something, but just not for me. My ego concluded my brain must already be balanced. Little did I know at the time...

It took me awhile to understand how the Universe works *with* me. For example, I've learned that if something comes to me more than once, then it's probably for me. When it came to India, I think I needed 5-7 promptings before I realized, "I think I'm supposed to go to India." It's nice to know that the Universe doesn't give up on us, even if we don't "get it" right away. Nonetheless, I wasn't completely up to speed on how this all worked when the Director of the Department of Corrections suggested that I look into Brain State Technologies. I assured him that I was already familiar with the work and that I had experienced the technology first hand. I neglected to share that I hadn't been as impressed with my training as he was with his own and the inmates who had tested it. It took almost another year for Brain State to come back to me.

The gentleman who originally trained my brain called and said something like, "I know you are looking for a career and I haven't been extremely successful with my brain training business. I'd like us to partner on this. I've been offered a six month contract in Puerto Rico. I'll bring the equipment to you, you can learn how to use it while I'm gone and then use your business background to build it into the success I know it can be." I'd exhausted my stock options and was getting a little concerned about how I was going to cover my financial commitments. But, I wasn't ready to do something I didn't fully believe in just for money. I told him I'd concluded that all modalities were helpful in their own right and I was looking for a modality that was a good match for me; something that would profoundly affect my life. His response changed my view instantly. "Angi, the best thing about this modality is that you don't have to address belief systems right away." He was right; my corporate identity was far more comfortable talking about a technology that works with the brain. It can be tracked and graphed, unlike other modalities that might seem a little more *out there* to some people, people like I used to be.

In that moment, I agreed to go to Scottsdale, to receive my certification. My expectations were blown out of the water when I truly came to understand how this technology works and how it benefits virtually everyone... including me. It became clear while I was there that previously I hadn't had enough sessions to have experienced a major shift. You see, most people need anywhere from 10-30 sessions, with the average being 10-12 sessions. I had formed my conclusion after only 7 sessions. Upon my return home, I completed 10-15 additional sessions. My sleep was the most obvious thing that changed. My entire life I have needed 30-90 minutes in bed before I am able to relax enough to even consider sleep. My brain activity painted a picture of a person with anxiety. Today, two years after completing those sessions, 5 minutes and I'm in the ethers. My dreams are more vivid and I can remember them if I choose. My meditations seem easier, deeper and more peaceful.

I am a firm believer that relationships are critical in our Spirit's path. Once the imbalance in my temporal lobes rectified, I have been far less reactive to others in trying situations. Words can't tell you how this improved my relationships. One client said that it's like a pause was created for her, between what was happening and her reaction to it. My experience is concurrent with that.

So, how does your brain affect the way you react to others? Traumas lead to an imbalance in brain activity. It makes sense that the brain would operate differently in times of trauma, right? Ideally, the brain goes back into balance once the trauma is over. However, it doesn't always. If left with an imbalance, you will likely experience inconvenient or unpleasant physical and/or emotional effects, such as sleep problems, depression, anxiety, focus, addictions, pain, memory loss, physical performance, health issues, etc. The effects of my physical traumas had left me with an imbalance that not only affected my sleep but also gave me a pretty snappy temper, which, incidentally, I thought I'd inherited from my father. I'd accepted it as part of who I am, not realizing it was merely a pattern that was running in my brain. Today, I can still get angry, but it is not my brain's automatic go to. I later discovered my father experienced some pretty dramatic physical traumas in his childhood, as well. Interesting. I experienced a whole new level of compassion for him when I realized he was likely stuck with effects of his imbalances. He was a personable guy, but he had a temper that could be scary at times. This alone has offered some spiritual healing within me.

You may be wondering what it is and how it works. Brain State Technologies uses a system called Brainwave Optimization with Real-Time Balancing™. I have taken the following directly from their website:

Your brain is the control center for everything you do. It drives your visual and spatial senses, attention and concentration, memory, language and your ability to reason and be logical. When your brainwaves are out of balance, so is everything else.

Just about every one of us has experienced a trauma or crisis that can throw the brainwaves out of synchronization. This can result in eating and sleep disturbances, addictions, feelings of hopelessness, anxiety, post-traumatic stress disorder, anger and irritability and physical pain and discomfort.

Brainwave Optimization with Real-Time Balancing (RTB)™ is an effective, holistic and non-invasive method that guides your brain back to its natural, healthy, balanced state.

Every series of sessions begins with a brain map. Our sensors are placed in strategic spots on your head. They collect information that enables you to actually see your brain. Our Brainwave Technologists will work with you to interpret the data and describe your brain balances and imbalances. We work with you to set goals and then, we work with your brain to restore it to its natural state of balance and harmony. The sessions involve translating your brainwaves into melodious sounds, allowing the brain to "hear" itself and guiding it into harmony.

Every brain is different. We don't train your brain to meet a standard or an average. Your brain is optimal when it arrives at its own unique state. Although there's a wide spectrum of time required to restore balance and harmony, most clients find a level of relief within just a few sessions. The average duration is 10-12 sessions, though your trainer will work with you to identify what it will take to meet your goals. Most find that once their goals have been met, there is little need for continued sessions. Some clients choose to visit us again during stressful life incidents or just when they are seeking deeper relaxation, clearer thinking or improved performance.

Using this technology in my business, Art of Attunement, I have worked with a diverse group of people. I'd like to share a few of their stories.

- The parents of a young man who was diagnosed paranoid schizophrenic were at the end of their rope; distraught and considering placing him in a home. After 25 brain training sessions, amino acid supplementation, dietary changes & cranial sacral sessions, he is employed, owns a car and has been approved for a home loan.

- A very talented & skilled UFC fighter was having focus issues right before he'd step into the octagon. Losing focus when he needed it most could have some pretty serious consequences for him. After completing 10 sessions, I got great joy watching his next pay-per-view fight and hearing announcers Joe Rogan & Mike Goldberg say repeatedly, "I have never seen him so calm & focused." He showed his skills as he submitted his opponent.

- A mother who lost her 24 year old son in an accident sought out Brainwave Optimization™ as a drug-free alternative when doctors began suggesting anti-depressants. She also hated the idea of traditional talk therapy. "I don't want to talk about it. I don't want to relive it. I've relived it a hundred times. I want to stop reliving it." On her 3rd or 4th day, she came in and said, "I now know why he died, how it fits into everything and why it was a gift from him. I still miss him but now I understand." We both believe he was in that room with us at times during her sessions.

- An adorable woman in her 60's became very depressed after a major life change. On her first visit, she told me when she woke up each morning that her first thought was that she hated the day. She hated it before it had even started. When she came in for her 5th session, she was singing and laughing down the hall to my office. She was taken off of anti-depressants. Her husband called me and said, "I don't know how you did it, but you gave me my wife back. Thank you."

- A 34 year old had become an alcoholic, after surviving an accident that had left him in a coma for 2 weeks. He was drunk virtually every day for ten years. Today he says, "I couldn't handle dealing with life and I drank because of it. Brain training gave me enough clarity to see the lessons of Jesus Christ. I'm carrying a B average towards my Master's degree, I enjoy people and I'm facing my life's tests without drinking."

- A gifted Healer who trains other Healers around the world was gifted sessions by one of her students. "This is helping me to reach places I haven't been able to reach. Beautiful."

- A very successful 32 year old entrepreneur called me the morning after his first brain training experience, "My wife noticed I was calmer, I slept like a baby and this morning I came into the office and solved a problem I've been dealing with for 3 months. This is incredible! I want more!"

- A woman in her 50's suffered neck & back pain due to her constant state of stress, despite attempts to relax. After 19 sessions, her pain suddenly disappeared and the stress that left her face was obvious. "At least thirteen people asked me what I'd done. Several asked if I'd had Botox!"

- A mother of two teens says, "I don't feel guilty about taking time to myself anymore."

- In the November 8, 2010, issue of People Magazine, Wynonna Judd credits her 55 lb. weight loss to Brain State Technologies. She says, "Now I eat 3 pieces of candy whereas before I would eat the whole bag!" She adds, "It balances me. I used to take medications in high stress situations, and I don't do that anymore." (Note: I did not personally train Ms. Judd. She trained at Brain State HQ in Scottsdale, AZ)

Please recognize that every individual's experience is as unique as their brain. Everyone is different and no two experiences are the same. Remember me; I didn't feel a thing initially. Hopefully, you are at a place on your spiritual path where you can recognize and appreciate that your experience isn't meant to be like anyone else's. It is uniquely your own.

I'm so thrilled to be involved with this technology as we begin to see how the brain can help us tap into our limitless potential, as human and spiritual beings.

To find a Brainwave Optimization™ affiliate near you, please visit www.brainstatetech.com

About the Author

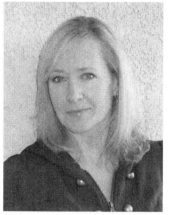

Angi Covington is a professional speaker, who has been a lifelong student of human behavior. Ms. Covington, a member of Mensa, is a go getter who's been recognized for her achievements in Corporate America. After receiving Oneness Deeksha, a consciousness raising energy, Angi had a series of profound spiritual experiences. She left the corporate world and began to fulfill her life's mission to help others.

Angi now serves as a Trainer for the Oneness University. She is committed to helping the Oneness Movement in its mission to alleviate human suffering. In Las Vegas, she facilitates Oneness Awakening courses, where new Deeksha Givers are initiated.

In addition to her work with the Oneness community, Ms. Covington is a business owner who works with clients to balance brain activity using Brainwave Optimization with RTB™, a drug free solution that helps with stress, anxiety, depression, focus, grief, sleep, mental clarity and a myriad of other issues.

Ms. Covington also has a long standing relationship with the Nevada Department of Corrections, where she is a volunteer. She teaches weekly classes, based on her book titled "7 Course Meal for the Soul" to inmates serving in prisons in southern Nevada.

Angi Covington can be contacted at:
www.artofattunement.com
www.7coursemealforthesoul.com
(702) 210-3383

The Seven Major Chakras

Joan S. Peck

When you were small and saw a beautiful rainbow after a storm, did it make you feel special and blessed...like a gift had just been handed to you? If it was a wonderful experience for you and you think about that time, can you almost feel the damp air surrounding you and smell that wonderful, distinctive smell that comes after a storm? If that is something that you can relate to, imagine how you will feel when you realize that you are just like that rainbow when you acknowledge your own seven major chakras that are part of you! Their colors, attributes and energies are very special gifts that allow an open pathway for living your life to your highest good.

So many of us struggle with life, and, sometimes, become exhausted with the poor choices that we seem to keep repeating. By dividing all aspects of living into seven sections of living, you have the opportunity to smooth out your life and stop the struggle that we all seem to be going through. You will learn to listen to your body and its energies the next time that you have to make a choice, and you will be able to choose more carefully because you will be able to sense with your body, mind and spirit those choices that will benefit you the greatest in all ways.

What is the purpose of the chakras? Why bother to learn about them? How can they help me? What happens if I ignore them? Isn't it hard to keep them in balance all the time? By learning the significance of each chakra, you begin to understand how the different emotions you sense and feel affect your body and daily living. You will realize how powerful these chakra energies are in assisting you in all the different aspects of your life. You will become aware of your own power in determining how well you live your life as this world opens up to you…a wonderful world of healing, joy and peace.

The word "chakra" is derived from the Sanskrit word meaning "wheel" or "disk." It is often described by psychics or clairvoyants as a spinning wheel of colorful light. The seven major chakras begin at the base of your spine as the Root Chakra and finish over the top of your head as the Crown Chakra. They are fixed in the central spinal column, and are located both in the front and back of the body and work through it. They work together and become your inner team to alert you when something in your life is out of balance. Now, all you have to do is pay attention to what they tell you! If you don't sense an imbalance in your life spiritually or mentally, the chakras shout out a blockage, usually through a physical ailment after you have ignored a "feeling" or "knowing" that you need to make a change in what you are doing or feeling. They, like the universe, want all the best for you and by understanding the particular energies of each chakra, they will work with you to ensure that you receive what you ask for.

Each of the chakras is the size of an orange and has a different color that vibrates and rotates at a different speed. All rotate in a clock-wise motion, both up and down your spine. The first chakra, the Root, rotates and vibrates at the slowest speed, representing the most human aspects, and the Crown Chakra rotates and vibrates at the fastest, representing the most spiritual aspects. The size and brightness of the chakras may vary according to individual development, physical condition, energy levels, disease, or stress. When balanced, the seven chakras help us maintain health, are vehicles to personal empowerment, and connect us to the divine.

Chakras are first mentioned in the Vedas, the ancient Hindu scriptures, between 1200 and 900 B.C.E. Although, the colors for each of the chakras were assigned much later and are a fairly new concept in comparison, they, too, are effective in healing your body. The understanding of the chakras was popularized by Sir John Woodroffe, who wrote under the pseudonym Arthur Avalon, in a book entitled, The Serpent Power – The Secrets of Tantric and Shaktic Yoga, first published in 1919. This is a guide to kundalini practice (the raising of the energy that lies dormant at the Base Chakra or Root Chakra).

Each of the chakra's energy centers are tied to and affect the different body parts that surround it. Each chakra has a center or attribute(s) that controls emotions, and identifies blocked emotions and physical problems. As you study each chakra, you will begin to see how the journey of the chakras is really a spiritual ascension, rising from the most human aspects of living to the most spiritual. Each chakra is important in your spiritual growth and each chakra works with the others to allow you to manifest what you desire.

The ROOT CHAKRA (security) is located at the base of your spine at the tailbone in the back and the pubic bone in the front. Its colors are red, brown and black. Its element is earth, the same element in the Astrological Chart for the Sun Signs Taurus, Virgo and Capricorn. This energy center is used for manifestation. When you are trying to make things happen in the material world, business or material possessions, the energy to succeed will come from the first chakra. This energy ties you to the physical plane which helps you see your ideas come to fruition. It is here where your basic needs are felt – primal instinct, survival, security, and safety. [The spiritual perceptions relate to commitment to life, trust in others and awareness of basic needs.*]

The SACRAL CHAKRA (creativity) is located two inches below your navel with its color of orange. Its element is water, the same element in the Astrological Chart for the Sun Signs Cancer, Scorpio and Pisces. This energy center governs your ability to relate to others in an open and friendly way. It is the great pleasure chakra where you can appreciate your sexuality and where the yin and yang resides. It is the creative chakra for birthing the young and birthing new ideas. This chakra provides you movement toward other things and where your self-worth resides. This is where you begin to develop your intuition. It is here where your basic needs are felt – sexuality, creativity, intuition and self-worth. [The spiritual perceptions relate to the development of trust in yourself and your own feelings, and the right to express and feel, and is the root of the right to be creative and expressive.*]

The SOLAR PLEXUS CHAKRA (personal power) is located two inches below the breastbone in the center behind your stomach. Its color is bright yellow. Its element is fire, the same element in the Astrological Chart for the Sun Signs Aries, Leo and Sagittarius. This energy center is one of transformation and is the center of your personal power and strength. It is also the center for astral travel and astral influences, receptivity of spirit guides and psychic development. It is here where your basic needs are felt – self-esteem, anger, ego, passions, impulses, and mental acuity. It is here where Truth lies. [The spiritual perceptions relate to the soul's ability to make an impact on the world and achieve success.*]

The HEART CHAKRA (loving relationships) is located behind your breast bone in front and on the spine between your shoulder blades in back. Its colors are green and pink. Its element is air, the same element in the Astrological Chart as the Sun Signs Gemini, Libra and Aquarius. This energy center is one of balance and healing, spirituality and unity. This is the center that connects body and mind with spirit. This chakra directs your ability to love yourself and others, to give and receive love. It is here where your basic needs are felt – love, compassion, healing and spirituality. [The spiritual perceptions relate to overall role of love in life and deals with issues about having a body and using it to achieve desires.*]

The THROAT CHAKRA (self-expression) is located in the V of the collar bone at your lower neck. Its color is light blue and its element is sound. This energy center is the center of communication and expression of creativity via thought, speech and writing. The possibility of change, transformation and healing are located here. This chakra can heal you when you let go of your anger. It is here where your basic needs are felt – self-expression and speech. [The spiritual perceptions relate to contact point for communication between the soul, mind and body. The place where the soul articulates its desires.*]

The THIRD EYE CHAKRA (self-image) is located above the physical eyes on the center of your forehead. Its color is indigo and its element is light. This energy center is one for increased intuition, imagination, visualization, clairvoyance and vision. The chakra assists in the purification of negative tendencies and in the elimination of selfish attitudes. Through the power of the sixth chakra, you can receive guidance, and channel and tune into your Higher Self. It is here where your basic needs are felt – intuition, extra sensory perception. This is the chakra connected to your Higher Self. [The spiritual perceptions relate to the origin of the abilities to register and establish the soul's vision of our life.*]

The CROWN CHAKRA (spiritual purpose) is located just behind the top of your skull. Its colors are white and purple and its element is thought. This energy center is one for consciousness and transcendence. It is the center of spirituality, enlightenment, dynamic thought and energy. This chakra allows for the inward flow of wisdom and connectedness with God. It is here where your basic needs are felt – divinity, peace and enlightenment. This is the chakra connected to your Higher Power. [The spiritual perceptions relate to the awareness of purpose and our own guiding principles.*]

We have talked about the importance of free flowing energy between all the 7 major chakras. You appreciate that when these energies flow, there is greater chance for better health, joy and peace. Now, let's study the blockages that can occur in your chakras. Any blockages that you may have are not there by accident. They are designed by you and put in place to protect you from what, at the time, you're not able to process.

They can be caused by psychological or emotional pain. Since all the chakras are tied together, a block at one will affect the functioning of the others, causing physical, emotional and/or spiritual distress.

According to Brenda Davies, M.D., the different types of blocks are:

1.   "Suppression of Feelings, which typically leads to depression and despair (usually a heart chakra block)

2.   Compression and Compaction of Rage, which is perceived as potentially destructive if it's allowed to erupt (usually a solar plexus block)

3.   Freezing of Feelings, that often results in a lot of tension and need to defend against any further possible attack (usually a heart chakra)

4.   Depletion of Energy and Abdication of Power, which renders the person apparently helpless and in need of much support from others, hence protecting them from having to accept personal accountability and responsibility (solar plexus and/or sacral block)

5.   Denial, which is usually a product of fear – here the person will often behave as though everything is fine while underneath there is chaos to such a degree that confronting it needs to be avoided at all costs to avoid possible breakdown (this can be present with a block at any chakra)"

According to the author, Cyndi Dale, "Blocks are points of resistance to our own well-being. A block is any physical condition, belief, feeling, or spiritual misunderstanding that prevents us from living our purpose. A block can be caused by a physical problem, false mental belief, unresolved feeling, or spiritual misconception, and is a problem because it inhibits the free flow of our natural energy and spiritual self."

Depending on the circumstances you find yourself in, you may use one of these blocks or a combination of them. All of us use blocks from time to time to regulate the flow of energy, depending on what we feel we can cope with. Sometimes, these temporary blocks can be a very helpful tool. Even body language can produce a temporary block of energy. All blocked energy can be cleared if done gently and with a genuine desire by the affected person to be cleared. Remember: no one has the right to remove your blockage unless you ask them to.

So what do you do with these blocks? How do you know if you have a blockage? What is the simplest way to deal with a blockage? Let me share with you my own experience. I have felt for as long as I can remember that no one is interested in what I say. In the past and even now, I catch myself describing a thought or a situation in as few words as possible thinking that what I say isn't really that important. I was thrilled to be able to say what I wanted in my books that I authored, taking time to say in words over and again what I believe is important about the chakras and how they affect our lives in a positive, beautiful way. After writing my books, it became obvious that I now needed to speak about them. I became determined to get over my blockage about speaking and the negative belief I had regarding whether what I said was important and worthy of being listened to by others.

I studied all of the aspects of the seven major chakras to see where my blockage might reside. I reviewed my childhood to see where I might have developed my negative belief about my speaking. It was interesting to me to come upon times that I remembered where I had no voice. I have an identical twin sister and we had our own "twin language," which only our older brother could understand. This lack of speaking clearly lasted into our first school years. Because my sister spoke more clearly than I, teachers and others would ask me a question, then turn to her for the answer. Therefore, what I had to say appeared to me to not be important. I also reviewed my past lives with a certified practitioner and became aware that I have had other lifetimes where I as a woman wasn't able to express some of my ideas and thoughts. When I speak today, I am very aware of my negative belief system and override it with positive affirmations and the understanding of where some of my old beliefs came from, and I can let it go. Understanding my chakras and their particular aspects has helped me address my issue and know that I have the right to be heard. And I am grateful for that.

Each chakra plays a role in the way you live your life on a daily basis. Now, that you have a general understanding of what each of the seven major chakras represents, you need to look at each one in relationship to how you are living them. By that, I mean, how you are living the "energy" of each chakra. We all want the best that life has to offer and to achieve that, you must look at your role to ensure that you are doing all that you can to make it happen.

Let's take a look at each of the chakras to see how you are "living" them. I have listed a few questions for each chakra knowing that there are so many more questions to ask yourself, which I leave up to you.

The Root Chakra is concerned with security and safety. What are you doing to keep yourself and your family secure? Are you financially secure and protected from losing every material thing? Is your residence safe and secure? Are you taking care of your body by eating for good health or exercising?

The Sacral Chakra is concerned with creativity and sensuality. Do you appreciate yourself for who you are? Are you happy with your physical form? Do you enjoy the idea that you can procreate? What do you do to enjoy yourself as a female or a male, whichever gender you are? Do you have good self-worth?

The Solar Plexus Chakra is concerned with personal power. Do you have great self-esteem? Do you feel empowered to help others? Do you believe that you can do anything that you set your mind to do? Do you believe that you have much to offer your environment and the world? Do you believe that it is important to help those less fortunate?

The Heart Chakra is concerned with loving relationships. Do you have someone special in your life? Is this relationship healthy filled with joy and love? Do you love yourself? Do you show your love to others in your life easily and effortlessly? Do you love unconditionally?

The Throat Chakra is concerned with self-expression. Are you able to easily share your ideas and thoughts with others? Do you express yourself in a healthy way? Do you hold your anger in your throat chakra? Are you able to be creative in all the ways you want? Do you have a desire to show your individuality in a creative way?

The Third Eye Chakra is concerned with self-image. Are you pleased with your image today? Are you careful to acknowledge your inner feelings? Do you honor your higher self? Have you developed your psychic abilities? Do you connect to the spirits who have passed?

The Crown Chaka is concerned with spiritual purpose. Do you know your purpose in life? Do you believe that we are all one? Are you happy with your belief system? Do you feel a connectedness with your higher power?

Take a notebook and list the seven major chakras leaving a lot of space to write between each chakra. Write down these questions and add your own. When you review what you have written, you will be able to see how you are living the energies of the chakras and will be pleased at all you are doing to live your life to its highest good and the highest good of all. You may come across some ways that you may want to change or ways that you may want to begin. As you know, you are in charge of your life; your journey is your own, and you create the way you live each day. So live a colorful life by understanding and appreciating your seven major chakras and all that they do for you!

About the Author

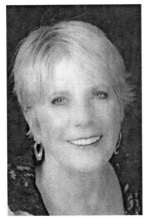

Joan S. Peck is the author of "The Seven Major Chakras – Keeping it Simple," "A Simple Approach to Living a Successful Life," and a featured author in "Life Choices – Putting the Pieces Together." She is a speaker and workshop facilitator, sharing how the chakras and their energies can take the struggle out of everyday living, and often comments, "Live the Chakras - smooth out your ride in life!"

Joan's passion is writing and editing. Ever since she was a child, she dreamed of writing and always put it off, thinking that "working" was the most important thing she could do. She has learned that living your passion is the most joyful thing you can do, and doing something you love brings all the best results.

Joan is working on a book on addiction with her son, who died of a drug overdose in 2005. It is a topic that fascinates her, particularly with the power that addiction has over so many. Joan resides in Henderson, Nevada.

Joan Peck may be contacted at:
www.bejeweled7.com
joanpeck39@gmail.com
(702) 423-4342

Channeling

Cheryl Johnson and Diane Johnson

CHANNELING

Channeling is a very personal and subjective experience. If you ask ten channels to define channeling, you could easily get ten different definitions. My own definition continues to evolve after almost 20 years of channeling.

I am a conscious trance channel. I began my studies around 1990 with one of the pioneers in the metaphysical movement, Reverend Don Weldon, who had been channeling since the 1950s and teaching since the 1960s.

Channeling is a phase of our return to knowing that we are one with all of life, including the Higher Power. In its current stage, it is usually viewed as connecting with a wisdom that is "above" or "beyond" our own. I believe that, as we evolve, we will begin to accept that the wisdom and love we receive through channeling truly comes from within Self as a natural byproduct of our oneness.

The primary purpose of channeling is to find a deeper connection with the Divine Wisdom that we are to make living easier, happier and more loving. I am convinced that we are powerful souls and have the answers to all of life's questions — once we clear the channels!

You may agree with what I present here, or not. That's okay. A wise teacher told me that when reading, we must read with discernment and without judgment. That means you accept whatever feels right to you and use it (discernment). Anything that doesn't feel right to you, you simply let go of without any emotional response (no judgment).

WHAT IS CHANNELING?

Channeling (also called trance channeling) is receiving information from the non-physical through means other than the five physical senses. This includes the use of any of your psychic abilities — in any way. You can channel with or without psychic tools, such as the tarot and the I Ching. As long as the information is coming through you from the non-physical and not from some memorized meaning, you are acting as a channel (or channeler).

At its best, channeling is connecting with the Divine Source to bring through wisdom, love and guidance as in the following channeled session.

The Empty Pitcher

There was a woman who spent every waking moment helping others. She threw a party for all her wonderful friends and family. She never rested or stopped to chat, hurrying to fill the glasses so that no one went without. Alas, when she came to her closest, most beloved friend, her pitcher was empty – she had nothing left to give.

Do not be this woman whose pitcher is empty. It is impossible for you to always be in touch with, or to always be there for everyone.

When will you replenish your supply? You need to fill your pitcher from the well of God's love and wisdom! You must have times of quiet meditation and reflection. In these times of quiet, what a joy this peace is that you feel! And in this peace, you find the answers that lie within the "I AM" center of yourself.

Can you see that it is to the highest good of all that you lovingly, firmly set boundaries for those who seek your help?

[There was a long pause as though the guide was looking for the right words.] "Lee, my dearest child..." her voice rose at the end as though in gentle question.

Lee replied, "Yes?"

Again a pause before the guide softly instructed, "Shut off the cell phone."

[Laughter broke from the group attending the channeling at the suddenly so down-to-earth advice.]

The guide laughed with them. "Shut off the cell phone! Draw the curtains over the windows! Don't answer the doorbell!"

At its worst, what some people call channeling can be expressing repressed parts of the personality, play-acting, ego-driven manipulation or self-delusion.

I Am Dracula

A television show invited people who claimed to be channels to appear. A young man and his wife volunteered, claiming the young man channeled Dracula. They said that they also used the channeling to enhance their sex lives. It was very exciting when Dracula "inhabited" the young man's body. You can imagine how thrilled the television producers were to have this ratings booster.

The host asked them to do a channeling on the air and the couple eagerly agreed. After a moment of silence, the young man introduced himself as Dracula. His voice had changed to a mild "I-want-to-drink-your-blood" Transylvanian-type accent as he boasted of his power and conquests.

The "channeling" went well until the host asked "Dracula" some basic questions about his personal life. "Dracula" couldn't answer the questions. Then the host asked him to speak in his native language. He couldn't. While the failure to speak a foreign language isn't proof that the channel is a fake, it did prove to be the final nail in "Dracula's" coffin.

HOW CHANNELING WORKS

Everything is made of energy — physical and non-physical. This energy is known by many names, such as Divine Source, Creator, God, First Cause, and so on. You are this same energy vibrating at different frequencies. It is only natural to communicate through this energetic connection — this oneness.

You may hear channels refer to individuals in the non-physical ("on the Other Side") who are helping them. These helpers are called by many names — teachers, guides, angels, Beings of Light, Higher Self/Superconscious, Jane, Dick or Larry. In general, the non-physical entity is referred to as a contact. Regardless of the label, it is important to remember that it is the same energy that you are.

Channels deliberately tune into this energetic oneness by entering trance. Trance is a different, yet normal, level of awareness that is known by many names, such as hypnosis and altered state. You relax the conscious level of awareness (the waking state) out of the way and go into the subconscious level from which you can gain access to the Superconscious level of Divine Wisdom. Once in trance, the channel translates the information being received from the non-physical into words.

The channel's depth of trance is a key factor in determining the behavior of the channel and what comes through. Some channels prefer light trance because they want to be more aware of what's coming through them or because they are so accustomed to communicating through the non-physical that a deep trance is not needed. Others feel that the deeper levels make it easier for them to "get out of the way" of the message. One level is not better than another; however, your experience will differ from level to level.

Light-trance channels retain enough of the conscious level of awareness to interact with you as they channel. At this level, channels may or may not close their eyes. Their voices and body movements are usually the same as in the waking state and they can remember some of what came through during the channeling session.

In light trance, the information received is presented in the same vocabulary and language the channel uses in the waking state. If the channel is well-educated, the message will be given in educated terms. If the channel is not well-educated, beautiful and deeply profound messages may come through in simple words and incorrect grammar. This doesn't make the message any less valuable.

It can be hard to tell when someone is channeling from a light trance. I've encountered this a few times. In one such session, after I had been channeling for about 15 minutes, my client said that the information was really helpful and made her feel much better, but that she would like to hear what the Other Side had to say about it. (I was, of course, very flattered that she thought such wisdom came from me!)

Medium-trance channels go deeper into the subconscious level and so are less aware of the world around them while channeling. They often close their eyes and don't remember much of what came through during the session. Their posture is usually very relaxed and they are not as active as light-trance channels. The tone and pitch of their voices and their vocabulary may change somewhat, but they still use the same language spoken in the waking state.

Deep-trance channels are usually not aware of their surroundings while channeling and do not remember anything about the channeling afterwards. Their eyes are almost always closed and they move little or not at all. The voice can change to a monotone and take on different rhythms, accents, or phrasing.

A channel working from a light to deep level of trance is called a conscious trance channel.

Somnambulistic-trance channels are rare. They are completely unconscious during trance and don't remember anything after the channeling. Their eyes may be open or closed. They allow the non-physical to take control and so their voices and vocabulary, as well as body movements, can be completely different from their waking state. They may even speak languages they don't know in their conscious state. These channels may be active like Kevin Ryerson or completely still like Edgar Cayce.

A channel working from the somnambulistic level is called an unconscious trance channel.

YOU ARE A CHANNEL

Now that you know how channeling works, you can see that you were born a natural channel because you are a soul — you are energy. In fact, you've already channeled many times! Have you ever had an idea or thought come to you "out of the blue"? This frequently happens when you're doing everyday tasks, such as washing dishes or taking a shower because they're automatic habit patterns requiring no focus. You accidentally went into the subconscious level. You accidentally accessed the psychic realm.

You Know You Can... So Why Can't You?

Even though you are prewired to channel, you may not be able to if you can't relax the noisy, conscious level of awareness out of the way. (This is a nice way to say that you need to get the chattering monkey in your mind to shut up.)

Negative filters can also block your ability to channel. You create through three levels of awareness. The conscious level is reason and logic. The subconscious level holds all of your automatic habit patterns, beliefs, and emotions and controls your physical body. The Superconscious level is the level of Divine Wisdom.

The beliefs, habit patterns and emotions that reside at the subconscious level act as filters. Divine Wisdom coming from the Superconscious must pass through these filters before manifesting in your life.

This is easy to understand if you compare it to sunshine and clouds. Everyone knows that the sun shines brightly during the day regardless of whether or not there are clouds in the sky. However, if there are clouds, the sun that is shining so brightly behind them comes through to us as dull light or rays here and there. In the same way, Divine Wisdom is dulled or distorted if it passes through negative filters at the subconscious level.

These negative filters can be created deliberately or accidentally. For example:

Deliberate Conditioning

Catherine came to me because she was experiencing "words floating into her head." She believed that we can receive direct communication from a Higher Power and the words she received always felt loving and proved to be very helpful. She couldn't understand why she felt so scared and guilty.

As I channeled for Catherine, she was reminded that she had experienced strict religious training from birth to about eight years of age. That religious training said that communicating with a Higher Power is a special gift belonging only to those chosen by the church. Anyone else who "spoke with spirits" was in danger of going to hell because they were either being fooled by Satan or committing blasphemy.

Catherine had changed her spiritual beliefs at the conscious level so she didn't think her early religious training mattered. However, that extended period of conditioning had instilled a fear at the subconscious level that was still active.

Accidental Conditioning

Henry came to me because he just knew he could channel, but he couldn't. In hypnotherapy (age regression therapy), he regressed to a number of incidents in his childhood. He had two older brothers who delighted in teasing him. Both of these brothers loved scary movies about psychic phenomena. Henry would watch the movies with them, get completely wrapped up in the show and forget all about his brothers. When the movie got to the scariest parts, one or both of them would sneak behind the couch and pop up and scare the dickens out of Henry.

As a result, Henry had developed an emotional connection of psychic with "scary." This created a block to Henry's ability to channel.

Anyone can learn to relax and any negative filters at the subconscious level can be changed. Whether you wish to become a channel or prefer to have someone else channel for you, you can enjoy all the benefits channeling offers.

BENEFITS

Through channeling you can receive assistance with everything in your life. For example:

Spiritual growth

When you look beyond the obvious benefit of receiving help to make decisions, you realize that the ultimate goal of channeling is communion and union with a Higher Power and your own power. As a channel or receiving guidance through a channel, you have the opportunity to connect with love and wisdom.

Making personal and business decisions

Don't expect decisions to be made for you. Channeled information is to increase your understanding of any situation in order to help you make the best decision for yourself. You may be made aware of things like recurring patterns, hidden emotional issues and past-life influences. Our Friends on the Other Side wish to empower you to live your life – not to live it for you.

Relationships

You can gain remarkable insight into why people do what they do and say what they say. This understanding can help you be more compassionate to others and to yourself so that you work through relationships in a more loving and enlightened way.

Predictions

Psychic predictions can be very useful guideposts. They can: 1) let you know that you're making good choices, thus encouraging you to"keep on keepin' on," 2) give you a heads-up if you're making choices that will result in a future you don't like, or 3) help you get through something you may not like but cannot change.

WHAT TO LOOK FOR IN A CHANNEL

You want a channel who:

- Respects you and all of life;
- Has a positive attitude;
- Shows a desire to help people help themselves;
- Makes it all about you (It is okay for a channel to share some of his or her experiences with you if they directly relate to your issues or are used to illustrate a point. However, any channel that spends time boasting about his or her works or dropping names is coming from ego).
- Encourages your independence (A channel who indicates that you may not go to anyone else for help is coming from personal need and greed).

Sometimes people go into a channeling session with the belief that "the Other Side always knows best," and that translates to "the channel always knows best." You can gain understanding, comfort, and higher vision through a channel, but the responsibility for your destiny rests entirely in your own hands.

When judging the quality of channeling, it's best to keep it simple. Ask yourself, "Is the message that I am receiving loving?" If the message is negative or destructive in any way, it's coming through some negative filters. Next, be sure that the information you receive helps you feel empowered to live your life with greater love and understanding.

What to expect

A channeling session can vary greatly according to the channel, the person receiving the channeling, the questions asked, and so forth.

The Tone and Feeling of the Message
The tone and feeling of the message can range from feeling protected and embraced by someone who loves you unconditionally to being advised and even kidded by a practical friend as in the example "The Empty Pitcher."

Content of the Message
Answers are always aimed at helping you make that next move, but they seldom come through as step-by-step instructions. Sometimes the answers you receive will require you to work through them—like solving a cryptogram.

A Song In His Head

A former student and very good friend wakes up with a different song in his head every morning. While taking my course on psychic development, he realized that the lyrics of the song were channeled messages. It was up to him to figure out which lyrics were the answers to his questions and how to apply them to his life.He said he felt such a complete sense of satisfaction from working out the rest of the puzzle himself that he wouldn't trade his method of channeling for any other!

Interpretation of the Message at the Time of Channeling
Sometimes the information that comes through isn't what we think it is.

You Say "potato"; I say...
Margaret came to me to channel her mother, who had died of an illness. (Channeling deceased loved ones is usually referred to as mediumship.) Margaret's mother had a wonderful sense of humor so the time was filled with laughter, as well as tears. As we were ending the session, Margaret asked her mother to give her a sign that she is okay and still around. Out of my mouth came the words, "I will send you flower."

Weeks later, Margaret called to tell me how her mother delivered on her promise. She was walking down the aisle at the grocery store, and for no apparent reason, a five-pound bag of flour fell at her feet. Margaret said she listened to the recording of the session again and the words that came out of my mouth were, "I will send you flour," not "I will send you a flower." We had assumed that the word referred to the universal symbol of love, not the basic ingredients for cookies.

A GLIMPSE OF HISTORY

Channeling has been around since man first gained consciousness. The ancient Egyptians had a highly-developed way of communicating with the gods; the Greeks had their Oracles and so on.

In more recent history, channeling first came to widespread fame (or infamy) in the 1840s through the Fox sisters. The Fox sisters claimed to communicate with the spirit of a murdered man. They duped thousands until 1888 when they publicly demonstrated how they'd been able to fake their powers for so long.
Thankfully, by the time the Fox sisters confessed, the channeling movement (then called Spiritism or Spiritualism) was well under way.

Many books of channeled information were written from the mid-1800s through the mid-1900s. Two of the most famous channels/authors are Helena Petrovna Blavatsky who channeled spiritual superhuman masters or mahatmas living in the Himalayas, and Alice Bailey, who channeled the Tibetan master Djwhal Khal (D.K.).

Channeling began to be commonly accepted and even fashionable in the 1960s and '70s. It was during this period that the name changed from spiritualism to channeling.
Controversial Episcopalian Bishop, James Pike, helped bring spiritualism to popularity after his son committed suicide in 1966. He went to several mediums to contact his son's spirit and participated in a televised séance with his dead son through the well-known medium Arthur Ford.

Jon Klimo, a recognized authority on channeling, started investigating and reporting on channeling in the mid-seventies and is still publishing findings.

Some of the more famous channeling partnerships of the '70s and '80s are Jane Roberts channeling Seth and J.Z. Knight channeling Ramtha.

In the 1980's, Shirley MacLaine put channeling in the spotlight. Shirley told the story of her spiritual journey and her contact with channels in her immensely-popular book and movie, "Out on a Limb."

Now, in the 21st century of mass communication, Esther Hicks channeling Abraham has a global audience. Television shows, such as Star Trek: Voyager and SeaQuest have aired episodes showing examples of channeling to millions of viewers.

SUMMARY
Curiosity continues to grow as more people discover the truth about channeling. The truth is that channeling is a natural ability. It is intended to expand your awareness of yourself and help you experience that you truly are one with all of Life—including a Higher Power. It's another step in your spiritual evolution. Through channeling or by receiving information through a channel, you can learn more about how to live a life filled with meaning and joy. The Higher Realms have a great sense of humor. As you allow yourself to laugh with them, you will truly "lighten up."

About the Author

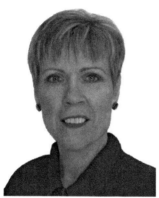

Rev. Cheryl J. Johnson, M.Msc., C.Ht. holds a Master of Metaphysical Sciences; is a Metaphysical Minister & Teacher; a Certified Hypnotherapist (aka Current- & Past-Life Age Regression); a Spiritual Counselor; a Dream Interpreter, and a Channel.

Cheryl considers herself amazingly fortunate to have studied with two renowned pioneers teaching metaphysics and hypnotherapy: Rev. Donald E. Weldon, mentioned in books by Ruth Montgomery, Dick Sutphen, and Alan Weisman; and Gil Boyne, mentioned in many texts on hypnotherapy and described by Sylvia Brown as "a noted instructor."

Cheryl uses a combination of modalities to help her clients:
- ➢ Metaphysics for the practical application of Universal Laws;
- ➢ Hypnotherapy to rapidly remove blocks;
- ➢ Self-hypnosis to relieve anxiety and reduce stress;
- ➢ Hypnotic Suggestion Programming to change negative programming;
- ➢ Channeling to bring guidance from the Higher perspective;
- ➢ Dream Interpretation to clarify guidance received through dreams;
- ➢ Courses to give the tools needed to live a happy, healthy, and prosperous life.

Cheryl J. Johnson can be contacted at:
www.cheryljjohnson.com
cheryl@cheryljjohnson.com
702-558-6889

About the Author

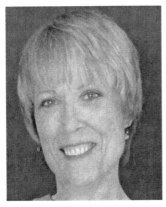

Diane L. Johnson has enjoyed many careers from traveling the world as a trilingual confidential secretary to working as a professional horsewoman. Diane is a conscious trance channel, an editor, and writer.

She holds a weekly group channeling session and edits all of Rev. Cheryl J. Johnson's written material. She is writing two works including a creative non-fiction book based on encouragement, counsel, and commiseration received from decades of channelings.

Diane began her metaphysical studies in the early-nineties with metaphysical pioneer Reverend Donald E. Weldon. After finishing numerous courses with him, she worked with Don preparing his memoirs for publication. Although Don crossed over before the book could be finished, Diane feels she was given the rare privilege of experiencing through him the excitement and trials of bringing channeling, hypnotherapy, and faith healing into the public eye beginning in the 1950s and spanning into the late 90s.

Diane used her knowledge of spirit-over-mind-over-matter to overcome cancer and mild traumatic brain injury.

Diane L. Johnson can be contacted at:
diane@scorpiotwins.com

Dreams

Reverend Cecilia Cattel Carrillo

"If you can imagine it, you can achieve it. If you can dream it, you can become it."

~William Arthur Ward

What is a dream? Dreams are a process that you experience when your body is at rest. You may be asleep or in a light relaxed mental alpha state similar to hypnosis or meditation. It is possible to experience visions, emotions, scents, tastes, and even sounds, all of which can seem very real. Sometimes, your dreams seem more real than what you may actually experience in the waking state. When you wake up, you may be relieved to find it was only a dream or, in some cases, you may be disappointed because it was something you really wanted to be true. Dreams come from your deepest desires and many times they are there to help you out of a dilemma in your waking life. Oftentimes, you can find the answers you need in the dream state, which can help you change your waking reality. This can be done when you learn to replay events in the dream and do them differently while you are still dreaming.

Dreams can instruct, predict or even take part in creating the future for you. They are a phenomenal healing tool when they release blocked emotions and anger or when they simply allow your mind to review unresolved events that can lead to resolution. Sometimes, dreams can predict the onset of a health problem so that you can correct it before it becomes a reality. Other times, there may even be a benevolent spiritual being helping you with your dreams to point out areas that you may need to address. A good aide is to place a journal by your bedside so that you can jot down your dreams and are able to interpret them after you wake up. Analyzing your dream reveals the language of your sub-conscious mind.

I have given names to various types of dreams that I have experienced:

One of the rarest and most powerful dreams is the Epochal Dream. This dream is special in that it can set the tone of your future and often shows you your purpose or destiny in life. Even though many dream images fade after a few hours, these special dreams do not. In fact, years later you remember them as if the dream occurred just a few minutes ago. These dreams often have the effect of placing people on the right track in their life. Inspiration and commitment on a higher level of goodness is often the result of this type dream. The message portrayed in this type of dream oftentimes is one of the most important things that you will remember in life and it can serve as a guide many years after the dream.

The Flashback Dream can have visitors or be without them. In these dreams, you might relive an event in your life that had a high emotional charge for you. You may remember the event as having actually occurred or not. Other times, the feeling of having been somewhere because we dream it often is termed "Déjà vu" (a French phrase meaning second view). It's interesting to note that science is working to find a place in the brain that relates to future knowledge as easily as they find memory in the brain.

The Healing Dream often gives you specific instructions or awareness that can bring a healing change into your life. You might be shown an area of the body or a particular body part with a general or specific problem. In some cases, there may be such a profound experience in your dream that you actually experience healing in your waking life.

The Inventing Dream is in conjunction with the Teaching or Learning Dream, and involves a process called Sacred Software. Inventive dreams often are intuitive answers and solutions to problems in any area of your life. From the mundane, such as how do I get my roof repaired, to the most creative problem, you can invent different scenarios in your dream that help you solve your problem.

Lucid Dream is characterized by an exceptional awareness of what is happening. When you are lucid dreaming, often you are aware that you are both dreaming and are the dreamer. This position splits your attention, and sets you up as the observer, with a parallel in waking reality. Some mystical traditions encourage you to get into the role of observer to gain a more practical attitude about your life, leaving out feelings and emotions so that you can observe and experience it with more objectivity.   When one is in a lucid dream, this happens automatically.

There are some exercises that can make you aware of lucid dreaming and even train you to dream lucidly. One such exercise is to look for your hand in the dream state. Now begin to manipulate your hand, perhaps by holding up one, two or three fingers or make a fist or just by holding your hand in front of you. The goal is to gain control over your hand in the dream state. Then you are aware that you are in a lucid dream.

The benefits of lucid dreaming are that you will have much more control over your waking life and can even transform it. You have a greater awareness that you create your own life by knowing that the energies you give out are those that will be returned to you.   Victims can become victorious, achievers can accomplish much more, and the Law of Attraction is instilled in a more practical way in the dreamer's life. Positive life changes can happen, literally overnight.

Nightmare or Frustration Dreams are very important, but can be disturbing. Often, these dreams point out a personal frustration that you are having difficulty overcoming. If you are shown a scenario as a helpless victim, it may indicate that you feel that way in reality, in your waking life. You can stop this dream if you face the one who is attacking you or if you change the situation in which you feel victimized. Remember, the dream is only reflecting your life and you have power in your dream to change the situation. By standing up to your personal demons, devils, attackers, and all the scary stuff, you become stronger in your waking life.

Psychic Dreams can be precognitive in nature where enough information is dreamt to give you an opportunity to alter the course of events. A fairly large percentage of dreams relate to precognitive events. Many times, the dream event occurs exactly one week, one month, one year or even several years later to the date of the dream. This is one reason it is so important to record the date of your dream in your dream journal.

The Repeating Dream may be the whole dream or only a fragment of your dream that plays over and over. Generally, there is some kind of problem or difficulty that the sub-conscious mind wants to bring to your attention and it keeps repeating the message hoping to get through.

The best way to stop a repeating dream is to analyze it and once you understand its meaning, make that awareness a part of your life, weaving it into your wisdom base of experience.   If the dream doesn't stop, or you can't figure its meaning, try changing the action in your dream. You are the dreamer, the scriptwriter, producer, and director of your dreams. You have much more power in your dreams than you realize. Dreams are of your creation; play with them and have fun creating your own outcome

The Sexual Dream is symbolic for whatever is happening in a sexual context in your life. For example, intercourse in a dream could mean verbal intercourse or a coming together in a passionate way or an exchange of ideas or energy. If the dreamer makes reference to being "screwed," this could have less to do with sex and more to do with being violated in some area of life. Some sexually explicit dreams are not at all about sex, while some other seemingly innocuous dream may actually be about a sexual relationship.

The Sorting-Out Dream occurs more than once a night and is there simply to help you sort out the events of the day. Often, these dreams are simple, visual and help you put events and thoughts into proper prospective.

The Teaching or Learning Dream may take place in a classroom or in ancient Greece or Rome or even in a spacecraft. You may have visitors in your dreams that are there to instruct you on various issues. Often, the information gleaned from these educational dreams gives you very practical real help in the waking life. These dreams offer immediate usable information to help answer current questions and problems. Sometimes, there is an avalanche of information given and you may unconsciously be storing some of it for future reference.

The Visitation Dream is where you are visited by another. It is important to note in your dream journal whether the visitor is alive or dead in the waking state. Sometimes the dead may visit you in a dream or meditative moment. It could be an important person participating in the drama of your life or even someone from your future, like a soon-to-be-born child. In this type of dream, there are teachers, guides, angels or masters who come to give you assistance. It is important to be able to distinguish whether the information they give is correct and helpful, or whether it is coming from your fear or your own darker and hidden personality characteristics. The visitor may be your weaker self or an angry and powerful side of you that you don't let surface in your awakened state.

Many visitors are guides or angels of a higher order that come to help and guide you, bringing knowledge or information that you cannot access in normal waking consciousness. Some people see religious figures and masters like Jesus, Buddha, the Virgin Mary, Sai Baba and many others. If you have a dream with a message from a master, it is considered a blessing.

Many of your dreams may take the form of several layers of the different types of dreams. You might have a dream that is an Epochal Dream that turns into a Lucid Dream and then a Visitation Dream. Each layer can be looked at and analyzed separately.

Dreams are a wonderful way to observe and track what is going on in your life, whether they have been obvious to you or not. Dreams are there for your use to better understand yourself and those around you and to make any necessary changes that will benefit you and those you love.

When you change your dreams, you change your life. ~ Cattel

I have a concept that I term SACRED SOFTWARE. Just as you can install software in your computer for a specific task you can do this with your mind, which works especially well in the dream state. Your sub-conscious can achieve results to situations by putting the problem in your mind before you sleep and letting your own unlimited creative process in your mind generate your answers or a solution. I call it sacred because a creative unity is usually inspired by a Sacred Source, generally your own repository of dreams. Occasionally, someone close to you can have a dream concerning you and come up with an answer that you may be seeking. It is as if the creative process is so abundant that there are many resources available to give you answers. If you don't get an answer one way, you'll get it another. There are many practical applications for this version of Sacred Software. Here are some examples:

Elias Howe invented the sewing machine. Were it not for a dream he had, it wouldn't have come to fruition. Howe had his invention nearly complete except for one thorny problem with the needle of the sewing machine. He dreamt that spear-carrying savages were leading him to death holding spears with an eye shaped hole near the point. After he awoke he whittled a model of the needle with an eye-shaped hole near the tip rather than the middle of the needle, which led to the solution of the problem and the completion of his sewing machine invention.

Robert Louis Stevenson dreamt the plot for "Dr. Jeckyll and Mr. Hyde," which made his book so infamous and still popular today.

Rene' Descartes was a soldier uncertain about his future. In a dream, he became aware that he was able to combine mathematics and philosophy. This ended up becoming a new discipline for which he spent the rest of his life engaged: Rationalism.

119

Carl Jung, a contemporary of Freud and one of the foremost proponents of archetypical symbology, had a dream of speaking with the masses, and not only to individual physicians. It was after that that Jung wrote his book, "Man and His Symbols" and made it available to the general public, something he had hesitated to do.

In 1920, Otto Loewi, had a dream that helped him design an experiment to prove a theory regarding how chemicals transmit nerve impulses, a theory he had conceived in 1903, but hadn't been able to prove until his dream of 1920.

The Periodic table of Elements was seen in a dream, almost in its entirety by Mendeleev as a way of cataloging atomic weights and substances in chemistry. This is currently in use worldwide.

There are many other examples. The ability to get answers in the dream state is remarkable. Whether it is something practical, like Elias Howe's answer to make the sewing machine needle work, or Otto Lowi's creative breakthrough about chemical transmission and nerves, dreams carry our hidden power up to the conscious level so that we have access to some of our greatest ideas and thoughts.

How can you activate the Sacred Software to be available to you?

1.   The first step is to have a real need, or sense of something hidden, that needs to be expressed, such as Otto Loewi needed to prove his theory that could change the face of science.

2.   The second step is to define the problem clearly so your subconscious mind can find a way to solve it for you…is there a money or time restraint?

3.   The third step is to spend a few moments visualizing what the solution would look, feel, sound, taste, and smell like to you. Use all of your senses; vividly imagine what it will be like for your quest to be answered.

4.   The fourth step needs patience on your part and the ability to put the puzzle together. While oftentimes the solution appears to be fully formed, other times, it comes in succeeding parts or in small segments, like so many little action steps. This can take time over several weeks.

For example, Napoleon Hill described in his tape series "You Deserve to Be Rich" how frustrating it was when he and his publisher were looking for a title to his soon-to-be published manuscript. In frustration, Napoleon demanded his subconscious to produce the right title. One morning, he awoke at 3 o'clock to the title "Think and Grow Rich." He knew without a doubt that this was the million dollar title he was looking for. By using his Sacred Software, his dreaming subconscious mind produced the solution he sought.

In the case of Otto Lowei, he waited seventeen years for the answer. Your goal by learning to use your own Sacred Software is to reduce the time necessary for your solution.

"Who looks outside, dreams. Who looks inside, wakens."
-Carl Jung

Let me demonstrate further by sharing some examples from two of my clients who were frustrated with some aspects of their life whose dream revealed the situation. They then were able to resolve their issues and make the necessary changes to live a way that was better for them.

CONI'S REPEATING DREAM

"I was in my car, but I was in the back seat and my husband was driving. That's what kept repeatin, for several years. We could be in rain or sunshine, snow or fog, but still he was just driving. Always the same basic thing – he was driving and I was in the back seat. Sometimes I'd be on the right, sometimes on the left, but always in the backseat.

Then the dreams began to change. Now, my son was in the front seat with my husband. For several years, I'm still riding in the backseat with my husband and son in front. Sometimes, my son would drive, yet I remained in the back. Later, even after I was divorced, the dreams continued. But now it was just my son up front in the driver's seat all the time and I was still in the back!

In class, you had me imagine what I would do if I wanted to change my dream. So I thought I'd try and drive the car. The next time I had this dream, I really got upset because I still couldn't drive. I just stood outside of the car and looked in!

After a few days, I had this dream again, but this time I got out of the car and walked away looking for a new car. However, there was a problem in that I was in the desert and there was no one around except my son, who was sitting in the car.

In the next class with you, you told me to try to see my hand in the dream. So the next time I had the dream, I tried to see my hand and had trouble doing so but ended up in the front seat. My son was still driving, and although I was in the front seat, I was very frustrated because I was never in the driver's seat of my own car!"

When Coni and I reviewed her dream, it was obvious how upset she was by not being able to drive her own car. When we related her car to her life and how she let everyone else control her, she was able to change how she conducted her life and live very differently than she had before. Vehicles, especially your car, in a dream state can often reveal how you live your life. When you journal your car dream, be aware of what you are doing in a car and write it down for review at a later time.

FLO'S VISITATION AND HEALING DREAM

"I have always felt dreams were a very important factor in our lives. They definitely provide messages to help us on our journey and are a very important factor in our lives and help us work out different issues that we are dealing with. Until recently, I never realized how effective dreams could be in settling issues with various people in our lives.

My Mother and I have never had a close personal relationship. When I was young, she and I had a bitter, full-fledged war raging at all times. As we grew older, it turned into a cold war. I knew we both wanted peace, but how do you rectify something that has been waging for 50 year? We had never been very good at communicating in a healthy way. I was planning a trip back to my hometown to see my children and also visit my parents, who were getting up in age. I said to several of my friends that one of the main purposes for my visit was to finally end the war with my mother. I was verbalizing my intention, which I wanted to happen with all my heart.

A week before the trip, I had the following dream. I was back in my hometown and driving a car. Some old friends pulled me to the side of the road, a couple I had known since I was 17 years old. I had introduced them to each other and even stood up for them at their wedding. They still lived in the same town in which I was raised and I hadn't seen them for years. In the dream, they stopped me and said, "I don't know how to tell you this but your Mother has just died".

I thanked them and said,"I need to get over to my old house." At the house, my Father was there with my children and other family members that would have been present in this situation. The most surprising person there was my Mother. She was just as real as everyone else there except I was the only one who could see her. I asked her "Why are you here?"

She said that once she had seen the other side she saw things completely different, so she wanted to come back and talk to me. I suggested we go into the back room and talk, which we did. She apologized to me for different things she had done and I apologized to her for the things I had done. Then I woke up.

Understanding the meaning of dreams, I knew this could be a prophetic dream and that the death could just signify a change. I went on my trip and when I got there I was amazed to see my Mother with a new attitude. It was exactly what I wanted, without the sarcasm that had been there in the past. It has now been eighteen months since the incident and we are still in the same wonderful place. Now, she always considers my feelings, as well. She has become the Mother I always wanted and, hopefully, I have become the daughter she has always wanted."

Give daily thanks to God for all things and use daily prayer to improve the quality and reception of your dreams.

How Can I Analyze My Dreams?

- Keep a notebook or digital recorder beside your bed. Record your dreams as soon after waking as possible.

- Suggest to yourself every night before you fall asleep, "I will remember my dreams."

- If you wake during the night, write down the main symbol; the entire dream will usually come back in the morning.

- Practice keen observation in your dreams through self-suggestion prior to sleep.

- Look for these components in your dreams: the setting, numbers, the people, the action, repeating patterns, the feelings and the words.

- Work on analyzing your dreams every day, otherwise their progression will be difficult to assess.

- If dreams are illogical, three reasons are possible:

1. Only fragments of the dream have been recalled.
2. Mental blocks have erased your recall.
3. The dream is reflecting something illogical in the dreamer's life.

• If you are unable to decipher an important dream, suggest to yourself before your next sleep that the dream repeat itself more clearly.

• Nightmares, which bring with them an inability to move or cry out, could indicate the wrong diet. To end nightmarish dreams, change your diet.

• Dreams that are unchanged through the years indicate some unchanging part of the dreamer's life. Through working with the dreams, powerful changes can happen.

• Dreams of ill-health can be either literal or symbolic warnings.

• When a problem confronts you, ask for guidance to be sent to you through your dreams. Many believe they have a dreaming guide or guardian and ask them for help.

• Title your dreams after they are recorded, for ease of recalling them later.

• Begin a dream dictionary, making your dream symbols your own. Although there are many dream books with a dictionary of symbols, they will only apply to you part of the time.

• Dreaming of a person named Bill could refer to "bills" that must be paid; dreaming of a bus could mean travel to one person but hard times to another because of a bad bus trip in waking life.

• Be practical in your interpretation. Always look first for a lesson. What haven't you faced or what have you been ignoring?

• Dreams are the reaction of the inner self to daytime activity, and often show the way out of a dilemma. So relate them to current activity, because dreams may be retrospective, as well as prospective.

• Dreams come to guide and help, not to amuse. They direct your attention to errors of omission and commission and offer encouragement for right action. They also give us the opportunity to pray for others and give them support in dealing with their burdens.

- If you receive an unusual message, reduce it to common terms. See if the symbolism of the bible or some other field of study can be helpful in interpreting the dream. For example, if you were an astrologer, a dream of a particular planet might be loaded with whatever that planet means to you symbolically. If you are a computer whiz, there are symbols particular to your work that might have relevance. What are the "buzz" words in your life and what do they mean?

- Look for past-life experiences in your dreams. Frequently, these are Lucid Dreams involving all the senses. These manifest themselves not only in color, but in the proper costume and setting of the period. They come to warn you against repeating the same old mistakes; to explain your relationships and reactions to certain people and places; to reduce your confusions; and to enable you to better understand life.

- Do not fear conversations with the dead in your dreams. If the communication is one-sided, it denotes telepathy. If both participate, it may be an actual encounter of bodiless communication.

- Dreams are primarily about you. Only a few are about others and relate to family, friends, and world events. Always ask "What part of me does this character represent" before you go looking outside yourself.

- Watch for E.S.P. (extra sensory perception) in dreams.

- Remember persistence is necessary to learn any new language, and dream symbols are the forgotten language of the subconscious.

- Pay attention to the actual words used when verbalizing your dream to others, and analyze your choice of words and why you spoke them.

- To induce lucid dreams, try seeing the dream characters and symbols as different aspects of you.

- If a devil, demon or scary figure appears in a dream, it may indicate a part of you that is cut off because it is scary or unpleasant to you.　These are called shadow parts of your personality.

I have included a DREAMPLAY SHEET for you to use to record your dreams. I suggest that once you complete a sheet for each dream that you want to record that you keep them in a special folder or notebook so that you can review them when you want.

In addition, I have provided detailed explanations to assist you in filling out these sheets. Enjoy the wisdom of your dreams and marvel in how fortunate we are to be shown messages in this way.

DREAMPLAY SHEET

Date of Dream   Time of Dream   Number of Dream

Numbers		
	❑	Title of Dream
	❑	People in this Dream I recognize
Symbols	❑	My Dream:
Colors	❑	Does this Dream relate to the events of the last few days, an earlier part of my life or a past lifetime? How about a possible future reality?
Emotions	❑	How do I feel about this Dream?
	❑	What can I learn from this Dream?
	❑	Do I feel any Part of this Dream is Prophetic?

EXPLANATION OF DREAM PLAY SHEETS

Following are a number of Dream Play Sheets. These are designed to maintain a consistent record of your dreams and assist you in determining interpretations valid to you. The use of these forms is very straight forward. Simply, fill in ALL appropriate areas and review.

Date of Dream: Enter the date you had the dream. Was it before or after Midnight? This will determine what the actual date was.

Time of Dream: At what time of night, or day, did the dream occur? Has a pattern developed? Some of the sorting out dreams tend to happen for me in the earlier part of my sleep cycle, while the insightful and prophetic dreams tend to occur in the later part of the sleep cycle, often the last dream before waking up to start my day. See if you have pattern.

Number of Dream: You may have had several dreams in one night. Which one of your dreams was this one?

Title of Dream: This item would be best filled out LAST, even though it is at the beginning of the sheet. After all else is filled in, a title can be developed or may be quite natural. Give your dream a title relevant to the dream. This will help you remember and define it better. It will also assist you in finding a specific dream if it is prophetic or needs to be referenced in the future.

People in this Dream I recognize: Write down only the people you recognize within your dream. Often, you will recognize a dream character as someone who is familiar, but one you can't place from where you know them. Play the "it feels, looks, sounds or seems like" game. The essence of this person may be someone you are yet to meet, or someone who reminds you of a person in your present life or your youth. He or she might be a compilation of several people, possibly from some particular area of your life, like family or job. He or she may be from your waking world, or one who has passed over, or one you do not know but have dreamed of before. Be willing to look at these people as symbols of yourself. No matter how a dream character acts, remember they are a symbol from your creative subconscious and they are a part of you. They are creations that respond to you.

My Dream: Write as detailed a recollection of the dream as you can fit into the provided space. If additional space is required continue on the back side of the same sheet, and add sheets as you need them.

Does this Dream relate…? Does this dream relate to anything within your world of existence? Current, past, possible past lifetimes or perhaps it is a dream of the future for you.

How do I FEEL about this Dream? What are your feelings and emotions both during and after this experience? Frequently, this contains the most important part of telling the message of your dream. As you write out your emotional energy of the dream, it may become crystal clear and you may really hear the message that the dream is trying to relate to you.

What can I learn from this dream? What do you feel is the message, lesson or insight you have received from your dream?

Do you feel any part of this Dream is Prophetic? This question may or may not be answered immediately. Possible future or past, dreams may need to be referenced. Waking life may need to be played out, and sometimes a dream occurs several years or months prior to an event formerly dreamt about. It is possible, with the evolution of your intuition, that you are able to perceive and make Prophecy. I found that this question seemed ridiculous when I first completed my sheets, but then I became amazed when I went through the sheets and asked myself this question, to find that I almost always KNEW when a dream foretold a future event.

To the left of the page is a separate column listing Numbers, Symbols, Colors and Emotions. In this column enter such things appropriate as reference material. Were there definite numbers or colors? What emotions did you have during the dream? What symbols did you perceive that are actual or inferred?

Numbers, often your personal numbers, will be repeated in dreams. Your birthday may become an address or phone number. The day of the month you were born may become an amount in a money symbol of a dream. Some people's lives seem to revolve around certain numbers and these are often woven into a dream. For example, let's say that you were born on June 6th, 1950. Sixes may figure very prominently and simply relate to you because you were born on the 6th day of the 6th month, and 1950 adds up to a single digit of 6 (1+9+5+0= 15, 1+5=6) also. Sometimes your Astrological Sign, or some other personal symbol, will relate directly to you. In one instance, a dreamer saw two snakes fighting and felt one was her husband and the other represented her. As it turned out both she and her husband were born in the Chinese lunar calendar Snake years.

Use the following PERSONAL DREAM DIRECTORY in front of your folder or notebook to easily find a particular DREAMPLAY SHEET with the recorded dream you are seeking.

PERSONAL DREAM DIRECTORY

A PERSONAL DREAM DIRECTORY begins the Dream Sheets. This will help you organize and quickly find specific Dreams. Be sure to enter into the Personal Directory every time you record a Dream, giving the page number to locate specific dreams in the future. Assign page numbers to added pages to continue your records in order.

Title	Date	Page #

You can also begin to complete your own symbol dictionary using different words and symbols from your dreams. List them like a regular dictionary using the alphabet and keep adding new ones in. This can be fun and very interesting.

I have used the references listed below and find that reading other authors' book regarding dreams can only increase your knowledge about dreams. Although some dreams can seem very straight forward and simple, most dreams take time to evaluate and analyze. However, I have found that it is well worth your time and effort to do so because the messages are there for you. The language of dreams will let you discover yourself through the doorway of your subconscious mind.

If you can dream it, you can do it." Walt Disney

REFERENCES:

Faraday, Ann   DREAM POWER, 1972

Goldberg, Phillip   THE INTUITIVE EDGE
                                Jeremy Tarcher, Inc. 1983

Petos, Lee   THE DREAM LOVER
                                Llewellyn Publications, 1991

About the Author

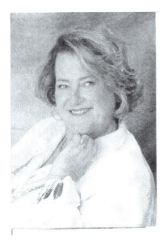

The following chapter on Dreams was written by Reverend Cecilia Cattel Carrillo a few years ago with the hope of having it edited and published. Unfortunately, Cattel died in March, 2010 before her dream could become reality. With gratitude and thanks to her friends, her material was gathered up and given to David Coffey and Regina Murphy to sort through and pull together, then given to Joan Peck for the final edit. Those efforts represent all the people in Cattel's life who loved her and appreciated her abundance of talent and encouraged her to write down some of her thoughts and experiences.

Cattel was born on June 31, 1951 in the Panama Canal area. She arrived in Las Vegas more than 30 years ago, and quickly became known as the Vegas Astrologer. Cattel was a certified hypnotherapist, a licensed minister for the Beacon of Light Church, and for three years served on the Board of Trustees to the First Church of Religious Science, aka Spiritual Life Center. Cattel lived a full life, and was a proud, foster mother to her son, Tha, in Cambodia.

Cattel was known far outside the Las Vegas valley for her radio show, "Stardate 2100," and assisted many all over the world that were in crisis and needed her calm, reassuring help. She was a featured author in the anthology "Life Choices – Navigating Difficult Paths," and wrote "We always have choices. Do we imprison ourselves, creating shackles around our heart, mind, or bodies? What we do with our choices can lead to freedoms, or most importantly our spiritual freedoms. Each time I give out a penny, or pay with Lincoln money, I send a silent prayer and intention...I give you this today to help you remember your freedom. "It is God given; never give it up for anything! Continue to make choices for freedom."

It is amazing how many times any of us can be talking about something, and then Cattel comes to mind wearing a smile on her face, and becomes connected to the conversation! She is sorely missed by all who knew her. But part of her legacy is this wonderful chapter on her version of Dreams, and we thank her for this.

Dream

Dream from your heart
It's always ok to hold on
Otherwise your hope dies
And your happiness is gone

Dream for yourself
It allows your faith to expand
It keeps you on your journey
It reminds you, that you can

Dream with your emotions
It's what takes you to the top
It's what brings life to your eyes
And won't allow it to stop

Dream as if you were a child
Being both, Innocent and true
Remembering, always the feelings
Keeping innocence inside of you

Dream with eyes that shine
Taking only what will bring you far
Never letting doubt to prevail
But always remembering who you are

Dream with ears that speak the truth
Don't tell yourself that you can't do whatever
Believe in the knowing of your faith
Hold on to it forever

Dream with your mind that lets you create
Inspire from your heart within love
Unlock your hidden gifts and shine
Always be thankful To God, above

Dream from the very essence of yourself
Teach others how to believe in the power
Remind yourself to hold it everyday
Never waste a day, minute, or hour

Dream with your imagination
See it bigger than beyond what you should
Tell yourself you can reach it now
But believe in the chance that you could

Dream from a place of beauty
See it all as magic, and explore
Be willing to experience all you can
Be safe to open and close every door

Dream, as if tomorrow never comes
Take the time to do it today
Let your dreams be whatever you want
Create whatever you may

Don't let a moment continue
Without putting forth your dream
For time is nothing but a waste
If you don't take time to dream.

~Donna Vicchiullo, 2011

About the Author

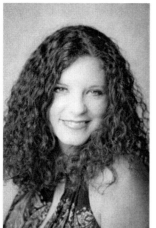

Donna Vicchiullo is an intuitive and a believer of following a spiritual journey to reach a higher self in one's life. On her own spiritual path, she became interested in connecting to her higher self through techniques and experiences of healing and energy work.

For the past 10 years, her desire to help other people, both physically and spiritually, led her to her own healing practices profession that include Massage Therapy, Reiki, and Spiritual Energy. She is available for private sessions.

Donna writes poetry, something that she has done most of her life, and is looking forward to publishing a book of her own poetry in the near future. She is a wife and mother of a 4 year-old daughter, and resides with her family in Las Vegas, Nevada.

Donna Vicchiullo can be contacted at:
www.donnastouch.vpweb.com
702 210-8077

Fairies

Danielle Dove

It is said that fairies are born when a child laughs for the first time. And the fairies would agree:

"We are born out of laughter! That is our responsibility - to make sure everyone is happy and merry."

In writing this chapter, I focused intently on listening to the small fairies that I could clearly see dancing around my desk through my third eye (with much excitement, my cat also saw them!). They had much to share about who they were in truth. Since Fairies and the rest of the beings from the Elemental Realm can be misunderstood, here is a viewpoint that they wanted to share with you, the readers of this book:

"We were created by God's laughter and now through all of you, we are able to exist to help the plant and animal world, and the fragile first years of babies and children. We guide them all safely when they are playing outside, we watch over them and help as much as we can. We are sensitive beings as well, but have been here for millions of years so we can transmit different knowledge, energies, and "beingness" into the human psyche to help you all with better flowing days. We love you all and support you so much. If only you could hear us better, we all could create vast abundance on earth for all to live happy lives. It isn't hard; we can help remove the weight of worry and fear that blocks the natural flow of your divine enterprises   here."

I was surprised that so much was coming through from these beautiful, little creatures. I took a break thinking that we were done, only to come back to find the ink of my fountain pen splashed on the desk and adjacent wall. I thought "How bizarre! They were careful enough to give me a sign without getting any ink on the carpet." I quickly cleaned it up and continued writing for them:

"[To the reader] we can guide you. Please read the chapter carefully, analyzing how you feel, and if any resistance were to come up, we can surely help you breathe through it. We thank you for listening; this means so much to us angels".

"Yes, we are angels! Even though we live mostly on earth close to plants and forests, we are still angels with wings, and we have special abilities that we love sharing with your world too!"

My understanding of the fairies and elemental realm is that they are the bridge makers between the people who live in closed houses, buildings and habitats - and the world outside full of green vegetation awaiting play and discovery. They are here to help us all remember to breathe in the light and colors that surround us and to touch plants with gratitude for their beauty. Whenever I have followed their guidance (and you can too!), every day feels as light and exciting as the first time that I fell in love.

It can really be a magical world out there if we would allow it to be. Serendipity will remind us that magic is real. Finding a long-lost friend spontaneously, rediscovering hidden talents, breathing deeper, wider, allowing more space within to flow, all of those gifts can come to us. Since we already have it all within – the last push is simply to allow. There is nothing to do, say or call, but to allow.

"Allow the energy to flow through you. When happy, you can fly, when unhappy, you can learn to release what makes you unhappy. It's easy, just allow it."

How did our planet become immensely abundant with a variety of species and color? Perhaps she has been "allowing" for that is all she can do. It doesn't take long to understand the entire earth system runs on organic, flowing relationships – such as the soil nurturing the seeds, and taking in the sun and rain. All of nature is always in a state of allowing. And isn't nature the richest of us all? Isn't nature constantly in a flux of abundance? It never lacks, but welcomes, allows and invites what it needs. When water is needed, the earth calls forward the rain and the clouds, the wind and all the elements to open up and receive. A forest left untouched in the Amazon can have thousands of varieties of fruits and is the home of many animals thriving from what was grown easily and almost effortlessly by the plants.

We are all like a forest...able to take in nourishment from Spirit, Nature, and Friends so that we may better grow, and ultimately have organic fruitful experiences, ideas, and creativity to share. If the forest stopped allowing, it would die. How often do we forget to "allow" as well, and end up feeling lack, fear and despair?

The fairies wish to do a healing for us now. They ask:

"Can you see yourself through our eyes for a moment? Imagine that you are indeed looking at yourself through our eyes .... Now, can you agree with us that you are such a wonderful magical being with energy at your own fingertips? We hope you have said yes! If not, we can help you get there; not to worry.

The first step is to ask yourself: Can I allow magic back into my life?

We say "back" into your life for it was there once, if not today. You remembered magic when something beautiful happened, when time no longer mattered and your feelings were so amazing you wanted to bottle them up to have them available for later. Magic is when you have a thought about someone and they soon call you – magic is when you no longer need to struggle to receive that which you are thinking of wanting. Magic is when you believe in magic itself – whatever you would like it to be."

I, myself, believe that energy is magic. It can enhance the quality of our lives, the food we eat and the beauty we see. Simply by sending love to someone, they can feel better! Isn't that amazing? Simply by blessing the land on which our crops grow, the energy of our loving intention can help food and flowers grow faster and stronger with more nutrients than if it hadn't been blessed (there is research done to prove this as well!).

Hugs are magic. Give more hugs, heart to heart, if you haven't received one recently. There are now groups of volunteers all over the world giving "free hugs." I've tried it for months now and it is a very healing experience for me. So much fun and "oneness" beyond words!

Hug your plants, your friends and family members, including your pets, holding the beautiful intention of blessing them with love as you do! We are all imbued with the purest, nicest energy of God's light and love and that of Mother Earth. We are spiritual beings but we also live on a planet in a body – we are denser than the fairies, yet we are so close to them in our abilities to spread light and magic all around. In essence, we can be just like the fairies spreading our magical "fairy dust," which for us might be a hug, a kind word, a smile, or positive thoughts to lighten up anyone and any place that might need it!

A journey home with the Fairies:

If you long to see the fairies and be closer to the earth, which many of us want, here is a little bit of advice for practicing "finding home" in everyday situations.

Learn to use your inner compass also called your internal guidance system.

The fairies suggest to allow (that word again) the sparkling light of our joy to tell us if we are going the right or wrong way.

"If something feels forced, it isn't the way home." they explained.

"Why is it so simple?" I asked.

"Simply because the true reality of home is comfort and coziness with an easy flow, where you can be yourself and still feel totally loved, accepted, and nurtured. So why would the way home be difficult, stressful, alone and dark?"

They have a point!

"If you feel this way, then you aren't heading home. Turn around, try something new because the way home is gorgeous, filled with flowers, blue skies, open-hearted friends and so much music you dance, dance, dance with arms open allowing, receiving, and welcoming!"

"This may take a few tries to start working. Please don't give up on your internal guidance system too soon. Look within and don't be afraid, but if you are, that's okay, too. You can breathe through your fear; it is only asking that you acknowledge it. Listen for a moment, and call upon your higher self. He or she will pick you up out of your fear, help you release your fear and like an old friend you will be able to say good bye to it easily so that you can journey onward, confident, trustful and allowing."

If you feel guided to work with the fairies, here is some more information to help you along your way. They can be hard to see or hear with your physical eyes and ears. Yet, there have been many sightings of fairies by people, especially children, in parts of the world where they are most common. That is not to say that they cannot be in your own backyard. If they know your heart is pure and you have good intentions in calling them forward, they will answer your call. The more you believe in them

("I believe in Fairies, I do, I do, I do!"), the more energy you give them to come closer to you.

Soon, you may see sparkling lights around you in a flash or an actual small fairy hiding in your backyard or on your morning walk. You might even see objects disappear only to reappear soon after once you explain to them you really do need your car keys to get to work – even if they are trying to get their message across that you should really stay home and take the day off to play. They are practical jokesters and love to lighten everyone up with their merry ways, but don't forget that they are very wise and always have your best interest in mind.

They know us all so well – they hear you when you cry, when you ask for help, and when you are afraid to receive. They can help you just as fast and efficiently as powerful archangels because they reside so close to us. You can work with all beings of light and love; there is no competition among them and they can all be with you simultaneously.

Fairies are not scary and never want to scare you. However, if you project fear unto them, the energy will feel like an attack and it will scare the fairies away. They are so sensitive. They can't be around smoke or pollutants in the home. It hurts their fragile wings. If you need to do a major clean up, simply warn them by talking out loud that you are about to spray chemicals and they really should step outside for a bit. Think of them as tiny sensitive beings that shy away from violence, anger and other destructive energies. Don't be afraid that they might not come back, they always will return to you.

Remember magic is always within. You are just as amazing as the fairy angels in your life. By allowing more of their magic and wisdom into your life, they will welcome you into theirs.

In the life of a "Day Fairy":

A Day Fairy wakes up gently, stretching her arms up with a smile, allowing the sun to warm her. She receives breakfast from the birds, seeds and fruits, and with a quick brush of her teeth with a green long leaf, she takes flight and oversees the plants assigned to her and any animals she is responsible for. She greets them all good day and, perhaps, even plays her music and sings to them, or spreads light from her hands to feed them spiritual nourishment. Do fairies meditate? Of course they do. It recharges their batteries. They meditate close to the ground or on top of trees, but they always flow energy from the light up above to the earth down below. Like a giant tree with huge long branches and strong deep roots, their energy acts as a conduit between the flow of sky and earth. Within minutes, they are full of energy imbued with the magic of God and Spirit. They say that without Spirit lightening them up, they wouldn't be able to fly as long or as well. They would ultimately get tired. Symbolically, it is the same for people. We may not see our wings, but we have them. If we get tired, we can't fly; so we all need to remember to charge up with Spirit, God and Earth and allow these three beautiful energies to re-enter our minds and body so the old can be released and the new can help our day flow better!

In the life of a "Night Fairy":

The Night Fairies have a different schedule. Some known fairies love to play, dance, be merry and laugh a lot. They are essentially the light in the darkness and are there to:
Keep children playful in their dreams,
Protect adults from making mistakes they'll regret in the morning,
Lighten up the day by having a really good night of fun play.

They understand that they may not be all that practical to the flow of life as are the Day Fairies, but they know that they were created for a purpose: "'LIFE." We live life at all times and creativity can happen at all hours. The night fairies are there for you if you are a night writer, or a musician, or dancer or work in the nightclubs. Don't be afraid because the fairies can protect and shield you, and help you stay "light" even in the dark. Remember to simply ask them for help, and call them forward, allowing them to come to you. Creating a fairy circle is another great way to invite the Day or Night Fairies into your life! (See below.)

Other Night Fairies fly above gardens and homes as gatekeepers, and act as messengers to other beings of light, such as Archangel Michael. In case there is a fight or a problem, they can report back to the angels of justice or the angels of healing to bring about resolution to a life threatening situation.

Night Fairies also work in hospitals quite often. Hospitals are places where much love and light is needed. They remind us all about the healing qualities of plants, which could assist the human body in its recovery alongside any prescribed procedure and medication from the doctors. The fairies do their best to brighten up flowers and plants around hospitals. They are grateful for those who take walks outside and admire the plants, the sun and the fresh air. For when we feel better, the fairies feel better, and earth feels better too.

Ideas for creating a fairy circle

Creating a fairy circle is easy and powerful! Fairy circles are an important tool to welcome the fairies through your intention and creation. You can create a circle out of rocks you find outside, flower or trinkets you own that are dear to you. It doesn't matter what you choose as long as you create the circle and pray over it for the fairies to come through. During my travels, I was guided to create a circle of angel cards or crystals wherever I stayed so that I could create an energy doorway for them to come through. I recommend you do the same wherever life takes you so your fairy friends can stay near you.

To see Danielle Dove's Fairy Circle, please visit :
www.youtube.com/user/healingdove

Meticulously, with their tiny arms and hands, the fairies can work on our energy when we call upon them for their assistance. Sitting by a tree outside, it is not uncommon to feel as though the tree wants to help us with our stress or worry. This is a practice I do often when I feel tired or "foggy." I ask permission if the tree would allow me to sit by it, and if I feel a heartfelt yes, I soon lean against it. Within moments you too may feel rejuvenated and much lighter. You may also feel the fairies around your heart, helping you release fearful thoughts. Like tiny workers they can get into the energy of our stress or heavy energy cluster and with love and light, replace the discord with harmony. The plant world is here to help us, as well. The fairies are its messenger and its caretaker, but it is important to follow your doctor's advice in using plants for healing.

I hope we all allow the fairies into our life to continue to bridge the world inside our head to the vastness of nature's world. They can help us live more spirit-filled lives. As we fill ourselves up with Spirit, we begin to notice events around us that we have attracted to help us find our way home. Every day is an opportunity to find home. Let's allow ourselves to be guided, and nurtured. We can start today. Right now! We can begin to use our loving intention to call back our innate powers and abilities, along with the strength and courage to take the steps to our bliss.

With the assistance of so many, you too, can become a Magical Being.

My own experience with the fairies
When I first read about the elemental beings and especially the people who had fairy-like qualities, I was sitting in the sand of a Malibu beach in California. It was my birthday...I was turning 24 on March 24, 2006.

142

Earlier, I had walked into the metaphysical bookshop, Malibu Shaman at Cross Creek, and picked up a tiny book by Doreen Virtue called Earth Angels. The day was spontaneous with a dear girlfriend visiting me from out of town. It was beginning to feel like a very healing week after a messy breakup just days prior, which had left me feeling sad and alone.

Yet, as soon as I opened Doreen's book, I felt an overwhelming sense that I was heading in the right direction. Her messages about the fairies, angels and other realms were bringing me back home. I slipped back into memories of my childhood. It explained why I loved being alone with animals around me, talking to the spirit of the forest. For many years, I was fortunate to have a horse to ride through the hills of Provence in the South of France until I moved to California in 1993. There is a magic to the forest that I will never forget because it is alive every day, growing, producing and renewing itself.

I learned that my sensitivities to food were normal since I had so many fairy-like qualities, and it gave me permission to explore another way of eating much closer to nature. I grew up eating very healthy and organic food, but I was still guided to go 100% raw vegan which I had started six months prior to my birthday. Of course, the fairies were delighted to see me stay on course and began to encourage me to start promoting gardens in school for children.

A few years after this first Malibu beach encounter, I realized working with kids brings much love to my heart. In 2009, walking through a grocery store in Las Vegas, a thought came to mind to ask about buying fruits wholesale. I didn't know whom to ask so when I saw an employee organizing some vegetables, I walked up to him, abandoning my own list of groceries, to explain I was "teaching a workshop to kids about eating fruits." The words came out of my mouth so fast I couldn't stop them. Was I teaching a workshop for kids on fruits? I had no idea...! It was indeed new to me...

I walked out realizing I had just been handed a new idea and a new assignment. Knowing the fairies tend to take care of the rest, I continued with my daily routine. Watering that new idea by exciting thoughts, I was grateful to think that the experience could happen.

Within a few weeks I was offering delicious (free) fruity workshops at multiple Whole Foods Markets in Las Vegas. Children of all ages came out to make it a meal! The colors popping from the table enchanted both parents and children. They came alive with the creations they could make and then eat. It was pure bliss to be able to share my love of natural foods with them, uncooked, unprocessed, natural sugars in high water content foods.

Since my first realization of the fairy realm, I have seen fairies many times, in many parts of the world. I will share with you a few stories, knowing that there are many more to come. Ask around; some people and children may be too shy to share their fairy stories, but with some kind nudging, they may open up!

Once at a home gathering in Santa Monica, California, I walked toward a group of friends and announced that I believed in fairies. Clapping my hands with excitement, my love for them came out spontaneously. I got strange looks from the people that night, but shortly after I understood why I felt guided to talk about them and celebrate them. Walking outside a short moment later with my soul sister Taylor, we saw a beautiful large flickering green light dancing in the dark blue sky right above us. "It's a fairy! It's a fairy!" Taylor exclaimed. I thought it was just a plane. Yet, I had to admit that it was a little too close to be a plane, and it was zigzagging in all directions. With a closer intuitive look, I could agree that it really was a happy celebrating fairy. We were both so thrilled to have seen it together! Our friend, Greg, who owned the home, got teary eyed to hear about a fairy near his home for he had been calling them and kept many beautiful plants alive in his home just for them.

It wasn't the first time an experience such as that one came to us. In 2008, we had gone to Hawaii together to attend Doreen Virtue's Angel Therapy® course in Kona. At the time, Taylor and I both were going through a period of healing past relationships. We needed a respite from hours spent inside practicing our new gifts of channeling. As I walked to the pool, I felt the urge to advance towards the black rocks on the edge of the ocean. Taylor was getting something to eat, so I went ahead without her. Within seconds, Taylor came up to the ocean and joined me. I grabbed her hand and announced loud and clear to the ocean and universe beyond, "We are Goddesses and we can be in relationships and excel!"

As though the ocean heard me, a huge dolphin jumped out of the water at that exact moment half a mile away from us in the deep blue water of Hawaii. Personally, I thought it was a fish, (again my eyes not being that great) but just to prove its point the dolphin began swimming directly towards us in and out of the water until he reached us at the edge of the cliffs. Our screaming and clapping had gotten the attention of the tourists at the pool, asking us if we had called the dolphin forward. I don't know who called whom first, but we all came together - dolphin, goddesses, and soul sisters - and declared our new truth and it was cause for celebration.

When we believe in God's helpers: fairies, angels, ascended masters and other divine creations, we give them energy which thins the veil between the two worlds so that we may feel God's love closer to us. Just as in a relationship with a loved one, you both need to give for the exchange to happen. It is the same with God's playful creation - love the fairies, cherish and honor them and they will work with you throughout your life as you journey onward.

Swami Ramananda says the three ways God loves to be worshipped is through dance, music and singing...all the ways the fairies celebrate life! If you are part of a religion that professes not to contact anyone outside of God or Jesus Christ, rest assured, you are safe to call forward the angels and the fairies. As long as we practice safe discernment, it makes our Father in Heaven happy to know we are welcoming pure beings of light and love into our lives. Learn to pay attention to the guidance you receive, but practice self-knowledge. Does the guidance feel it comes from a positive source outside yourself or a negative one within your mind? If you would like to learn more about how to hear your angels, please study Doreen Virtue's book by that name: "How to Hear your Angels". It is a great little book that I have found very valuable in my classes.

If you love dolphins, mermaids or unicorns, these beings are also from the elemental realm. Connect to them for they will bring much love and healing into your life. The animal world is so sensitive to us and knows so much more than we have understood. There is always more to discover. Be open to inviting all the answers to your questions into your life, they will come!

Much love and blessings.

About the Author

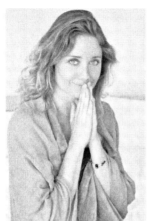

Danielle Dove, Angel Therapist® Energy Healer, and co-founder of Healing Dove Therapy™, was born and raised in France until the age of 13. She moved to the U.S. to continue her education in the States leading her to attend UCLA with a B.A. in Environmental Studies '04. Throughout her childhood, she grew up close to nature on a small farm in the South of France.

Her ability to hear and channel messages began as a child when she could hear "downloads" of scripted messages whenever she slept or spent time alone with her horse. Thereafter, 3 sudden deaths over the span of 8 years led her to ask many questions. She was able to use her gift to receive answers, which led her to the path of a healer and a channel for God and His Angelic Realm.

As a devoted Light Worker, she works in the United States and Europe spreading the healing light to all who seek the same healing and answers that she had needed many years before. In 2011, she is birthing her first child, as well as birthing a new certification program for Light Workers interested in turning their gifts into a fulfilling career. Her philosophy in life is to Love All and Shine Brightly.

Danielle Dove can be contacted at:
www.healingdove-therapy.com
www.danielledove.com

Feng Shui

Are You Ready To Move Forward

Magdalena Brandon

Let's go on a journey. Close your eyes and visualize your home. Do you know why you hung that mirror in that particular spot? Why do the red walls make you happy? Are those furniture pieces too big for your living room? When walking into your bedroom, is there a sadness that comes over you? When sitting in your family room, are you relaxed? Can anyone afford not to know about Feng Shui? If you are looking for answers to these questions, then please read on...

Having been an interior designer for over 25 years, I was introduced to Feng Shui a few years ago by several Feng Shui Consultants, who wanted my expertise in selecting paint colors for their clients. As we worked together, it was intriguing to me how Feng Shui worked. Listening intently to their comments and suggestions, I became aware that I had been practicing the art of Feng Shui intuitively for years without any formal training. I became certified in Feng Shui in 2004, my intuition was magnified and I gained an even greater understanding, awareness and knowledge of the workings of Feng Shui. This gives me the ability to have complete clarity with my clients, and know that we will accomplish their intentions.

Feng Shui (literally translated as *wind-water*) is an ancient Eastern philosophy gaining a huge following in the West due to its beneficial and

147

amazing results. Today's westernized approach to Feng Shui enables you to balance your hectic life, and create a sanctuary in your home and office. Using Feng Shui in your environment enables you to create a happier, healthier and more prosperous life. Feng Shui works with the energy surrounding you, or "Chi," and allows this energy to flow freely and fill your life with positive results. Working with a Feng Shui consultant empowers your environment and allows the Universe to work for you rather than against you. Simple techniques are applied to allow "Chi" to travel through a space without obstacles, thus creating a fluid journey through life. If intention is clear at the time Feng Shui enhancements are made, the results are dramatic!

Harnessing the power of positive energy in your environment and allowing it to support your intentions and dreams in life is the art of Feng Shui.

The Bagua means eight sides that relate to nature, man, family, relationships, and all eight aspects listed below. It is used to both guide and interpret a person's life and problems, and is used as a cure to resolve them. As you can see on the Bangua Map (pg. 152), each area is outlined showing the quadrant, which element is predominant and the colors to use for paint, accessories and artwork.

Currently, I am working with a client who was at the end of her "rope." She had no feelings of hope; felt she had a hole in her soul; suffered physical health challenges, and was very unhappy with her life and where she was headed. After several failed relationships, she is single, has cats for her companions, and is passionate at what she can do for other people regarding health and nutrition through diet and exercise. A mutual friend recommended my services to her, and told her that I could help her create a more harmonious environment, more wealth, the possibility of a fabulous relationship, and support her body in healing itself. We set up a time for our first meeting.

Before I meet with a prospective client, I have guidelines that I use to help me:

- <u>First Impressions</u>. I become aware of first impressions, feelings and messages that I receive upon arriving at the site. These "hunches" that I sense most likely are something I have to focus on, and signal a main Feng Shui issue.

- Alterations in my "Chi". By keeping my senses alert, I note anything that alters my "Chi" through my five physical senses. If it catches my eye, it alters "Chi," if it catches my nose, it alters "Chi." Always remember that "Chi" is the leading factor affecting human life. Translated as "breath," "Chi" is energy or force that creates mountains and volcanoes, directs streams and rivers, and determines the colors and shapes of trees and plants.

- Stay open. I keep open to receiving messages from the environment as I approach my destination. I take some time to listen, be silent and allow my intuition to guide me.

- Communicate and listen to my client. When I meet with the client, it is her turn to tell me what is going on in her life and home, and what she wants to accomplish.

The consultation with my client began with us touring her home and taking notice if there was clutter that had to be removed. Most of us consider clutter to be stacks of junk lying around. In Feng Shui, clutter can be more than that. It can be stacks or piles, numerous "little" things, clothing that doesn't fit or must be repaired or having **too much**, in an area **not big enough**.

My client had several areas in her home that had clutter. Because the releasing process can be challenging, getting rid of the clutter became her homework assignment. I suggested that she play music during this process because it can set the tone and allow her to get into a rhythm of de-cluttering. She will complete her work with four options: she can trash it, organize it, donate it or give it to someone who will benefit from it, or she can either sell or return it.

As she went through this process, the energy produced from removing her clutter was unbelievably powerful. It became clear to her that having this clutter had produced a lethargic, tired feeling and kept her feeling depressed while living in the past, and even had produced health problems.

Don't let this happen to you! When you de-clutter the areas in your home or office, here are the 10 steps that will support you during the process…the same 10 steps I gave to my client.

1. Hold and honor items – thank it for the place it held in your life; then let it go.

2. List objects that you have in each room. Does each object have a place and is it something you absolutely love.
3. Don't buy anything without getting rid of something.
4. Sell things before buying another.
5. Burn items in a ritual.
6. Give things away before you bring in new things.
7. Limit your surface areas to 50% covered.
8. Say NO to objects given to you that you won't use or don't love.
9. Don't store objects for yourself or others – use it or lose it.
10. Move things around at least once a year. This helps the energy move and not become stagnant.

After my client completed Phase I (De-clutter), the next step was to determine where she was in her life, what her biggest challenges were, and the reason she wanted me to Feng Shui her home. Previously, I had asked her to write down her intentions before we met to discuss them. As we talked, it became clear that she wanted to be in a romantic relationship, wanted to create more wealth, and wanted to expand her career. In order to be effective, her intention had to be 100%.

As we started this process, we found that the energy in her home was stuck. She had many silk plants, keepsakes from the past, artwork that was negative, furniture that had to be moved, and new furniture to be purchased. What does all that mean?

First, the silk plants were dusty, dried out and old. They had to be removed or if kept, had to be cleaned. Because there were silk plants in every part of her home, it was a huge challenge for the "Chi" to keep moving. Many of the keepsakes from relatives and friends had negative meaning to her and were in two important areas of her home, the Career and the Health of Home. The "Chi" was blocked in this area and it didn't surprise me that she was having health issues. Are you able to see how this relates to the Bagua Map? My client was able to keep an open mind, take notes and get to her true feelings.

We then moved to the area concentrating on relationships. This was extremely enlightening as her master bedroom was in that area. At first glance, she did not have anything that represented pairs, such as matching nightstands, lamps, artwork, etc. The bed was under the window and had to be moved immediately because the bed should be the most comfortable place to lie down and relax. Having the bed under the window allows her to hear traffic noise and sirens, and the experience will affect her mental stability, her heart will beat faster, and she will become more excitable. This has a great negative impact on the balance of the nervous systems. The room was very "cold" and had no personality. Since a romantic relationship was number 1 on her intention list, this was a priority! In order to have better "Chi," it was necessary to have this room changed to include the following:

1. Matching nightstands
2. Pair of lamps
3. Pair of live plants
4. Replace or repair the smoke detector
5. Bring in symbols of love
6. Display artwork with pairs i.e., pair of butterflies, birds, flowers, etc.
7. Introduce a water feature
8. Bring in colors of red, gold and green
9. Soften windows with fabric

Next, we moved into the Wealth corner of her home which is the Living/Dining Room. We had to focus on creating a huge energy shift! There was no life in that area...her walls are white and she did not have the budget to repaint them yet, so we had to create other solutions. Existing in the room were silk plants, dining room furniture and an armoire. By bringing in soft, flourishing, live plants along with water flowing, it increases the "Chi." You can also use tall columnar shapes, vertical stripes and greens, purples and reds to accent.

We next focused on her Career area because she had indicated that she wanted to bring in more modalities to support her clients' outcome of better health. The Career area is her staircase and her guest bedroom. The staircase is sharp and steep and has limited space. The guest bedroom was being used as a storage area. What can enhance this area is flowing water or pictures of water and glass or mirrors. The colors suggested for this area are shades of blues and black.

As we walked through the rest of the home, more notes were taken, and we itemized all the areas that required purchases, keeping in mind to use what items we had before making unnecessary purchases. We moved existing artwork, cleared the clutter from the bookcase, and moved furniture. Next, we began to shop for items, making sure that we were in alignment with what was within her budget. She was the ideal client because she was ready for change and ready to move forward, trusting that what we were doing would support her intentions.

After shopping for a few hours, we came back to put it all together. What a transformation of energy! You could feel the shift, breathing became easier and her cats were happier...they became playful, showed more love, and did not hide when people visited.

The artwork was hung, the master bedroom was transformed, the living room/dining room was coming alive! We used the mirrors that my client had sitting in her garage not being used to hang on the wall of the stairwell, along with some candles, and added a plant on the landing. This helped deflect the bad "Chi," brought the heavy "Chi" upward, and brought good energy to this space.

I also walked the property outside, paying close attention to the shape of the lot and pathways, landscape, roof line and condition, streets, telephone lines or transformers. The exterior of any house is always ongoing and we made some changes to support the shift of energy. We used wind chimes, potted plants both in front and back of the house. The rest of the landscape project will be completed by next spring.

Did Feng Shui help my client? Within a few weeks, she began dating a number of men, and finally settled on one that she liked the best. Her whole being has softened, and she has become more approachable. This is helping her create more relationships that will bring potential clients into her business. She is continuing her education and looking at alternative healing methods for increased health for her clients.

There are different schools of Feng Shui and I am certified in the Black Tantric Buddhist (BTB) Feng Shui. This school was brought to the United States in 1980 by Professor Thomas Lin Yun. He addresses the way we deal with our immediate environment and how it shapes our lives. Feng Shui attempts to define what elements in your environment depress or elevate you. It also identifies design problems and offers simple "cures" to balance and enhance your surroundings and your life. He eliminated the compass orientation of the Bagua and included form school principals in his teaching. Rather than relying on compasses and mathematical formulas, Professor Lin Yun taught a more spiritual approach, emphasizing intuition and conscious intention. Today, many practitioners follow his teachings and some have modified them further. I find this western approach more compatible with our lifestyle in the United States and with my own beliefs.

Here are the four major components of Feng Shui:

1. "Chi" Flow – Chinese believe that everything is filled with power, energy and spirits…animals, plants, rocks, minerals, water, thunder, lightning, weather systems, etc. The goal is to arrange rooms and furniture in the most beneficial way to achieve maximum harmony with nature. According to Chinese beliefs, once this is achieved, prosperity and happiness will follow.

2. Bagua – Represents eight areas for different aspects of our lives. The Center of the Bagua represents complete balance and having endless possibilities.
   - Wealth and Abundance
   - Fame and Reputation
   - Relationships
   - Health and Family
   - Creativity and Offspring
   - Knowledge and Self Cultivation
   - Career and Life Path
   - Benefactors and Travel

3. Yin & Yang – The Yin represents all that is still, receptive, cool and contracting by nature. Yang represents all that is active, creative, hot and expanding by nature. When we go too far in either direction – imbalance and disharmony occur. To live in harmony is to be in balance with the natural earth forces of Yin and Yang to create healthy and prosperous lives. The balance of Yin and Yang is the ultimate goal of Feng Shui.

4. Five Elements – Along with the Yin and Yang, the 5 elements are an additional way of analyzing and harmonizing the "Chi" of a person or a house. "Chi" can be divided into five elements: metal, wood, water, fire and earth. The five elements can be associated with colors, times, seasons, directions, planets, body organs, and so on. For example, water is associated with black – the deeper the water, the blacker it is; also, it is associated with winter and north direction. Fire is red, summer and south. These elements mutually create and destroy each other in a fixed order.

   For example:
   - Wealth area is associated with Wood
   - Fame area is associated with Fire
   - Relationship area is associated with Earth
   - Health and Family area is associated with Wood
   - Creativity and Offspring area is associated with Metal
   - Knowledge and Self Cultivation area is associated with Earth
   - Career area is associated with Water
   - Benefactors and Travel area is associated with Metal

As a Feng Shui Specialist, I pay close attention to the balance of the 5 elements. If the occupants of a home are experiencing difficulties in any particular area of their lives, I look to see if the elements are out of balance in relation to their proper position on the Bagua Map. (see Bagua Map).

Today, mastering Feng Shui requires many years of training, along with an intuitive talent. Keeping it simple for my clients is my intention. Here are some of my suggestions:

1. Keep clutter to a minimum. This includes boxes of "stuff," too much furniture, and piles of magazines, mail, or newspapers.

2. Harness your "Chi" by using cures such as mirrors, wind chimes, water features and crystals.

3. Make sure there are no mixed energies in your home. For example, having clothes in your closet that don't fit; exercise equipment that is not being used; an open door that leads from the bathroom to the bedroom; your "office" located in the dining room or the bedroom.

4. Evaluate your rooms. You might have furniture in your home that is either too large in scale or you have too much in one room. Or there might be a color imbalance – either all the walls are white or there is one color throughout.

5. Check surfaces. Have surfaces such as kitchen counters, tables, night stands, etc. covered less than 50%.

6. Use the space you have. Lack of use of a space such as a guest room, dining room or bath should be used on a regular basis.

7. Keep the electro-magnetic fields to a minimum, especially in your bedroom. These include clock radio, television, telephone, and cable. Having all of these items in one room will disrupt concentration and/or sleep.

We all seek to have in our lives peace, love, happiness and success. Have you ever wondered why some people seem to have it all and success comes easy to them? Without even realizing it, you may be holding yourself back from all that you deserve simply because of blocked energy or "Chi." I encourage you to read and understand Feng Shui. I know that it can seem a bit confusing, and I will make myself available to help you or find a Feng Shui Specialist in your area. Remember, "If you do not change direction, you may end up where you are heading!"

BAGUA MAP

Wealth
Wood,
Green, Red,
Purple, Blue

Fame
Fire
Red

Relationships
Earth
Red, Pink, White

Health & Family
Wood
Green

Earth
Yellow

**Creativity/
Offspring**
Metal
White, Silver,
Gold

**Knowledge,
Self
Cultivation**
Earth,
Yellows, Greens,
Dark Blues

Career
Water
Black, Dark Blues

**Benefactors,
Travel**
Metal
White, Grey,
Black

|| || ||

Main Entrance or Door

About the Author

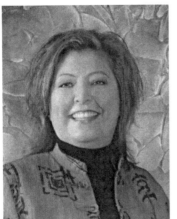

Magdalena Brandon has always had a passion for color and design and began a career as an interior designer in 1984 and opened my first retail store in Las Vegas, NV in 2000. Her articles have been published in the Las Vegas Home and Garden Magazine. She also is a Feng Shui Specialist and understands the importance of balance and harmony, not only in ones' environment, but also for Mind, Body and Soul.

She started coaching professionally in 2006; prior to becoming a MMS Certified Coach, she discovered that it was because of her ability to listen to her clients and ask them questions that created the unique relationship that she has with them.

Magdalena is a creative, passionate, ethical business professional who always has fun no matter what she does! She enjoys supporting others in achieving their objectives, be it creating a beautiful home or creating a beautiful life, internally and externally.

Magdalena Brandon can be contacted at:
www.magdalenasvegas.com
magdalena@magdalenasvegas.com
(702) 218-5415

Goals and Affirmations

You have the Power to Create Your Future

Judi Moreo

Many of us think we have no control over our lives. Failure to accomplish what we want in life is a result of failing to believe in ourselves enough. We let doubt sneak in and then we make excuses about our ability, time constraints, training and talents. Doubt creates stress, panic and anxiety.

Sometimes, people succeed in a conventional sense, but lack happiness because they aren't doing what they really want. Instead, they attempt to fulfill the desires and goals of someone else rather than meet their own needs and goals. Perhaps, they have fallen under the influence of a parent or a spouse. How can they feel passionate about something they don't really want? They may have even stopped making any effort toward their real goals because of a fear of failure, a fear of rejection or lack of self-worth. If only they would pursue their own interests and use their natural talents, they would be sure to succeed.

When you know what you want and take action in the direction of your goals, it gives you a reason to get up in the morning. When the goal is your own and you work toward it, you have more energy and your days become exciting.

Consider how much time you have left to live if you live to an average life expectancy of 77 years. How old are you now? We are all born into greatness and through our upbringing or life circumstances, we sometimes allow life to pull us down into mediocrity and something less than we desire. That's not necessary. Decide now how you want to spend the remainder of your time on earth. If you are feeling as if life is passing you by and you don't feel a burning passion inside of you urging you to fulfill your life's purpose, then something is wrong! Ask yourself these questions:

When was I the happiest in my life?

What things made me happy?

How much time do I spend now doing the things I like to do most?

How often do I feel that I am not accomplishing anything?

Then:

Make a list of what your childhood dreams were.

Make a list of your wishes as they are now.

Make a list of all the things that you do well.

Make a list of all the things you'd like to do.

Once you have evaluated yourself, you will have an idea of what is missing, what's desired and what's next!

Start now to establish concrete goals for yourself within the framework of your true talents and interests. Determine what your needs, wants and desires are --for now and for the future. You can't gain control over your life without knowing the direction in which you want to go and having a plan of action to get you there. Goals focus your energies in one direction…toward your vision. Defining your goals will put your imagination to work. You will start to concentrate on what you really want rather than just getting by day after day. When you decide what you want in specific detail, then your mind will start to formulate a plan to get it. Define your goals!

You need to know what you want. In goal setting, it's okay to be selfish! Do you have any childhood dreams that remain unfulfilled or any cities that you have always wanted to see but never visited? Consider all the material things you want, the lifestyle you desire, the places you would like to go or things you would like to do and incorporate them into your goals. What is important to you? What are your most important values? When do you feel most needed and appreciated? What do you love to do? What gets you excited?

Set definite goals for things you want to have and to do. Write down that dream you have been carrying around in your head. Don't believe any desire is too great or out-of-reach. Be descriptive. Writing down your goals will help you acknowledge them, commit to them and then act on them. When you put your goals in writing, add every detail. Write down the size and name of that new boat you've always wanted. Describe your new home's square footage and its location. Finally, use positive phrases. Instead of "I want a new home" write "I am enjoying my new beach house by (write in a specific date.) Be honest with yourself. Don't write down things you think you should want or things other people have told you to want. Goal setting is what you do for yourself, not something to do to please others. Write down only what you want; then, write down what you are willing to do to get it. It may take time to achieve your goal, so make it meaningful and fun.

You may not even be aware of how easy it will be to achieve your goals when you start to *believe* you can, and take steps in the direction of your goals. Action is what it will take to make your goals a reality and writing them down is your first action. Then you need to focus on the goals and work toward them...one step at a time. Don't worry about knowing all the steps at the beginning. Just start. With each step, you'll see how to go further and that will increase your self-motivation.

Self-motivation is the bridge between thinking about your goals and accomplishing them. Self-motivation is the desire you have to achieve or obtain something and it is essential to have it if you are to succeed in any endeavor. It isn't something that comes naturally for everyone. However, it can be learned and developed. It is the inner desire that keeps you always moving forward in spite of discouragement, mistakes and setbacks.

You can build this desire and achieve your goals by staying focused forward and allowing only positive thoughts to dominate your thinking. You must believe you are a success for success to come your way.

Planning your future

Set goals in the eight major areas of your life:

1. Career
2. Finances
3. Health
4. Relationships
5. Recreation
6. Education
7. Community
8. Spiritual

Each area of your life should be planned keeping in mind how you will achieve the goals you are setting. Write steps or sub-goals to use as check points so you will be able to tell whether or not you are making progress. Ask yourself questions that pertain to each area of your life. The answers will define your direction and goals. Once you begin, you will be amazed at how quickly things start to happen for you.

SMART Goals

Once you have given considerable time and thought to the evaluation of your life, you will have the vision and the big picture. Big picture dreams are wonderful because they inspire and excite. It's up to you. It is now time to turn your dreams, intentions and desires into firm achievable goals. Writing your goals out, using the SMART method is the first step to living your dreams. SMART goals make it easy to stay on track and resist temptation that may attempt to sidetrack you in directions you don't want to go.

SMART Goals are **S**pecific, **M**easurable, **A**greed upon, **R**ealistic and **T**ime framed.

Specific

Be very specific when writing your goals. Detail every aspect. Writing down your specific goals clarifies exactly where you are going and how you will know when you have arrived. Assess where you are now in relation to where you want to go. By evaluating your current position, you will be able to measure the distance between where you are and where you want to go and write sub-goals for the steps you will need to take. Also, you can identify changes you may want to make along the way. Take a close look at your current title, income, residence - anything that reaching your goals may alter in the future. With a realistic assessment of your current situation, you will be better able to set achievable goals.

Measurable

Regular assessment is how you measure progress. Set a timeline and determine checkpoints in order to keep track of your progression toward your goal. Remember, big visions take time to materialize. Identify several smaller goals you must accomplish to reach your big one. As you reach each small goal, reward yourself and move on to the next. It is important to celebrate your successes as you go. Recognizing your achievements along the way will help you keep a positive attitude throughout the journey.

Measurement is how we keep track of our progress and how we will know if we begin to veer off the charted path. In this way, we can immediately make any adjustments needed.

Agreed upon

If there are other people whose cooperation you need in order to reach your goal, you need to get their agreement early in the journey. If they don't agree to do their part or to support you in achieving your goals, your journey will be more difficult than need be or it may not be attainable at all.

Realistic

When your goals aren't realistic, you are setting yourself up to fail before you have even started. Your goals must be high enough to motivate you and yet realistic. If you don't believe they are realistic, self-doubt will set in and undermine you causing you to become immobilized. Ask yourself if your goals will create conflict in any other areas of your life. How far are you willing to go to get what you want?

Ascertaining what you want requires self-examination to determine the extent to which your skills, beliefs, values and attitudes relate to your objectives. You will be more likely to succeed if your objectives evolve from your natural abilities and a positive attitude. Achieving your goals requires a high sense of priority that will require belief and discipline. Make sure you have given yourself realistic time frames and resources to accomplish your goals. Don't be concerned with how realistic these goals appear to anyone else. Just be sure you believe you can do what you have set out to do.

Time framed

If you don't have a time designated as to when you will accomplish your goal, you probably won't accomplish it at all. If it doesn't matter when it gets done, it usually doesn't get done. Start your plan with the final objective and work backwards, making sure to allow enough time for each step. Knowing not only what you intend to accomplish but when you want to accomplish it, keeps you focused as well as letting you know if you are ahead or behind your intended schedule. Time lines are set as a means of breaking projects down into smaller, bite-sized chunks so you don't feel overwhelmed. They are not meant to stress you out or make you feel guilty. They are observable criteria that ensure your steady progress rather than leaving it to chance. Good intentions are nice, but a good plan is powerful and a timeline is essential to your success.

Get a clear picture

In addition to the SMART method for setting goals, there are other things that you can do to assure success. Cut pictures out of magazines of the things you want to have and the places you want to go. Paste the pictures next to your written goals or someplace where you will see them daily to imprint them on your mind. Affirm positively, out loud, that you will achieve them.

List the benefits

It is important to identify the benefits you will derive from attaining your goal. Make a list of any way you will benefit from each of your goals either during the process or after attainment. Focus on your rewards. Why should you be motivated? What positive consequences will you enjoy when you put your plan in motion? Visualize the rewards that achieving your goals will bring. Visualize clearly and vividly. Make it such a clear picture that you'll do almost anything to be a part of it. When you drive toward that image, you are motivated.

When you set goals, you are no longer leaving your future to chance. You are actually choosing to make changes in your life. Be prepared to feel a little uneasy at the prospect of doing things you haven't done before, and give yourself time to adjust to new situations. When you do things you haven't done before or attempt things you've only dreamed of, you often feel fears...fear of getting lost, fear of not knowing what to do, fear of looking stupid, fear that you are not "good enough," fear of rejection and many more. It's natural to feel fear. Identify and understand your fears. Only then will you be able to defeat them. Recall job changes, moves or other upheavals that you have experienced in the past to remind yourself that you adjusted then and can adjust now as well. Take action. Action cures fear. Once you begin doing something, it becomes easier and your fears disappear. Take changes one day at a time and stay positive by focusing on the reason for them. When you are able to cope with changes whether you make the choice to change or the changes come unexpectedly, you are taking charge of your life and your future.

Set priorities

If you plan your days and your activities, ranking tasks in order of importance and taking care of the most important things first, you will have fewer crises in your life and you'll get more positive results. Priorities are also a psychological trigger to action. If you don't have pre-set priorities for your day, you could spend your entire day trying to figure out what to do next, as well as allowing anyone and everyone to interrupt you and keep you from accomplishing anything important. You will appear disorderly and indecisive.

With clear cut priorities, you can get your day off to a fast start and stay on the right path throughout the day gaining momentum as you go. Sir Isaac Newton formulated the laws that govern momentum: "A body at rest stays at rest," and "A body in motion stays in motion." It is far easier to keep working once you are on a roll than it is to get started in the first place. Working your priority list, when you finish one task you will move right into the next. It will be easier to make decisions as well, because if it's not on the list, unless it is an important emergency, it doesn't need to be done until the priorities are finished.

People who set priorities usually accomplish more in shorter periods of time.   This allows them to avoid workaholic behavior and live a quality life.

Identify possible obstacles

If you have big goals you will probably face some adversity along the way. Make a list of any people, habits or other obstacles that may stand between you and your goals. Then decide how you will handle them. In addition to the obstacles you recognize now, consider potential changes and what obstacles those changes may present. Find out what resources are available to help you overcome obstacles. Consider opportunities for training, learning or acquiring new technology as well as meeting and networking with new people. Take advantage of any opportunities. The road to your goals may not always be smooth, but the bumps and potholes you foresee will be easier to overcome than the ones you don't expect.

Review your goals regularly

The things you do every day will either take you closer to your goals or lead you away from them. Discipline yourself daily to do the things that need to be done to accomplish your goals. If you are going to be successful, you must stay focused on your vision. Be sure to post a written version or a picture of that vision in a place where you will see it often. Be sure to review your goals frequently in order to stay motivated. Look at the pictures you have in your book and write in your journal each day what you have done that day to accomplish your goals. As you review your goals, measure your progress and make any changes necessary in your strategy. You become what you think about, so make a mental picture of each goal and carry it around with you.

Journal for Achievement

Journaling is another avenue for success and is a very personal undertaking. Whether you choose to write daily or weekly or whenever the mood strikes you, there are some guidelines to follow that will help you stay on target. Writing it down gives you an opportunity to see what you are thinking. It gives you a chance to clarify your thoughts and become more precise. Reviewing past entries can give you a chance to celebrate how far you've come.

It is not important how much you write or whether you write daily. It is important that you write as often as possible. Whatever you write should be positive and definite. How you write is as important as writing. Avoid negative words like "not", "won't", "don't", "can't ..." The more you program your thinking with positive, definite statements, the easier it is to become the change you are seeking. Journaling should not be a diary of daily events, hurts and challenges, but rather an achievement journal intended to be a record of your steps toward achieving your dreams.

Whenever you write, date your journal entry. Don't forget to put the year on your entries. When you look back over your old journals, you will be able to see where you were at specific times in your life. Dating your entries will also help you chart your progress toward your goals.

Be sure to give yourself gold stars or stickers for your accomplishments. Rewarding yourself for a job well done feels good.

Affirm Your Success

Affirmations are one of the most important elements of goal achievement. To affirm means to "establish or pronounce," something to be true. An affirmation is a powerful, positive statement that something you would like to have happen has already happened. It is a way of making your mind and subconscious believe that what you are imagining can be reality.

Most of us have dialogues going on in our mind almost constantly. We talk to ourselves about anything and everything. Our thoughts, feelings, emotions, questions, judgments all run through our minds like an endless movie. Yet, how often do you really think about what you are allowing this endless dialogue to say? Is it negative or is it positive? What you are thinking influences your feelings about what is happening in your lives. And since your thoughts create your feelings, your feelings influence your behavior, and your behavior brings about the results you have in your life, then you can safely assume that your thoughts create the way you respond or react to just about everything that happens in your life.

Many of us are not aware of the kind of thoughts we habitually think. Many of your thoughts have been programmed into your mind by your previous relationships with parents, teachers, friends, spouses, and others. Many of your thoughts come from your culture or your education.

These thoughts have become like tape recordings playing over and over in your mind and they influence who you are and what is happening in your life.

Affirmations are positive statements that we consciously make to ourselves to reprogram our subconscious mind. Since we can't erase the old tapes, we must simply record over them. The practice of doing affirmations causes your mind to transform what you think about your life. You can replace any old thinking with new, more positive thoughts.

When you write or speak an affirmation, you need to be very specific. Some important things to remember about affirmations are:

You must never attach a negative word to the words "I am." Don't say, "I am no longer fat."

Say instead, "I am at my perfect weight." Wording it this way creates a positive picture in your mind.

Don't use negative words in the affirmation. So instead of saying something like "I don't overeat anymore," say instead, "I eat only the foods in the amounts that my body needs and can process."

Don't put things out into the future such as "I am going to go to Paris someday." Instead state the affirmation as if it's happening to you right now. "I am enjoying my trip to Paris." This is acknowledging that you must first be able to see it in your mind, in order to bring it about in your life circumstance. In other words, you must believe it to achieve it.

Keep your affirmations short and simple. Affirmations that are too long and too wordy lose their meaning and their impact. Plus, they are hard to remember. Affirmations need to be said over and over. The shorter they are, the easier they are to remember.

Make sure you are comfortable with the affirmation. If it doesn't feel right, it won't work for you.

Your affirmation should convey a strong feeling to your subconscious. The stronger you feel about it, the more impact it will have.

Affirmations are tools to help you create a new perspective which will in turn enable you to have more satisfying results in your life. They are not used to change something that already exists. They are used to replace something or create something new.

When you are using an affirmation, try to create the feeling that what you are saying is true at this moment. Temporarily set aside judgments and imagine yourself in the moment of what you would like to believe. Experience the feeling of what it would feel like if it were true right this moment. The more you feel it, the more able you are to bring it about.

Goal achievement is easier if you will use daily affirmations. You can use affirmations alone or you can combine them with your journaling process, your meditations, or your daily prayer. Even churches have found affirmations to be very powerful. On Sundays, my church uses the following affirmation to end the service.

"The Light of God surrounds me; the love of God enfolds me; the power of God flows through me. Wherever I am, God is, and all is well."

This affirmation sends me out into the world for the week feeling powerful knowing that I am not alone. It is easy to remember, so I can repeat it to myself throughout the week. It is easy for me to believe because I was raised in a Christian home. It resonates with my soul.

Start now. Don't wait until you have the perfect circumstances. There will never be a time that is "exactly right." Get in motion as soon as possible. If you have a habit of procrastinating, now is the time to break it. Act now! Stand up to your fear. Take the first step toward the first goal on your list. As your momentum builds, so will your motivation. Keep your time lines in mind to remind yourself time is ticking away. Don't make excuses for waiting and putting things off. When you have fear, you may feel frozen. This is when you should "Just do it." Take some action. The price of inaction is high, so never put off until tomorrow what you can get done today. Do something toward your goals. They will never become a reality if you don't take the first step. Action is the key to taking control.

Translate your personal and professional wishes into goals today. Align your goals with your purpose, pursue your vision with passion and soon you will *know* that you *can't* fail, because you have unlimited possibilities and the power to create your future.

About the Author

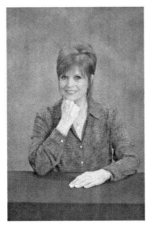

For over twenty-five years, Judi Moreo has studied the lives and habits of highly motivated and successful people. She has translated the mystery behind the illusion that only a chosen few are allowed success and has become a respected authority on high-level performance, personal development, and self-esteem.

Judi Moreo is a Certified Speaking Professional. This is the highest earned designation of the speaking profession. Fewer than 10% of the speakers in the world hold this distinction. Ms. Moreo has spoken in 27 countries on four continents. In addition, she is the author of nine books including her award winning book, *"You Are More Than Enough: Every Woman's Guide to Purpose, Passion, and Power"* and its companion, *"Achievement Journal."*

Her passion for living an extraordinary life is mirrored in her zeal for helping others realize their potential and achieve their goals. With her dynamic personality and style, she is an unforgettable speaker, inspiring motivator and an exceptional coach.

Judi Moreo may be contacted at:
judi@judimoreo.com
www.judimoreo.com
www.youaremorethanenough.com
Turning Point International
P. O. Box 231360
Las Vegas, Nevada 89105
(702) 896-2228

Healing Animals

Maria Hosmer

When I started writing this chapter, I needed to be reminded not to attach myself to the outcome…that it would take on a life of its own. All I can do is follow what spirit guides me to do and release the outcome knowing that all is as it should be. This is something I find very difficult to do! Being the "control freak" that I am, this is a huge life lesson for me. "Let go and let God"…especially when I offer a healing for an animal or a person. However, I'm like everyone else and appreciate the work being validated. So I will explain what I do and why I do it and trust that it will turn out as it should be.

I am a healer. That is my function and my passion. I am an animal lover. They are my life's work and with that I have a sense of responsibility for their well-being and a duty to their spirits. As a dog trainer, I knew training them to be obedient was not my only concern. My main concern was to help them live in a human world without forgetting for a moment that they are living, breathing, soulful beings. Among my other practices, I have found that Reiki can be of great benefit to them.

Sometimes, healing animals with Reiki can be confusing to the animal's guardian because the treatment is done by moving energy…which is not easy to see. In addition, the results of the treatment aren't always obvious until later, and it usually requires more than one session. It is all about the intention… which is always about love, and healing for the highest good.

Reiki on animals is performed much like we do on humans with the exception that the animal determines the length of a session or even if they want a session in the first place.

Do you understand the advantages of your pet having a Reiki session? Has your pet ever had one? Do you understand that both you and your pet can have a session at the same time?

Reiki is life force energy. Reiki never harms and the intention is healing the mind, body and spirit. It can be done hands on or even at a distance. We are all connected, and when I give a treatment I receive one, as well. Needless to say, we all help one another in the exchange of energy.

Let me share with you how I started this. I had been hearing about Reiki for several months before I actually got involved with it. I learned of a certification class being offered so I signed up, and after I completed it, I felt like I had come home. I was destined to do this! The more I experienced the changes in my own well-being and spiritual growth, the more I wanted to share it with everyone.

The benefits to the people I helped to heal ultimately got me thinking of how I could incorporate it into my dog training business. If it was so beneficial to humans, why couldn't it be just as beneficial to their pets? And to my own pets? I realized that Reiki may be able to help alleviate some of the emotional and behavioral issues many of my clients' pets were displaying.

Spirit then guided me to an animal Reiki certification program that was being offered in Northern California and the rest, as they say, is history.

The hardest part, I have come to find, is trying to explain Reiki to my clients. I imagine it sounds kind of "out there" to some of them, especially when I tell them the healing can be done hands on, or it can be done from across the room, or that the pet doesn't even have to be in the same room! Reiki energy flows through everyone and everything and goes where it is needed for the individual's highest good.

I experienced firsthand the effect Reiki had on a Terrier that was very hyperactive and could never seem to relax. She was also recovering from knee surgery and her guardians needed to keep her quiet.

I began the session sitting on the floor with her. She turned herself into me and backed into my lap and received her treatment hands on. After about fifteen minutes, she retreated to her bed that was about three feet away, and for the rest of the session she laid there watching me.

The next day I called to see how she was and was excited to hear she had slept for about five hours after I had left and was behaving much calmer.

The most powerful experience to date is when I attended the certification class in Northern California. The sanctuary where it was held is home to dogs, cats, and geese, as well as goats, pigs and horses. I have great respect for horses and admire their beauty and strength. They are powerfully energetic.

I had been looking forward to working with the horses since I arrived and now I was in the pasture with them. There were three of them, and they were very calm as I entered. With instruction from my teacher, I stood still as they slowly but purposefully approached me. I felt scared and exhilarated at the same time. I began offering Reiki to them and I could feel the energy flow between us. It vibrated from my fingertips to my elbows. The sheer power of it brought tears of joy to my eyes. I had never felt anything like it then or since.

Although Reiki can be enjoyable to some animals, others may find the energy to be too much for them. I have found this even with my own pets. I have a Miniature Schnauzer named Cricket. Cricket came into my life with a host of health problems that conventional care, while relieving her symptoms, were not addressing the causes. I found a remarkable holistic veterinarian that has worked miracles with her. Cricket is, at this time, 7 years old and has such a beautiful spirit that you swear when she looks at you, she is looking into your soul.

Cricket still struggles with mild infections which we treat homeopathically, and since Reiki has had such promising results, I wanted to offer a healing to her. I still remember the first time I offered it to her. I thought, "This is going to be great! " We were both on the couch; it was nice and quiet, the perfect setting for a session. I started with a hands-on approach and you would have thought someone had pinched her! "Alright, maybe I startled her!" I thought. I tried again by putting my hands just above her, making sure not to touch her. She jumped again! With one last try, I offered it to her from across the room. She leapt off the couch and walked into the other room. To this day, she will not accept Reiki.

Not such the case with my black cat, Bean.

Bean came into our lives after my husband, Jamie, and I were married. We were living in Florida at the time when we walked into a pet store. I still do not remember why we went in there, but nonetheless we did. (Knowing what I know now, it was obviously meant to have happened!)

There in a cage, was a single scrawny little black kitten. I walked over to her and poked my finger in the cage which she immediately swiped. I said goodbye and turned to walk away, when her tiny paw with little needle claws caught my shirt as if to say, "Where are you going without me!" Well, out we walked with kitten, food and litter tray in hand.

As a kitten, Bean was very affectionate. She always slept on top of my hair, which was very long at the time. She would play fetch with a wadded up piece of paper, and loved to join us for breakfast, especially if we were having melon.

As a grown up kitty, Bean will have none of those juvenile antics and prefers sleeping in the closet at night. She rarely comes to anyone for affection... that is until I started practicing Reiki.

Bean is fifteen and has had a bladder stone. She occasionally has bladder infections and I am not aware of them unless she has an "accident" outside her litter box.

She began coming back onto the bed and I was so happy thinking that maybe old age has mellowed her out a little. The times that she did come up, she would sniff my hands, which I found to be rather odd. She continued to do that a few more times and I just put it out of my mind. But, on those mornings, I would find that she had an "accident" outside her litter box.

We went off to the animal hospital where their tests showed what I already suspected, she had a bladder infection. She received antibiotics and for a while all was well. A few months later, she began coming up on the bed again. Again, she sniffed my hands, but this time I thought I would try and offer her some Reiki. I placed my hands on her and she started to purr. After about ten minutes, she jumped off the bed and this continued for the next several nights. She has not had any "accidents "outside her litter box since.

I have to include one of my dear friend's dog in my list of animals that enjoy Reiki. He enjoys it very much. When I go to visit, I always have to make time for a treatment however long or short it may be. He insists on it!

He is a very gentle, very large dog. I do not think he realizes just how big he is, because if he could, he would sit on my lap for a treatment. Instead he opts to just back himself into my hands and settle in for a while. When he has had enough, he turns his massive head as if to say "thank you." He is the most appreciative dog I've ever met!

The most interesting thing about working with animals and healing animals is that it is a magnificent way of healing ourselves. There are many programs and services that prove the healing power of animals on humans. These programs have shown to restore emotional and spiritual connections for both human and animal alike.

Several prison programs are in place, which use dogs to help rehabilitate inmates. There are dogs in these programs that benefit from rehabilitation, as well, as they are dogs that require special care and attention. Many of them are shelter dogs that if not for the help they receive from the inmates, may have had to be euthanized because of behavior problems or overpopulation.

There is an exchange of healing for both sides. The inmates may achieve a sense of pride and achievement as they see the progress being made with their dogs. They are entrusted with the responsibility of another life and are gifted with the unconditional love animals are more than willing to give. The dogs do not judge them regardless of their present circumstances.

The dogs flourish with structure and socialization with constant supervision and care. Those that may have been abused or neglected may regain their trust in humans again. It is a bittersweet day when a dog from the program gets adopted, but another opportunity to learn that love is just a wag away!

Hospitals and hospices have made therapy animals welcome. They bring their own special brand of love and healing to all who come in contact with them. If only for a few moments, a patient can make genuine connections with the animals and the animals bring them comfort when they need it most. The animals seem to know just what to do and exactly who needs special attention.

There are reading programs where dogs are brought in and the children are encouraged to read to them. This may help the child develop their reading skills in an environment where they do not feel they will be ridiculed if they make a mistake.

Service dogs can give a physically challenged person a sense of independence and companionship. They see their owners through eyes of courage and devotion, not with pity or judgment.

I have shared how the power of pure, loving energy can bring about significant change in the lives of humans and the animals in their care. Animals have such a great deal to teach us. They have the ability to bring even the most stoic of us down onto the floor for a wrestling match or a good belly rub. Feathers and fur brushed across our cheek make us giggle and brings a tingle to the backs of our necks. Flying across a field on the back of a horse leaves us breathless as we feel our life blood pounding through our veins. And just the sight of a baby animal can make us smile even on our worse day. Now that is power.

Healing can be achieved in ways we do not even imagine. It can happen with a kind word or a gesture. It can come in human or animal form. For me, it comes in animal form.

I come from a large family and my parents worked very hard to support all of us. With five boys and two girls to feed and clothe, it could be difficult at times. My mother was exhausted most of the time and she did the best she could in the way of attention. She found me to be a very sensitive child and tried to find a way to relate to me. The one thing she was absolutely sure about was my love for animals. So any time someone was looking for a home for a dog, or a kitten or even rabbits, she would bring them home for me.

That was how our relationship worked. If I was disappointed over something, I might get a dog. If I became sick, maybe I'd get a kitten. If we had an argument, she might bring home a bird as a peace offering. That was her way of trying to make me happy.

I think back to all the animals I've had in my life and thank each one of them. I would not be the person that I am today without them.

I feel the same way about the animals I have presently. I believe they have all come into my life for the same reason. They are here to give me the unconditional love I crave and they have taught me to give it back. They have come to heal the girl I once was, who felt like she was not worthy of love. To give the woman she became, a sense of purpose and confidence. They have forced me to learn new things and to believe in myself. They have come into my life with health and behavioral issues because they knew I would move heaven and earth to find the best ways to heal them. Reiki is just one of the ways I feel I can give back to them for all they have done for me.

I have had my own spirit healed with the help of my animals. They have taught me not to take myself too seriously. When my spirits are low, I love to just sit in my backyard and watch the birds hop around on my wall or pecking at the ground. Most of all, I love watching my dog, Jack, play ball by himself.

He is obsessed with his ball and always brings it to me as soon as we get outside. There are days that I'm not in the mood to throw it back so he plays by himself. He takes his ball and tosses it in the air and catches it every time. He could go on like that for hours. Suddenly, he'll stop and just race around the backyard like someone touched his back end with a hot poker. I watch him do this and it looks like he's having more fun doing nothing than I've had doing anything.

In that moment I get a glimpse of pure joy. Joy as it was meant to be. Joy that is simple and all-consuming without a thought of anything else but what is happening right now. I watch Jack, finally exhausted, lie on the grass as he suns himself. His eyes are half closed and his tongue is hanging out. He'll suddenly flip over and start rolling around trying to scratch an imaginary itch. His legs are now above his head kicking at the air and at the sky above him, seeing if he can kick the cloud away that is blocking his sun. When he's all through, he absentmindedly chews on a piece of grass.

It does my soul good to watch Jack. I want to be more like him. He is teaching me to appreciate the moments as they come and to bask in the sunlight of pure joy.

Now that I have shared this chapter with you, I hope it has helped to shed some light on the healing power of Reiki for your animal companions, as well as for yourself. My wish is that this chapter has made you look at the animals in your life a little differently. To see them for the angels on earth they were sent to be. Take a moment and really look deep into their eyes. I know you will see beautiful souls with a mission. They take their responsibility seriously and the only thing they ask for in return is that we honor and heal one another.

I believe by doing so, that all shall be as it should be.

About the Author

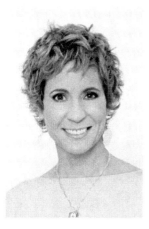

Maria Hosmer was born in New York before moving to Las Vegas in 2000. She was a singer for many years before her love of animals took her on a journey that led her to her true calling.

She has been a professional dog trainer for over 8 years, teaching obedience and behavior modification. She is a strong advocate for returning our animal companions to a more natural state of being. She is also a Reiki Energy Healing Practitioner, Essential Oils Advocate, Flower Remedy Consultant, Animal Nutrition Consultant, and utilizes these modalities within her practice.

Maria attended Clayton College of Natural Healing and acquired credits in animal acupressure at the Animal Acupressure Training Academy in Northern California.

Her love of animals is only surpassed by the love for her husband, Jamie. She is the proud guardian of her companion pets Brady, Cricket, Jack, Grace, Bean, and Mia.

Maria can be contacted at:
www.dog-e-mom.com
(702)448-5398

How To Live A Spiritual Life Through The Use of Crystals and Gemstones

Susan Goecke

The practice of using crystals and gemstones for health and healing dates back thousands of years. It's easy to comprehend this because crystals and gemstones have been around in their same form and evolved forms for millions of years. Most are found in our mountain ranges while some have fallen to earth through meteors. Naturally, our earth's structure has changed since its origin and so has the evolution of the crystals and gemstones in which it houses. As the earth's surface has been disrupted with earthquakes, erosion, and other natural phenomenon, the way crystals grow and where they can be found has evolved over the course of earth's existence.

Ask most children if they enjoy playing with stones and most will say yes. Bring a child into a store that has a bucket of pretty, polished stones and surely most will insist they bring a few home with them for their collection. Collecting and playing with stones is very natural for young children because young children are natural healers, especially those ages seven and younger. This is because their cord to Heaven is still intact and they are consciously connecting to their higher selves and listening to what their spiritual, physical, and emotional body needs. Playing with stones increases their vitality and is a very beneficial practice for relaxation and rejuvenation for youngsters. Looking back at your own life, can you remember having an affinity with stones?

Living a Spiritual Life is both easy and difficult as we maneuver our way through changing times, uncertainty, and life's challenges. Living spiritually is easy if we allow ourselves to raise our vibrations and practice modalities given in this book. Living spiritually is sometimes not chosen because it is easier to lower our vibrations to meet earthly needs and not heavenly alternatives. I find working with gemstones and crystals to be a very simple way to raise our vibrations because crystals are readily available and a tangible object we can rely on.

The easiest way to find your special crystal is through your own intuition. Ask yourself which crystal calls out to you. Does a crystal jump into your hand? There are several reasons a specific crystal might call out to you. A crystal's color, shape, and texture might be the first thing you notice when in their presence. However, the energy you receive from the crystal itself speaks a whole other story. Generally speaking, a person might be drawn to a certain crystal because his or her own physical, spiritual, and aura field might be lacking a certain energy the crystal will provide. However, depending on the situation, a person might be attracted to a crystal because their very being resonates to the crystal's energy and it enhances their situation. A person might also react negatively to a crystal for the same reasons if they are not ready to accept the energy the crystal will bring to them.

Why are crystals such powerful healers? A crystal is made up of a crystalline structure that has been growing in and on Earth's surface for millions of years. A crystal holds memories, knowledge, and vibration of the Earth throughout time, and a person who holds the crystal can tap into the infinite wisdom of the crystal to receive information and healing.

A person's body consists of seven chakras, or energy centers, which run up and down the spine to the crown of the head. Each chakra is linked to a color, emotion, relationship, and cellular memory. The crystal a person chooses will correspond to the chakra in need of healing or enhancing. It is easy to remember the colors associated with each chakra because they match up to the colors of the rainbow. For example, the first chakra is at the base of the spine and it relates to the color red. The sixth chakra is at the forehead and it matches the color purple. If you are aware in which chakra needs healing, choosing a crystal in its specific color range is helpful.

Let's start with the **root chakra**. The root chakra is our most earthy chakra and is associated with family relations, tribal beliefs, safety, and security. It is the chakra that grounds a person to the Earth and is associated with the lower part of the body from the base of the spine and down. Since, the root chakra is associated with the color red, the gemstones that vibrate to the root chakra are red, black, or gray. Good examples are Garnet, red jasper, ruby, obsidian, and onyx. These stones have the ability to draw negativity out of a person, as well as protect the person from negativity. For example, garnet is a deep red color and when the person wears or places a garnet stone near their thyroid, a feeling of draining out of the body occurs, as well as intense heat. Obsidian is very useful for protecting environments from electronic toxins. I like to place a black obsidian stone near the computer in the house. It also acts as a grounding component. A person may be drawn to red or black stones if they are struggling with family relations, security, or have safety concerns.

The second chakra is called the **sacral chakra**. The sacral chakra deals with creativity and growth. This chakra vibrates the color orange. Beautiful orange stones are carnelian, amber, orange calcite, peach moonstone. These stones have various properties that protect the part of the body below the naval and the hip area. This area of the body has to do with emotions of confidence and relationships not related to the tribal family. Peach gemstones, such as moonstone and Morganite, are very effective for this chakra because they have a calming effect on the body. This effect helps the subtle body relax and instill in the person a greater sense of relating to others, and encouragement to expand and grow.

The third chakra is the **solar plexus** and is the area above the navel. This chakra includes the stomach and all the digestive organs. The solar plexus deal with personal power and vibrates to the color yellow. A person's relationship with him or herself is shown here. A wonderful stone to enhance personal power is Citrine, which is also known to reduce anxiety. Another effective stone for personal power is Tiger's Eye, a very casual stone that can be worn daily. The pretty brown color is very soothing to the area. Other yellow stones are amber, yellow jade, and rutilated quartz. Rutilated quartz is a filtering stone and helps a person release negative emotions buried deep within.

The fourth chakra is known as the **heart** center and resonates to the color green, and the color pink, as it relates to gemstones, also resides here. The heart deals with emotions attached to love, self-love, and compassion. The most common heart chakra gemstone is Rose Quartz. Rose Quartz has a very gentle energy that is suitable for anyone and most children resonate and are drawn to it. Another heart Chakra gemstone is Malachite. Malachite is a deep green stone with black bands running through; this deep color shows how strong the energy is. Malachite is very good to boost up the immune system of a person and also to consciously connect to others. Other heart gemstones include, but are not limited to, Jade, Rhodochrosite, Kunzite, and Emerald.

The **throat chakra** revolves around a person's will, honesty, and truth. This chakra resonates to the color blue. A popular throat chakra gemstone is turquoise. Turquoise is known as a Shaman's stone, has mystical qualities, and is very popular in Native American Communities. Turquoise is also a very good stone for those born under the Scorpio astrological sign as it helps ward off a loose tongue. Another popular throat chakra stone is Larimar, known as the dolphin stone, because it helps the wearer reach the fifth dimension. Wearing Larimar brings about the feeling of being at the sea and swimming with dolphins. Larimar is a fast acting stone and resonates with a person's energy field quite rapidly. Sodalite is another common fifth chakra stone; it's energy has the ability to help a person release control issues. Sodalite is a very effective healer's tool as many people like to hold onto controlling others and situations. All of these stones relates to the throat chakra because they relate to truth, honesty, and will. A person's will is most important because without that, nothing would be accomplished!

The sixth chakra is known as the **third eye** and resonates to the colors of indigo and purple. The third eye is the center of intuition and is susceptible to headaches; migraines occur due to chaos of the mind. Amethyst is effective in releasing migraines because an amethyst geode has many inclusions that draw pain and confusion away from the site. Lapis Lazuli is also effective in opening the third eye. The color of the stone and the vibration Lapis resonates to help clear blockages relating to intuition. Other stones include ametrine, which also has third chakra vibration, lepidolite, and purple agate.

The seventh chakra is at the **crown** of the head and is the connection a person has to God, angels, and the Heavens. This chakra is known as the most heavenly chakra, and resonates to white light. Clear quartz is an appropriate stone to use on the crown chakra because quartz is pure light and encompasses the full spectrum of the rainbow. This is very important because when placed on the crown, white light filters through the top of the head and lights up all the chakras. A beautiful rainbow is now activated throughout the physical body. Other seventh chakra stones are Angel Aura Quartz, Topaz, Selenite, Herkimer Diamond, and Mother of Pearl.

Quartz points are also very effective when pointed into the side of the hand between the pinky and the wrist. This point clears up negative emotions and helps release the mind and body during times of stress, anxiety, depression, and anger. Quartz points direct energy to the spot it is pointed towards.

Gemstones come in many different colors, shapes, and sizes. Picking the right gemstone for you is easier than you might think. The choice really depends on what feels right. It is vital to remove your mind as much as possible when making your decision. Sometimes, crystals will appear in dreams, making it even easier to find your personal stone.

Below is a guideline to refer to if you are quite stuck. You can refer to this list to help you make appropriate decisions while choosing stones to enhance your life. After each stone, a basic description of the stone is described, and the stone's properties and zodiac signs are listed.
Gemstone chart:

Agate: various colors; slow growing stone which helps encourage stability for a person; enhances mental function; useful in resolving disputes; A wonderful stone for Gemini's

Amethyst: The stone of Archangel Michael! Amethyst opens up intuition; clears headaches; helps wearer have a deeper sense of faith; for the Piscean

Angelite: Pale lilac-blue in color; The stone of Mother Mary; helps bring peace during violence or war; contains protection from the angelic realm; stone for Aquarius

Aquamarine: Light aqua in color; Legend says that aquamarine came from a mermaid's jewelry box; contains power of the sea; aids in phobias regarding travel and swimming; treats neck and throat problems and reduces swollen glands; stone of pure love; encourages peace; Piscean stone

Carnelian: Orange stone; increases confidence and self-worth; enhances creativity; depression releaser; for the Capricorn

Citrine: A yellow stone which increases power within the core of a person; fills the belly with the power of one thousand sons; increases prosperity; heals the stomach; excellent for Gemini

Coral: Pink, red, or cream in color; symbolizes joy and happiness; protects against negativity; helps osteoporosis and fertility issues; benefits Scorpio and Taurus signs

Fluorite: A purple, green, and yellow stone; balances the mind; helps break patterns of thought; helps release addictions; great for allergies; diminishes insomnia; beneficial for eyesight and bones; excellent stone for Pisces

Garnet: A deep red stone which helps wearer feel hope where there is no reason to hope. Garnet absorbs negativity from holder of the stone; makes wearer more stable on their feet; for the Leo

Hematite: A shiny black stone that helps ground the energetic field of the wearer. It is useful for regulating the blood and blood pressure; for the Aries

Jade: A green stone; signifies wisdom gathered in tranquility; recognizes self as spiritual being on a human journey; reduces eyestrain, prosperity stone; good for channeling ancestors; improves health and past-life recall; Star sign is Aries

Labradorite: Silvery gray in color; Highly mystical and protective stone; deflects unwanted energy; accesses spiritual purpose; symbolizes fantasy and creativity; relieves stress, regulates metabolism; stone for Scorpio

Lapis Lazuli: Indigo in color; increases intuition; also effective in dealing with grief; stone of Egypt; effective against depression; for the Sagittarius

Larimar: Aqua blue color; Dolphin stone; radiates love, peace, and tranquility; assists in angelic contact; helps regulate bipolar disorder and self-sabotage; beneficial for bones, arthritis, and sciatica; A stone for a Leo

Leopard Jasper: Pink stone; Improves the power of endurance; calms wearer yet stimulates the imagination; increases bond between wearer and environment; helps detox the liver, gall bladder, and bladder; relieves abdominal pain and reduces tension; excellent stone for Gemini

Moonstone: Creamy white, purple, peach in color; hormonal balancer; calming stone for a woman as it helps a woman's body trace the vibration of the moon. A great stone for the Cancer sign.

Malachite: A green stone with black bands; emotional balancing stone; drives out ego; helps with depression and manic depression; beneficial for Scorpios

Onyx: A black stone; known as a magic stone; deflects negative energy; grounds energy; increases awareness of visions and dreams; increases concentration; great for a Capricorn

Phrenite: Light green with black specks; Stone of Archangel Raphael; stone of unconditional love; enhances prophecy and inner knowing; stone for a Virgo

Pietersite: Deep brown stone; Helps wearer soar spiritually and find time within oneself; Helps to weather the storm; reminds wearer they are spirit on human vacation; Stone for Sagittarius

Sodalite: Dark blue; helps release control issues; helps tone down voice; for the Cancer

Tiger's Eye: A brown and gold stone; enhances personal power; strengthens resolve; improves insights; softens stubbornness; increases self-confidence; for the Leo

Topaz: Clear stone; Creates awareness for the wearer; encourages "I am" instead of "I do;" cuts through doubts and uncertainty; activates cosmic awareness; promotes truth and awareness; for a Leo or Libra

Turquoise: Shaman stone which activates the power to heal; clears throat chakra; gives wearer a feeling of safety as this stone serves as an amulet of protection; for a Scorpio

Rose Quartz: A pink stone that holds the energy of love or self-love. This stone opens and heals the heart; for a Taurus

Unakite: A green and peach stone; Symbolizes union between Venus and Mars, husband and wife, long term partners; helps to communicate to an unborn child; promotes harmonious relationships; for Scorpio

There are different things to be aware of when selecting your crystal or gemstone. Place your hand near a selected stone and ask yourself what you feel from it. Does the stone make you feel good? Do you feel energy coming off of the stone? Does the stone feel like it has dead energy? Testing the energy of the stone is easy and you will intuitively know if the energy is right or not. Sometimes if the energy of a stone is very powerful, my knees will buckle! On other occasions, I feel that the stone needs to be reenergized. Whenever you bring a stone home with you, the stone should be cleansed and energized. This is most easily done by rinsing it off in purified water and then placed in the sunlight before 12:00 pm. This is a general cleansing technique. However, some stones can be recharged and energized in other ways. For example, moonstone is best recharged during a full moon during the nighttime. Larimar should be charged in water under the moonlight. Quartz should be charged in the sunlight in greenery.

Some gemstones have been through some trauma and have picked up very negative energy. This can also be called dead energy. If cleansing and clearing don't do the job, I recommend burying the stone and placing the stone back into the Earth for Mother Earth healing. Of course, that is the worst-case scenario. One time I entered a new crystal store while on vacation. Right up front was a large sphere that took up half of the lobby entrance. Normally, a stone that large would make my legs weak and induce a slight headache because of how powerful the energy would be. To my surprise, I felt nothing! I left the store and later found out that crystals were brought into that store illegally. That made perfect sense to me since I had no reaction whatsoever at all to that crystal. That is a good example of when a crystal should be reburied in the earth with hopes of being reborn.

Crystals are wonderful tools to help a person lead a more spiritual life. Not only are they breathtakingly beautiful, they are the holders of timeless information and the vibration they give can heal people on so many levels. Crystals and gemstones are also readily available and easy to keep on hand. They can easily be put in your pocket, worn as jewelry, or kept on a nightstand or coffee table. Choosing, clearing, energizing, and treasuring a special crystal or gemstone is an easy way to do something special for yourself. The intent to care for and allow the magic of your stone to work wonders in your life is a great start to living a more spiritual and fulfilling life.

About the Author

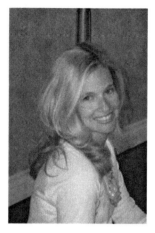

Susan Goecke has had an affinity with crystals and gemstones since she was a little girl. Surviving three near-death experiences brought her very close to the angelic realm. She has personally met her guardian angel in the physical realm and is able to maintain close relationships to her guardians through the use of crystals and gemstones.

Susan makes gemstone jewelry that has been channeled in by Archangel Raphael. Reiki and angelic energy is infused in the stones so the wearer receives constant healing from the angelic realm. Each piece is created with intentions of emotional, spiritual, and physical healing. Susan is also a certified yoga teacher and uses crystal healing with her students during their yoga practice.

She currently resides in Las Vegas with her husband, four boys, three cats, and two dogs.

Susan Goecke can be contacted at:
www.Angelicallyguided.com
angelicallyguided@cox.net
(702) 327-8126

Hypnosis

Cheryl Johnson and Diane Johnson

HYPNOSIS: Silly, Scary or Spiritual?

You're sitting in the theater, excited and leaning forward. The stage is full of hopeful volunteers all hanging on every word the hypnotist says. The hypnotist whispers a magic word into each person's ear. The next thing you know, burly, 200 lb. football players are wearing frilly tutus and dancing ballet – with each other!

At the whisper of another magic word, some guy screams like a girl because his belt has turned into a snake. He has to take the belt off because it's a snake – but he can't touch the belt because it's a snake — but he has to take it off because... Frantically hopping and spinning around, he looks like he's trying to run away from his own rear end!

Or you find yourself at the movies with your eyes glued to the screen. A mad scientist (you can tell he's completely daffy – his eyes are buggy and his hair is sticking out like he just stuck his finger in a light socket) waves a watch in front of a helpless victim. Motionless, his victim stares through glazed eyes, seeing nothing as the mad scientist intones, "You are now in my power. I have hypnotized you and you will do whatever I say." Like a robot, his face void of expression, the victim rises and goes forward to do the insane scientist's dastardly bidding.

Yikes! With press like this, it's no wonder hypnosis is so misunderstood.

What's In a Name?

Hypnosis (also known as hypnotic trance) is a natural, altered state. It's that euphoric, floating feeling you experience for an all-too-brief moment before you drop off to sleep. It's also when everything around you disappears as you become more and more deeply immersed in your daydreams, or in a good book or movie. The body, mind and emotions all merge into a deep, satisfying relaxation as you shift your focus from the outer world to your inner world.

Hypnotism is the science of applying techniques to induce the state of hypnosis, although the two words are often interchanged.

Self-hypnosis is (Wait for it...) hypnotizing yourself.   With proper instruction, anyone can hypnotize himself or herself.

A **hypnotist** is trained in the techniques of hypnotism to help others enter the state of hypnosis. The hypnotist simply helps you control your own ability. Say for example, I do a progressive relaxation. If you want to go into hypnosis, you will; if you don't, you won't. It's up to you whether or not you accept the suggestions of relaxation or any other suggestions. (Hypnosis isn't mind control. In real life, the helpless victim in our movie would snatch the watch from the mad scientist, bonk him on the head with it and demand that he seek professional help.)

Hypnotherapy (also called past- and current-life age regression therapy) is a rapid, short-term (quick results) modality. Through the hypnotic technique of regression, you access memories that are keys to the hidden negative beliefs or blocks residing at the emotional (subconscious) level.

A **hypnotherapist** is trained to use proven therapeutic techniques, along with the state of hypnosis, to assist in making permanent changes to deeply ingrained, and often unknown negative beliefs.

How We Create Our Lives

In order to understand how hypnosis works, it's important to know the basics of how we create everything in our lives.

We create through 3 levels of awareness:

1. The **Superconscious** is your Divine Self, also known as the Higher Self or Divine Consciousness. This is the level that contains all answers to all questions.

2. The **subconscious** holds all of your memories, is the seat of your emotions, holds all of your beliefs, and runs all of your automatic programs (habits). It's also your gateway to the Superconscious.

3. The **conscious** is the level of reason, logic and willpower.

The raw creative power of the Divine Source flows from the Superconscious level of awareness through the subconscious level of awareness to the conscious level of awareness.

Have you ever asked yourself…

- "Why does this keep happening to me?"
- "Why can't I have/do/be what I want?"

Emotion-based beliefs buried in the subconscious hold the ever-searched-for answers to these questions.

The beliefs at the subconscious level are what you **feel** is true about life and yourself at your deepest (usually hidden) level. These beliefs act as filters that shape the raw creative power flowing from the Superconscious. You originate in Spirit as perfect as a Michelangelo painting. By the time the creative power is filtered through all the negative beliefs, your life is a Picasso abstract.

These beliefs are the cause of all of your automatic responses (also called programs or patterns or habits). They are automatic reactions that you don't control at the conscious level of reason and logic.

All of your beliefs have been created through your reaction to everything and everyone around you from the moment you are born — or earlier.

Button...Button...Who pushed your button?

You're born with everything going for you. The Superconscious is in open dialogue with Divine Source. The subconscious is already running its first automated functions for survival – lungs pump air in and out, the heart swooshes blood back and forth, back and forth.

Then, it starts to get sticky.

Because the conscious level of reason and logic doesn't kick in until you're five or six years old, beliefs are formed based on repetition and the emotional responses of a two- to four-year-old child. That is to say with **no** reason or logic!

We breath, walk, write (and we all know people who drive) without thinking about it.

The programs in the subconscious are like shortcut buttons on a computer. Once you program the computer to take a certain action when you push a specific button, you get exactly the same response every time you push it. The same thing applies with automatic programs at the subconscious level. If you want something different to happen when you push that button, you have to make the changes in the computer's programming, your subconscious. You have to reprogram the response that comes when something "pushes your button."

Most of us aren't even aware that those buttons exist because we started programming them so long ago, and because we've been taught to ignore our emotions in favor of reason and logic.

These automatic programs dictate your life. They can lie hidden in the subconscious for years or lifetimes.

A Matter of Life and Death

It's the responsibility of the subconscious to *run already-existing* programs based on already-existing beliefs — not to *change* them — so any new idea that comes into the conscious level of awareness that does not agree with the beliefs already accepted at the subconscious level are rejected.

The subconscious always has a "good" reason for keeping negative programs. All programs exist to help you survive as in the following example.

Nan had a very harsh childhood. Every time anyone paid attention to her, she was blamed, ridiculed, hit and humiliated. This young lady was extremely overweight and plain. She never wore makeup and sometimes forgot to wash her hair.

After she escaped her abusive environment, she decided that it was her turn to shine. She tried all kinds of diets and exercise programs. She would do great for a while, and then stop exercising and start eating "everything in sight."

Nan, like so many dieters, would become discouraged and impatient. She would experience uncontrollable cravings for the very foods that she had been avoiding.

During a hypnotherapy session, Nan realized that she had learned to be as inconspicuous as possible to survive her childhood. The belief was formed at the subconscious level that people noticing her meant pain. Attention was dangerous. The protective "camouflage" of excess weight and being as unattractive as possible kept her safe from attack.

On the conscious level, Nan knew that she was safe because her abusers were no longer around. The reason she would do okay for a while is because you can create a certain degree of change through willpower from the conscious level. However, when her weight loss began to threaten the subconscious belief that a certain amount of excess weight was needed to be safe, that belief kicked into high gear to stop the dangerous changes – loss of weight could mean loss of life.

When you give your best efforts and don't get positive results, it's a sure sign that there's a belief running at the subconscious level that's in conflict with the belief at the conscious level. That's clear in the above example where consciously Nan believed she was safe to change her image and start getting attention, but the subconscious belief was still that attention was dangerous.

In a battle between beliefs at the two levels, the beliefs at the subconscious level will always win. They have to. They have been in existence and have been building energy far longer than beliefs at the conscious level and the subconscious runs the survival center.

The strongest willpower in the world won't beat the instinct to survive.

Hypnotherapy

I've been a practicing hypnotherapist since 1993. My work is based on the Truth that you hold the answers to all of your questions and problems within you. Every session has proven to me that the power to change your life lies **within you**.

In my opinion, the fastest and most powerful method of gaining benefit from hypnosis is hypnotherapy experienced with a qualified hypnotherapist.[1]

I work with most hypnotherapy clients an average of two to six sessions. You experience relief from the very first session because the work is done at the emotional level where the problems exist.

As the hypnotherapist, it is my responsibility to assist you in finding your own answers – your own wisdom. When you go into hypnosis, you set aside the conscious level of reason and logic and go straight into the subconscious level so you have access to the hidden programs and beliefs that block you from knowing oneness with Spirit and living a life filled with lots of love, money, and fun.

Once you change those negative beliefs, Presto! You have access to the unlimited potential of the Superconscious.

Hypnotic Suggestion Programming

---

[1] Hypnotherapy is a specialized method of creating change at the emotional level. Be sure the professional you're working with has had proper training. Check to see what school he or she attended, what the curriculum was and how much actual supervised practice was included. For more on this, visit my website www.cheryljjohnson.com.

Perhaps the best-known therapeutic application of hypnosis is hypnotic suggestion programming.

A suggestion is an idea that stimulates emotional reaction. An idea that doesn't stimulate an emotional reaction is just a statement. In other words, if I give you a suggestion and you don't accept it, it's not really a suggestion to you. You must accept it and give it emotional impact in order for it to be a suggestion.

While in hypnosis, you hear suggestions for desired behaviors and emotions. Hypnotic suggestion programming works the same way you taught yourself to tie your shoes or to write – through repetition. You listen to the suggestions over and over again. Because you're in hypnosis, the suggestions go straight to the subconscious level where the negative and positive beliefs exist. Further, because emotion drives the subconscious, the stronger the emotion that you attach to the suggestion for the desired behavior, the more powerful its impact and the more likely it is to "stick."

As the following story shows, the proper wording of suggestions is extremely important.

A hypnotist was working with a group using hypnotic suggestion programming for weight loss. After two months of listening to the suggestions, everyone in the group was slimming down. The hypnotist decided to tweak the script in the hopes of getting even faster results.

*By the end of the next two months every member in the group had gained weight in the hips — only the hips. The hypnotist checked his script and found the problem: The original script contained wording about a slimming energy **moving** all through the body. In the revised script, the word "**spreading**" was used numerous times and with great emotion in the part describing the energy moving through the hips. The word "spreading" caused the hips to "spread"! He changed the wording and the problem was solved.*

So, if you decide to work with suggestions, get proper training and/or check with a professional.

Hypnotic suggestion programming and self-hypnosis work much more quickly when used with hypnotherapy.

It's a Win-Win!

The list of benefits possible using the state of hypnosis is almost endless. Some of the most common uses of hypnotherapy, hypnotic suggestion programming, and self-hypnosis are to:

- Pass exams
- Lose weight
- Stop smoking

Daddy's Girl

Mary came to see me to help her stop smoking. Mary was in a loving relationship and was extremely successful in business. In fact, she had been able to accomplish anything she put her mind to – except to stop smoking.

Mary had enjoyed a close relationship with her mother and her father. From our conversation, it was clear that she loved and respected both of them very much. Her father had passed on many years earlier, but her mother was alive and the two were still very close. Mary looked like her mother, dressed like her, talked like her, and even had the same career her mother had had. She mentioned that her father had smoked, but she couldn't really remember because it had been so long ago. At the time, it was no big deal that he smoked because that was before there was proof that smoking causes cancer.

While in hypnosis, Mary quickly regressed to a very young age. She flung her arms around her beloved daddy's neck and said, "Daddy, I'm going to be just like you!" Mary described the "wonderful" smell when she hugged him. It was the smell of cigarette smoke. The emotional level had created a link between smoking and loving daddy. To stop smoking would be to break her word that she would be just like him.

Through some simple therapeutic techniques Mary discovered for herself very important ways she was just like her dad. She had his strong sense of right and wrong, his mischievous sense of humor, and his "full speed ahead" approach to life. The emotional belief that she had to smoke to be just like daddy was changed – she was just like daddy anyway – so she was able to stop smoking.

- Release anger
- Reduce stress
- Improve sleep
- Enhance memory
- Improve health
- Explore past lives
- Sharpen study habits
- Heighten self-esteem
- Attract healthy, loving relationships
- Increase abundance
- Learn to meditate
- Increase concentration
- Remove emotional blocks
- Increase psychic sensory perception
- Enhance problem-solving abilities
- Gain greater control over bodily functions
- Eliminate fears and phobias
- Heighten levels of creativity
- Remove blocks to spiritual fulfillment, such as unworthiness, fear, etc. and reconnect with your divine nature
- Get to the cause of and eliminate psychosomatic illness

Hysterical Partial Paralysis

A young woman came to me for assistance with hysterical partial paralysis. She would occasionally lose the use of her legs. The episodes appeared to be random with no obvious triggers. After a while, the paralysis would disappear and she could walk as if it had never happened. Her doctors were convinced that there was no physiological cause.

In hypnosis she regressed to several lifetimes where she suffered injuries to her legs, some resulting in paralysis. Each of those lifetimes was filled with intense hardship and emotional suffering. She worked and never rested. While in hypnosis, she pinpointed the fact that the partial paralysis in the current life happened whenever she was so busy that she went into complete overwhelm. She realized that her body was telling her to slow down and be nice to herself. She needed to change her frantic schedule to stop the symptoms.

As a result of the session, she started making dramatic changes to her lifestyle.

In a phone call about six months later, she mentioned that the partial paralysis had started to come back a few times. I asked if she would like to come in for a second session to make sure that didn't happen again and she laughed. Imagine my surprise when she told me that she wanted to keep it!

he said, "It only happens when I forget to make time for myself. I use it as a warning signal now. If I start to feel the funny tingling in my legs, I take some things off my to-do list and set up some fun and relaxing things for myself. Then my legs are just fine!"

DID YOU KNOW?

Did you know that the word "hypnosis" is a misnomer attributed to the Scottish surgeon James Braid around 1842? He thought the trance was a "nervous sleep" so he used the Greek word "hypnos" which means sleep. He later realized that the state is not sleep and tried to change the name, but the terms hypnosis and hypnotism stuck.

In temples of ancient India, Egypt, and Greece, hypnotic-like inductions were used to place an ailing person in a trance and hypnotic suggestions were used to affect cures.

Austrian physician Franz Anton Mesmer brought hypnosis to the attention of the medical community and Western scientists around 1770 with his technique which he referred to as "mesmerism." Though hypnotism became the official term, still hundreds of years later, you can hear someone say, "She mesmerized him."

In the early 1800s, Abbe (Father) Faria declared that the results of hypnosis are "generated from within the mind" by the power of expectancy and cooperation of the patient. Still, it wasn't until 1956 that the Roman Catholic Church lifted its ban on hypnotism, allowing for its use by health care professionals for diagnosis and treatment.

Surgeon James Esdaile operated on patients using what he called "mesmeric sleep" as his only anesthesia in the 1840s.

Modern pioneers like Ormond McGill, Milton Erickson, and Dave Elman continued the efforts to demystify hypnosis and uncover its unlimited potential.

FROM SUBCONSCIOUS TO SUPERCONSCIOUS

In 1932 David Anrias channeled the book "Through the Eyes of the Masters." In it Master Morya states "... the world in general is destined to evolve through the study and then the control of the subconscious mind. Hence some sort of training must be evolved to enable people to accomplish this."

Control of the subconscious can be accomplished through hypnosis. The more you work with your subconscious, the more you can realize your oneness with Divine Source and begin to live directly through the All-knowing, All-powerful Superconscious.

About the Author

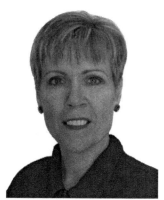

Rev. Cheryl J. Johnson, M.Msc., C.Ht. holds a Master of Metaphysical Sciences; is a Metaphysical Minister & Teacher; a Certified Hypnotherapist (aka Current- & Past-Life Age Regression); a Spiritual Counselor; a Dream Interpreter, and a Channel.

Cheryl considers herself amazingly fortunate to have studied with two renowned pioneers teaching metaphysics and hypnotherapy: Rev. Donald E. Weldon, mentioned in books by Ruth Montgomery, Dick Sutphen, and Alan Weisman; and Gil Boyne, mentioned in many texts on hypnotherapy and described by Sylvia Brown as "a noted instructor."

Cheryl uses a combination of modalities to help her clients:
- ➢ Metaphysics for the practical application of Universal Laws;
- ➢ Hypnotherapy to rapidly remove blocks;
- ➢ Self-hypnosis to relieve anxiety and reduce stress;
- ➢ Hypnotic Suggestion Programming to change negative programming;
- ➢ Channeling to bring guidance from the Higher perspective;
- ➢ Dream Interpretation to clarify guidance received through dreams;
- ➢ Courses to give the tools needed to live a happy, healthy, and prosperous life.

Cheryl J. Johnson can be contacted at:
www.cheryljjohnson.com
cheryl@cheryljjohnson.com
702-558-6889

About the Author

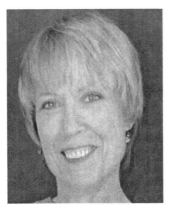

Diane L. Johnson has enjoyed many careers from traveling the world as a trilingual confidential secretary to working as a professional horsewoman. Diane is a conscious trance channel, an editor, and writer. She holds a weekly group channeling session and edits all of Rev. Cheryl J. Johnson's written material. She is writing two works including a creative non-fiction book based on encouragement, counsel, and commiseration received from decades of channelings.

Diane began her metaphysical studies in the early-nineties with metaphysical pioneer Reverend Donald E. Weldon. After finishing numerous courses with him, she worked with Don preparing his memoirs for publication. Although Don crossed over before the book could be finished, Diane feels she was given the rare privilege of experiencing through him the excitement and trials of bringing channeling, hypnotherapy, and faith healing into the public eye beginning in the 1950s and spanning into the late 90s.

Diane used her knowledge of spirit-over-mind-over-matter to overcome cancer and mild traumatic brain injury.

Diane L. Johnson can be contacted at:
diane@scorpiotwins.com

Kinesiology

Elta Rahim

I am sad, or more correctly, I was sad. I was born in the 50s in beautiful, but cloudy Seattle, Washington where many people had SAD. Seasonal Affective Disorder (SAD) is also known as winter blues, or winter depression, and is a mood disorder in which people that have normal mental health throughout the year experience depressive symptoms in the winter. As you may know, Seattle is rainy, overcast, and cold for most of the year - the perfect storm for SAD.

I believe we choose our "family" - parents and siblings – and I fully accept the interesting experiences I had growing up....all of which led me to learn, and now share with you, a miraculous healing system called PSYCH-K.

My father, mother and brother all worked for The Boeing Aircraft Company when I was growing up. My father was a brilliant engineer; my mother was an inspector, and my brother was a genius. I was not. I was and am the gal who the song, "Girls Just Wanna Have Fun" was fashioned after. My parents thought I was "different" and not in a good way. As long as I can remember, they tried to change me, and did the best they were able to do.

I had a very confused and unhappy childhood. I attempted suicide twice and spent time in a mental institute. In my younger years, I was put in jail in Georgia for standing up for black people and was jailed in Texas for speeding. And many other negative experiences kept happening.

I can't imagine a healing, seminar, teacher, book, or experience that I have not tried to make myself "healthy." Then, I hit success with the book, **"The Missing Peace in Your Life"** by Robert M. Williams, M.A. published in 2000.

While living in San Francisco, I came across a flier about "the missing peace" and wanted to know more. I attended a two-day workshop, and finally, finally found something that worked. Not only did it work for me, but it was possible to *prove* that it worked and I needed *proof* that something was shifting, something was changing, and I could finally be "well." It turned out that I wasn't that "sick." Using Kinesiology, I was able to access the decision making part of my brain, the subconscious and super conscious, the essence of this modality.

Yet, still the inner conflict that I could not quite put my finger on remained. Why did I sabotage my work, my relationships, myself? Why did I feel as if I had to feel bad or stressed? I felt broken and deep down did not believe that I deserved to live, share my truth or even be happy.

I learned that if you don't change your subconscious brain, life just continues the way it always has. Your subconscious has one job - to take care of you - and the way it learns to care of you is by your reactions to what happens to you from age one until the age of three or four. Your subconscious monitors the operations of your body, such as your heart rate, digestions, and more. It thinks literally, is timeless, has expanded processing capacity, and can be long- term memory, holding thousands of events at one time.

Your conscious mind sets goals, judges results, thinks abstractly and is time bound, thinking in the past or future and has short-term memory.

In order to change...one has to access and speak with the subconscious. With PSYCH-K, you can do that. PSYCH-K is a user friendly way to "rewrite the software of your mind and change the printout of your life!" as quoted by Rob Williams in "The Missing Peace in Your Life."

PSYCH-K is way beyond affirmations, will power and positive thinking. Using "muscle-testing" to detect the presence or absence of stress (inner conflict) with a simple "yes" or "no" question that is well-formed and positive is the only way to contact the subconscious. Remember, the subconscious only knows the "now" and it is essential to speak to your subconscious in the present tense. For example, "I deeply appreciate and accept myself," not "I would like to deeply appreciate and accept myself." "I would like to" is future based, and the subconscious will just go back to doing what it was doing because you have not engaged it in any way.

With the PSYCH-K system, we work with 7areas in life which most people would like to improve: Grief/Loss, Self-Esteem, Relationships, Spirituality, Personal Power, Health/Body and Prosperity. In spite of the fact that we have hundreds of "questions" to pose to the subconscious, we invite you to form your own personal questions as well. We offer sessions in a safe setting whether it is a two or four-day seminar or a private session.

Having worked with dozens of people myself, as well as with several PSYCH-K practitioners who have helped thousands of people, I find this modality the easiest, fastest, most eloquent change system I have ever seen. You only need a well-formed question and a person to press down on your arm for muscle testing to receive a "yes" or "no" so that you know the next step to take.

Let's pretend you are at the psychologist's office. You have just spend several hundred dollars and many months discussing what you believe to be "wrong" with you. The psychologist says "That is interesting. Tell me more." You do and you relive the experience, which may or may not have been disturbing.

With PSYCH-K, you don't have to relive anything. PSYCH-K is easy in that way. This modality has hundreds of well-formed questions for use to keep it easy, but you are encouraged to make up your own. One thing that I have learned in my practice is that you may have come to my office to work on your self-esteem, yet the more questions that you are asked identifies that you are really there to work on grief and loss, or relationships.

My job is to stay "curious" making sure that the questions asked of you stay positive and that you "stay in your body." It is fun to watch the subconscious try to get out of the work...the eyes start to wander or you might get tired or thirsty. No worries. We take care of all of that with a little water or a "timeout" and then we are good.

When doing a session, you first test for the belief using the simple, magical "lie detector" of muscle-testing, the PSYCH-K way. If you test "weak" to any question, you just complete what is called a "Balance." There are several different types of Balances, and sometimes you even get to create your own balance. However, we usually use the simple Resolution Balance or my personal favorite, The New Direction Balance, both simple techniques.

First, you muscle-test to establish communication,(like or dislike) then pre-test a belief statement, get permission and commitment. Something else that is very important and unique about PSYCH-K is that we always ask permission. We are asking your "higher self" or your subconscious before we make a change. What you may think is good for you to change may still have a lesson for you within it and changing that belief before the lesson is learned may not be a good idea.

Most of the time, we are able to get agreement between the person who wants the change and the subconscious. When we don't, I have found that for the most part, the client is tired or has had enough for that day, or for reasons unknown to the client or me, it just isn't happening.

When you have permission and agreement, you complete the Balance, which does just that, balances your right and left hemisphere of your brain using easy body movements. And the change lasts forever or until it is no longer needed! I have tested myself on changes I have made years ago, and they are still there.

After the Balance, you have changed a belief and you are tested again to make sure that is true. You confirm completion by post-testing the belief statements, and then allow yourself to celebrate!! Many times, all of this can happen within approximately 5 minutes although it can take much longer for a client to go through the process, which is fine. Isn't it worth whatever time it takes to change a belief that has cause havoc in your life for years? You bet it is!

Why do we believe that it is good to celebrate? We are working with the four-year young brain...that is who you are speaking with when you talk to your subconscious, the child who took this belief into their being, not knowing that it was destructive. Therefore, it is important now to reward the child within. Dance, laugh, or do whatever feels right. It is my favorite time!

If you are still looking for the missing peace in your life, may I offer this to you...Try PSYCH-K! Visit the site. www.PSYCH-K.com to find a practitioner in your area as we are all over the United States, as well as internationally..

About the Author

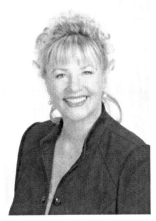

Elta Rahim is a certified Psych-K facilitator and helps people break-free of the limiting beliefs that are barriers to their happiness and success. She has worked with speakers, who were afraid to speak in public, authors with blocks, and people who just want to be or do a little better living their lives.

Elta is the National Director for iZIGG, a phone text marketing company.

Elta lives in "lively" Las Vegas, Nevada with the man of her dreams, her husband. She spends many summers in "sweet" Seattle, Washington with her daughter and son-in-law.

Elta Rahim can be contacted at:
www.eventsbyelta.com
elta@live.com
Elta Rahim702-767-4525

Lightworker

"You are the light of the world"

Danielle Dove

Awakening to the power of light work has the potential to change your life forever. It is a fantastic subject, simply because it includes everything and everyone, no matter what religion you practice, no matter what your beliefs or origin might be, whether you're a healer yourself or simply like the idea of working with "light" or "energy." It is inclusive of everyone for the very good reason that we all come from the light and are of the light.

We are all light beings! If you wonder if that's true, go look at your baby pictures or any newborns you know and notice how much light you see radiating from their faces. At birth, we are all light beings with a purity of soul that is evident in young children. As light beings, the potential of being at awe with life never diminishes. This potential can become forgotten when children become adults. Yet, the light never turns off. It can't turn off – it is energy, and as with the empirical law of physics,*"energy can neither be created nor destroyed: it can only be transformed from one state to another."[2]*

And that's exactly some of the duties of Light Workers: to transform light and energy into whatever he or she intends and focuses on.

---

[2] Wikipedia, the free encyclopedia *Conservation of Energy,*
http://en.wikipedia.org/wiki/Conservation_of_energy (Nov 29, 2010).

(The key to being a powerful Light Worker and staying one is to remember to keep one's inner light of awareness shining brightly.)

Light Work can be marvelous. It can bring relief to someone who suffers from an illness; it can awaken the thought pattern that created the disease; it can heal past life karma, and on a more grounded level, it can protect businesses from negative energies and financial losses, among many others.

Energy work and Light Work in and around buildings where people spend much of their time thinking, arguing, developing, selling, or buying can be of great help since all of that energy adheres to people after they leave, and take it home with them.

If enough Light Workers could get together and spread their love and light cleaning out old energies from buildings, businesses and people, we would feel better, have fewer illnesses, and make wiser decisions out of love, and a lot less out of fear.

Not all Light Work is energy work per se. For some it's writing and spreading incredible knowledge (such as Eckart Tolle), sometimes it's Angel Therapy® and healing with the angels (Doreen Virtue), for others it's publishing new age books (Louise Hay), for some it's social movements (Martin Luther King), and for my greatest teacher, it was Divine Romance and Self Realization (Paramahansa Yogananda).

Historically, the one I refer to the most when I try to explain Light Work is simply Jesus Christ, originally called Yeshua. He was the ultimate messenger and Light Worker. He traveled spreading God's truth, as well as healing people through the power of his mind and intention. He would connect to Source and telepathically through his own thoughts and knowingness, decide the person to be healed and trusted that it was so! He transformed energies through the power of his mind as well as the laying of hands, which overrides all mental and physical limitation that any sick person might have had.[3] Now, it takes practice to strengthen one's mind to have the power to ignore what is (the disease or lack) and transform it into health or abundance; but it's not impossible, and many people have been able to heal others. It's a God-given ability we all have.

---

[3] Paramahansa Yogananda, *The Second Coming of Christ: The Resurrection of the Christ within you: a revelatory commentary on the original teachings of Jesus* (United States: Self Realization Fellowship, 2004), 334; 415-429

Light Workers come to earth with a deep knowing of their mission and they can be found among us in all areas of society. They come with a kind heart, a deep knowing of the truth and vigor to fight injustices and falsehood. Yet, anyone who learns a little bit (or a lot) about energy work and practices the tools can help in wonderful ways. Would you like to learn how to ease tension in a room? How to relax and calm someone down and restore them to their natural state of love? How about protecting and shielding yourself and those you love with an energetic shield? These are but a few examples of what a Light Worker can learn to do, and the list is unlimited! What's most important is that you understand how you can work with light in your own unique way and share that knowledge and skill with those around you.

Recognizing Light Worker traits in adults

I have seen similar traits in adults and children I have helped who could be identified as "Light Workers." This list is not exhaustible or complete in any way; it is simply to offer guidance.

Sense of independence and leadership
Highly self-sufficient and creative
"Out of the box" ideas for how to fix or heal the planet/society
Energy workers – Reiki masters; massage therapists; nutritionists; spiritual teachers with a sense of wanting to lead and organize and change the status quo
Always different as a child, yet felt very connected to a force outside of oneself, as though being watched over
Writers – usually love to read or write
Care greatly about the wellness of others
Genuine and gracious
Could have had a slight torment or experience with the dark side but not afraid of it (either through direct contact such as an addiction or through relationships with others…etc.).
Determined and focused to better themselves
Can suffer from burn out if they do not learn to balance their personal lives with their sense of duty

Recognizing Light Worker traits in children

You may use these descriptions to see if you were one yourself early on or if your child might be one as well.

A *Light Worker child* can often be a tad bit antisocial and extremely sensitive to others. They may either be very shy and quiet or loud, and at times, even angry, but either way they don't seem to totally fit in.

The signs can be very subtle: as babies they grew fast and wanted to do everything on their own. Later, they would spend a lot of time alone daydreaming, or they would walk meditatively or even sit down to meditate all on their own. You, as the parent, might have heard them talk to their "imaginary friends" asking big spiritual questions, or seem eager to learn from you. They may seem wise beyond their years and that wisdom is often what separates them from others their age. They can't relate, and they are in a hurry to get on with their mission. They want to do well and they try extra hard to please, yet can rebel extremely strongly towards teachers or authority figures who they may perceive as not always authentically truthful.

Gifted children who demonstrate early signs of intuition and telepathic gifts are often here to help the world become a brighter more peaceful place. They love you as parents, but they also care about achieving their mission. That's the programming they were born with so try and not take it personally when they seem distant or preoccupied or want to leave home as soon as they are able to. They are extremely advanced souls who have a lot of work to do, and may not need to relate to family dynamics, as well as non-mission oriented Light Workers, yet will always be loving, caring, and generous with their time toward the family, as much as they can.

If you know your child is a Light Worker, I encourage you to talk to him or her about Spirit or what their own idea of God is. You will be surprised by the knowledge they were already born with.

A Light Worker child may miss "home," which ultimately is God's purity and light. So, if your child acts out in anger or seems unusually lonely, he could simply be home sick. Invite him to meet spiritual teachers and other safe young people who meditate, eat a more sensitive meat-free diet, and prefer peaceful human exchange. Your child will recognize these energies as "'home" and feel better right away. I have seen it many times with children that I meet. Often, they are just looking for energies that are "safe" and tranquil, which they will absorb and transfer through their words and emotions, rendering them much more peaceful. (*To the adult Light Worker, please consider yourself as that child and nurture your own needs the same exact way; it's never too late to offer to yourself that which you've longed for!*).

Many Light Worker children and adults are also very good at fitting in. They can have a wide range of friends from all walks of life. They love everybody and learn from everyone. They are the least discriminating for they see through people's physicality and understand the light is in everyone.

Young Light Workers may not relate to the materialistic world, although to fit in, they will pretend that they do enjoy it and want to be a part of it. Later, when your child is old enough, allow him or her to create a means of income if he or she desires. They came with so much to learn and teach that they may be eager to be independent. I highly recommend that if you think your child is a Light Worker to read up on it; the books will come to you, if you are willing to be guided. Then, share the knowledge you've learned with your child and other adults around you.

A Light Worker child wants to help and heal others, so one great way to bond with your child is to allow them to help you. If you are sick, ask them if they would place their hands on the part of your body that's ill. You usually should feel instant relief, but be patient; your child will love helping you, but it may take a few tries for him or her to remember all of their healing powers. They are natural born healers and guides, and with you as their parental figure, I trust they are in great hands to grow their light into incredible miracles.

Light Worker Initiation:
You have learned so far that you are already a light, but what does it take to turn that light into an action verb: to be a "light *worker....*".

Through my work as an energy healing and Light Worker, I have outlined the steps one can take to begin the initiation process. If you are reading this chapter and your pulse is quickening and it's exciting you to know that you are a light being here to work with the light, then welcome! It is so good to meet you and to offer this chapter to you as a gift for your ascension.

As an adult Light Worker, you might have had some instances where you encountered spirits, saw them, felt them or had a strong knowing of a spiritual life outside of you... do not be afraid, call on the highest light which I know to be God, but you can call it whatever you are comfortable with, and ask for the highest messengers to come to you now. Once you establish a good connection with your guides and angels, you're covered. But they are not allowed to intervene until you ask for help, so lower your guard and be willing to receive a little help...it won't cripple you in any way, but actually strengthen you.

Next, I suggest you increase your inner sense of breath. Take yoga, walk or run daily, do whatever you can, but get breathing! That's the prana energy we all need within ourselves to receive pure energy. Prana means life force or breath in Sanskrit. If you feel guided, explore ways to research Prana energy. Simply reading on a new subject you have never heard of before will help develop new brain cells for your mind to welcome the information. Keep growing, your potential is unlimited!

Next, I encourage you to seek other Light Workers in your community. You will make the best of friends and relate on such wonderful topics. It's important for all Light Workers to know they are not alone. Even if your mission feels like one to be done solo, trust that a good foundation of spiritual friends like you could really help you in times of healing.

Play together, read each other's oracle cards, meditate, take energy classes, learn about angels, do anything that gets you into a mode of playing and celebrating life together. That is also energy – and when a Light Worker is happy, the work gets so much more powerful!

Being guided: The Treasure Map:
Imagine from now on that your life is one amazing great big treasure hunt and every encounter, every book, every movie can have that clue you need to awaken to the next level (this is why Light Workers need to learn to play, relax and turn their mind off as well through games and sports; otherwise; it can get to be too much.)

Since a Light Worker is here to help spread a message of healing or heal people directly through energy work, then a Light Worker is also one who learns to heal himself or herself quickly. That is why the treasure map is important and staying open minded is key to seeing the signs.

You might have been guided to let go of relationships that are not helping you grow. I encourage you to trust that letting go is safe. A French author said, "The best way to reconnect to your destiny is through solitude." and sometimes that's all it takes, some quiet time alone, reflecting, healing, letting go.

I don't recommend extreme solitude, but a Light Worker does need a lot of time alone to think and reflect and be guided. Once you open up your gifts of telepathy and intuition, you can be in constant contact with the angelic realm and ascended masters or your guides from your own planet so as to never feel truly alone.

In the life of a Light Worker:
The road to your awakening may have been challenging and bumpy, but trust that it was all to serve you. We live in a world of duality as long as we are acting from a place of ego, but as soon as we remember our true nature – love - then the ups and downs of life can end. There is so much a Light Worker needs to learn about how to be guided, how to open up to understanding signs and messages, and how to work with energies, it can seem overwhelming. So I share with you a few examples in the life of a Light Worker.

Energy work and Meditation:

Meditation for a Light Worker is not only union with God - it's also calibrating your internal computer to be one with Divine Consciousness – it is about welcoming the Truth of your day.

Am I moving in the right direction out of faith or fear?
Do I really need this 9-5 job when I am so unhappy in it?
Can I believe in my gifts, and slowly but surely, step out of my day job?
Can I be intuitive enough to know when my guides and angels talk to me to hear a yes or a no?
Am I willing to be led?
Can I let go and delegate to my guides and angels what I need?
Can I find balance between receiving information and taking an active role to fulfill my heart's desire?
Can I love myself enough to work towards achieving the greater good?
(Define what your own greater good is for yourself).
Can I get myself out of apathy if that's where I have been stuck?
Am I willing to pray and ask for help and receive that help?

Light Workers have to be strong-minded since it is from their thoughts that their powers manifest. This can be achieved either by effort with affirmations or by reading self-help books or meditation. Either way, there is always a sense of magic about their thoughts: either what they say manifests, what they write becomes true, or what they intend falls into place. A Light Worker has lots of tools in his or her toolbox and part of the initiation is to discover what your own tools are.
What am I really going to be good at? *Could it be that what I'm already really good at doing has always been inside of me? Could it be that it is the same thing that can help me find true happiness in the world?*

WHAT CAN HOLD BACK A LIGHT WORKER
Through my healing practice, I have seen these thoughts hold people back and I offer you some guidance on how to heal them as soon as you can.

1. "I have big dreams but I don't think I am worthy of them or could even do it..."

If the thoughts you have about yourself and your ability to achieve your dreams limit you in any way, I encourage you to pray and ask for help. You will be guided to a healing method, a book, or a teacher who can help you eliminate the limiting beliefs. You can also find the thoughts that hold you back while in meditation and choose to let them go spontaneously!

Also, remember your divine inherent connection to All That Is. If you feel intimidated by your dreams, simply remember, it is the incredible mass of energy that has created all of life that will act through you and direct you, one baby step at a time.

"It is not I but the Father, that doeth these good works" – Jesus Christ

2. Getting too caught up with the status quo and mainstream media:

"I have to get a job, and get that car, and the credit card to do what everyone else does to fit in."

Practice self-awareness:
Are you too engaged with the status quo or what's on TV and what other people's beliefs are? A Light Worker has to ignore the outer manifestation of the world since it is only the reality of other people, and most are caught up in endless cycles of pain and pleasure.

To be able to invite a new energy into that world, one must leave "what is" to find something that works to help you change your own world. It is insanity to think one can keep doing the same thing over and over again expecting different results.

You cannot accept everyone's beliefs that times are hard because it means you are making the economy your source of wealth instead of keeping the power where it belongs...in God's hands. Especially for a Light Worker, it is of utmost importance that you always keep your focus on doing what you love, knowing the money and physical needs are always taken care of. A Light Worker working for money is sure to lose it all very quickly. The physical reality of money is the effect of the actions you've taken – the cause. If you take those actions out of a need for money – it comes from lack. Lack creates more lack. But, if you take action doing the work you love, already feeling abundant, then the energy multiplies and all that you need comes to you.

When you keep your mind off this world and focus instead on the reality of God's infinite unlimited power, then you are open to receiving help and abundance from all sources – not just one - your boss or your spouse or your society. *(Please note baby steps are greatly respected; it is progress not perfection that is important here, so take your time! It's ok!).*

"I am in this world but not of this world" – Jesus Christ

3. "A sense of inferiority"

Whenever you feel out of sorts within a group of people, or don't belong there and you feel inferior, get out...redefine yourself and call on God to help you release the shyness. If you feel inferior to anyone, that's your ego lying to you, seeking to separate you from others by saying that you're either better than they are or you're not good enough. Learn about *The Power of Now* by Eckart Tolle and the way our pain body wants to recreate more pain through relationships. The worst thing for a Light Worker is to get caught up in the earth drama and forget who he or she really is. If you think you are in a co-dependent relationship or find yourself surrounded by friends who drain you, call for help and be willing to let them go until you've regained your strength.

You need to learn what your unique connection to Divine consciousness can create through you – those are your unique gifts you are here to share with the world, so please, don't lose hope. Take one day at a time.

LIGHT WORKERS ARE HERE TO:

Develop their own ability to connect to the light
Continually expand their inner light to help others
Heal and neutralize negative energies
Heal others and themselves
Create new ways to help the planet find long-lasting peace

It is so important that a potential Light Worker remembers who he or she really is...you are much more than a just a body! You are an amazing mass of energy that has come to earth to shine brightly and defog the world of falsehood. Sometimes, it's on a universal level, and sometimes it's on a much smaller, local level. Either way, I guarantee you that it's an incredible journey to be on and one where it only gets better every day.

Becoming a Light Worker has been a tremendous experience for me. I've likened it to "getting loved up into wholeness." Just like puzzle pieces coming apart and back together into a new mosaic of colors for each day that I surrendered to the present moment, whether it was comfortable or not. Each time Life inspired me with epiphanies and self-realization that have served my wellness every day.

The signs I was allowed to see – the books that fell off the shelves as I'd walk by them or those that seem to "light up" on their own for me to read; the development of my intuitive gifts as I journeyed onward seeking truths behind each encounter, each seeming catastrophe, which always revealed themselves to be blessings in great disguise.

I knew that every request I said out loud or intended was creating my reality of tomorrow. Life would then follow by presenting me with new friends, opportunities and ideas that I could take along with me as answers to my prayers.

Ever since I was a little girl, I always had a strong knowing that I was here to grow big and take care of others, whether it was my older sister, my mother or the world at large. I would telepathically always be asking my angels or God for help without knowing at that age what I was actually doing. When good things happened, I would bow in deep gratitude, even as a child, thinking "thank you" already knowing that there was a force outside of myself bringing about good in the world.

The journey continues to amaze me. Today, I have a spiritual practice and a form of healing therapy which all began from an innocent prayer that I repeated each time I visited Yogananda's Self Realization Fellowship Temple: May I help awaken Thy love in all hearts.

Thy love is God's love. It is the Light of Consciousness that can cut through fear, anger, grief, despair, and even violence within our own self, neighborhoods, countries, or nations. Ultimately, it is the light that once awakened in someone never goes away, but actually helps the world heal, one person at a time, one moment at a time.

I am grateful to say that with prayer and intention come realization. In 2011, Healing Dove Therapy™ was born to certify other talented healers and practitioners who have the same wish as I do to open up their healing wings and fly spreading God's love. The healing methodology comes from the hundreds of private sessions, channeling, and workshops I was lucky to facilitate. More information is available on the website, as well as in an upcoming handbook and workbook, oracle card deck and divination board game.

If you feel guided to learn more about the Healing Dove Therapy™ Certification or to take a look at our active practitioners, come stop on by, send us a note, tell us about your own experiences. We'd love to hear from you and stay connected.

There are always workshops, classes and retreats taught regularly all over the world to bring you meditation, healing, a spiritual family and new found hope in who you are and what you can do in this world. You are an unlimited being living in an unlimited world. Make it count!

About the Author

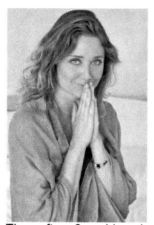

Danielle Dove, Angel Therapist® Energy Healer, and co-founder of Healing Dove Therapy™, was born and raised in France until the age of 13. She moved to the U.S. to continue her education in the States leading her to attend UCLA with a B.A. in Environmental Studies '04. Throughout her childhood, she grew up close to nature on a small farm in the South of France.

Her ability to hear and channel messages began as a child when she could hear "downloads" of scripted messages whenever she slept or spent time alone with her horse. Thereafter, 3 sudden deaths over the span of 8 years led her to ask many questions. She was able to use her gift to receive answers, which led her to the path of a healer and a channel for God and His Angelic Realm.

As a devoted Light Worker, she works in the United States and Europe spreading the healing light to all who seek the same healing and answers that she had needed many years before. In 2011, she is birthing her first child, as well as birthing a new certification program for Light Workers interested in turning their gifts into a fulfilling career. Her philosophy in life is to Love All and Shine Brightly.

Danielle Dove can be contacted at:
www.healingdove-therapy.com
www.danielledove.com

My Spirit

My spirit is liquid silver
Hiding in mountain streams and creek beds
Witnessing Native American rituals
Thunder voices calling over pounding drums
Visions of nature's carved crayon canyons
Embedding in my spirit rock

Time is mine now
But time does not own my spirit
It is only an altered perception
For if my spirit is to survive the test
I must not create barriers of illusion
I cannot hide from the eagle
For fear does not abide in the spirit
Who has been bitten by life, yet lives
To capture its personal wind song

My spirit is a vortex
Of my imagination, my simple soul
Wading through the swirling waters
Of my dark side
Washing clean the bruises of time
To fill my pristine spirit
With glowing angel light
Etched in love stone
Flowing like liquid silver
Down around and into my spirit's eternal memory…

~Carole J. Hannon, Ph.D. 2012

About the Author

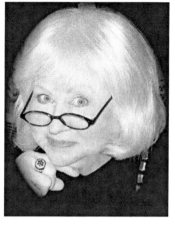

Dr. C.J. Hannon, long term President of *Turnstyle Consultants,* serves as media research, management, communication, training consultant to varied private industry, government and educational organizations. Early in her career, she developed a special series of workshops for Women Managers in the business community. It is estimated Dr. Hannon has interacted with more than a million people on a small group or workshop basis.

Dr. C.J. Hannon received her Ph.D. in Communication from the University of Oklahoma, winning the prestigious Affleck-Carroll Award for the most significant contribution to family issues research. Her dissertation is ranked in the top ten for research in this area. She keeps her finger on the pulse of ever-changing and diverse cultural issues as an Adjunct Professor (UNLV, Regis University) and as the Creative Media Director for *Maple Street Greeting Cards.*

Dr. C.J. Hannon was born a poet. She has authored two books of poetry, entitled *Thorns Have Roses* and *Free.* Her third book of poetry, *Remnants of a Rainbow,* is soon to be published.

Dr. C.J. Hannon can be contacted at:
Carole J. Hannon, Ph.D.
2362 North Green Valley Parkway #49E
Henderson, NV 89014
www.maplestreetgreetingcards.com
drcjhannon@netzero.net

Manifesting

Doreen Lavender Ping

Wouldn't it be wonderful to receive anything just by asking? Is it possible that you can create magic just by what you think and say? Have you seen others create abundance and wonder how they did it?

Life is a process that requires us to be aware every day of what we are creating through our thoughts, words, actions, and feelings. Once you understand just how easy this can become, you will always know that you can have anything that you desire as long as it does not purposefully hurt another soul.

This process is called MANIFESTING. It's a way to create what we want, and to be able to actually experience results through simple tools and methods.

For many people, they pray and ask their creator for what they want. The problem, however, is that when it does not appear, they think that they have done something wrong or that they are not worthy.

A child will repeatedly ask for the same toy over and over again until finally a parent will just break down, and get the toy. Children learn quickly that they just need to keep asking. In life, however, as adults we learn that it's not that easy. The continuous asking does not always reward us. I have found that repeatedly asking for the same thing just signifies that you don't trust that you can have it in the first place.

I would like to share with you how I learned to receive what I desire in a simple, yet defined method. I call it the **Miracle Formula**. Throughout my life, I determined what I wanted by first looking at what I did not want. For example, if I am driving to the mall to Christmas shop, I don't want to drive around looking for a parking spot, only to find one at the very far end of the parking lot. That's what I don't want.

Then, I determine that I want a parking space in the front rows of a certain area of the mall. That's pretty simple. Then, I ask the Universe for this parking space quickly and easily. As I'm driving, I give my thanks in advance and drive directly to that area. I don't doubt the results or the speed in which I will find the empty space. The result is that there is always a space. In fact, my friends refer to me as the "parking space queen" as they know I always manage to manifest a space.

Here is the six step formula to manifest what you want. Let's use, for example, that you are manifesting the purchase of a new car.

1. Determine the type of cars that **you don't want**.

Perhaps, you are tired of spending money on high maintenance costs and fuel bills. Therefore, you no longer want an expensive luxury car. Although you like the feel of the high-end cars, your lifestyle has changed, and your needs and priorities have shifted.

2. Write down the major specifics of **what you do want** in this new car.

For example, your family has grown and you need more room and safety features for passengers. Greater gas mileage is a factor now that you are driving 30 minutes to work each day. Price range is important as you are now planning ahead for your children's educations, and monthly payments must be in a certain range for your family budget. It's not necessary that you determine the exact model and year, but have a general understanding of what models would fit into your family's needs. Remember: "The spoken word is powerful, but the written word is law." That's why it's important to write it down.

3. **ASK the Universe for what you so desire**.

When we repeatedly ask the Universe for the same thing, it shows that we don't trust that we will receive what we are requesting. So, ask only ONE TIME.

4. Every day **give your thanks** in advance for the divine completion.

Assume the Universe has heard you, and you are trusting in receiving what you asked. Begin to see yourself driving your new car. What color is it? See yourself driving to work. How does it feel? Recognizing the feelings that you attach to the end result is really important in confirming this process.

5. Begin to **take action** to find this car.

Miracles happen every day, but you must be "present" to receive. Take the action of looking on the internet and in the local newspaper, shopping at different car dealerships, and telling your friends. You never know who or what will bring you the answers. If you stay home, and don't try to investigate, there's a greater chance you won't find your perfect car. Taking action says to the Universe that you are truly serious about what you are manifesting. At times, we get tested to see if we are sure. In other words, perhaps a car might become available that does not meet all your needs. Will you settle for something that isn't exactly what you are manifesting? Perhaps it has all the requirements, but the price is $1,500 higher. What decision will you make? If you have thought out the process in the beginning, and determined what you want, then you should not settle for anything less or for more money. This is the Universe's way of testing you to see if you will accept less.

6. **Don't allow fear or doubt** to come into your thoughts and words when the **timing** isn't as fast as you had hoped.

Perhaps the car that is just perfect for you is still on a transport truck and has not arrived in your city, as yet. We never know why there are delays, but remember it's always in divine timing. Don't allow fear or doubt into your words or thoughts. It's like telling the Universe that you don't think you are worthy to have this new car.

When you allow yourself to be in fear, the Universe thinks you have changed your mind on what you want. Then nothing happens. The result is that you must start the formula all over again.

Using this method of manifesting over time will result in positive results. The more you use it, the greater you will trust the results. Using the formula for a parking space during the holidays is just the beginning. It's a simple example, but so powerful. Then as you trust more, there will be more depth in your understanding, and you will allow the Universe to gift you with the unexpected magnificent abundance of all that is.

Remember: "Today is the tomorrow that you created yesterday." Each day is built on the power of the previous day. Days fold into weeks and weeks stretch into months. Before long, you have created years of successful manifesting.

What other methods can be used to manifest what you desire? Your words are powerful, and it's important to understand that your thoughts create an energy that is then transferred into words. Sometimes, you can actually limit yourself in what and how you can receive. You never want to put a cap on the abundance that you desire. Someone told me years ago, when my first book was published, that he hoped I would sell one million copies. I replied that I never wanted to be limited to only one million. How do you not limit yourself?

Look at the words you are speaking. Try using the phrase "in excess of" in asking for what you desire. For example, if you were to say, "I am manifesting in excess of $15,000 per month." That way, the Universe can bring you the avenues that will not hold you back. Let's say an employment opportunity is coming to you that would pay $15,500 per month. By using the words "in excess of" you are allowing yourself permission to receive this monthly income. Without the added phrase, you are limiting yourself to not receiving this income, and possibly not receiving the new position. Would that actually happen? If your intention is only to accept $15,000 per month, the Universe will know that you cannot allow yourself anything greater than you requested.

Look at how you limit your life right now with your thoughts, then words, then feelings to your words, pronouncing these words to others, as well. There is power in what you say. When you share this limitation with others, it gives them an opportunity to attach their judgment, creating more limitations and negativity.

In addition, use the words "quickly and easily" in your manifesting sentences. Here's an example, "I am manifesting in excess of $15,000 per month quickly and easily." In other words, knowing that time is undetermined, this opens the door for the abundance to be received without delays. I have a saying "If you get stuck, let it go. If it flows, it's a go." Again, this same thought brings in the abundant flow. If you are manifesting, life is flowing, and you begin to look at obstacles only as items to be redefined in your thoughts and eventual words.

The beauty of this is that you get to create what you desire. Now, begin to view your life in a different way. Using these simple tools will help you to create, accept, and manifest your total well-being. Use these methods every day and see results. Watch along the way for signs that you are not in the flow. In other words, if people are presenting chaos or drama to you, perhaps you are getting caught in an energy that is not yours and not for your highest good.

One of the best ways to release this unforeseen chaos and drama is to send back the energy. Have you ever walked into an office or store and felt the negativity? Have you listened to a friend discuss a situation in the most harsh and inappropriate manner? Your friend begins to feel better, but you begin to immediately notice that his or her negativity seems to stay with you. The good energy that you were feeling is now covered up with this aura of negativity that just doesn't seem to go away.

You never want to send back negative energy to anyone, but clearly you don't need or want to hold onto it, as well. Sometimes, you are able to recognize where the negativity came from, and other times you are not aware of why you feel agitated, restless, or depressed. Everything in your life can be flowing smoothly, but suddenly your demeanor begins to change, and you unknowingly have picked up someone else's negativity. So, how do you release or send back this energy?

The Universe blessed me years ago with this lesson. I had gathered a group of spiritual sisters in my home for an evening. Towards the end of our time together sitting in a circle, I walked behind each one placing my hands on their shoulders, blessing them with a channeled message. As each left that evening, one of them told me her right hip had been painful for months. She said it was now gone and she felt so much better. I was thrilled for her recovery.

The next morning I awoke with pain in my right hip. At first, I was not aware that it came from anyone else. For days, I just thought I had slept on my side and had pinched a nerve. As time progressed, I realized that my pain was not normal. I had obviously picked up this energy from someone else.

I began using the techniques of yoga, meditation, and chakra balancing to release this imbalance in my hip, but nothing eased this pain. I even visualized this area of my body with bright golden healing energy. It felt better, but did not completely go away.

Nearly eight months went by when many of my spiritual sisters returned for another evening together in my home. Toward the end of the night, I was guided by the Universe to have everyone sit in a circle to embrace the loving energy that we were all creating. I was again directed to hold my hands on each shoulder and channel another message. As I walked over to the woman who originally had the hip pain, I spoke an unknown affirmation and then a message for her. I repeated this affirmation and a personal message for each sister.

The next morning, I awoke with no hip pain. Several weeks later, I received a call from the sister that originally had the hip pain. She wanted to tell me that she finally realized what she had been doing to create the hip pain that she had suffered for months. No, she did not get the hip pain back, but she did have the understanding of why it had been created in the first place. She had been unable to move forward in an area of her life.

In order to retain or regain your balance, the negative energy received from someone must be forwarded back to them. However, we do not want to send out negative energy, because it is important to remember "What goes around comes around."

The following affirmation is for you to be able to send back energy without it being received as negative energy.

(Person's name) I do NOT accept your thoughts, words, actions, feelings, and energies. I send it all back to you surrounded with the White Light of Love and Protection, to be dissolved within the Universe.

Thank you. Thank you. Thank you.

Since this affirmation is surrounded with love and protection, the person receiving it will not be harmed in any way. It does, however, give back the responsibility of what was given to you either purposefully or inadvertently.

We all must be mindful of what we send out to others. If you direct respect and honor to others, you will receive back the same. When you live in a circle of harmony and balance, anyone that comes in contact with you will automatically have the opportunity to see, feel, and sense your well-being.

Now, watch and enjoy the transformations that will occur in your life, and the renewal of positive energy. Manifesting becomes a way of life. As you begin to see and experience the rewards, you will take greater steps in what you can achieve. Eventually, you will do it all the time without consciously thinking about it. That's when the magic truly explodes!

As you begin to manifest, write the results down in a journal. Include the process of the **Miracle Formula**. Begin each page of the journal with what you are manifesting. Using the formula, write down what you **don't** want. Then include the aspects of what you **do** want. When that is completed, write your question ONE time.

Set up a column or section for all the action items that you are taking to complete this goal. As far as timing, record the date you first began to think of your question. Then, list the date that you actually first wrote your request.

In addition, record the timing of when it was completed and any thoughts that were repeating in your mind that could possibly have altered the results. Recognizing any brief negativity will then help you avoid these problems.

Sometimes we are not even aware of simple statements that trigger delays. Here are a few things to notice:

1. Listening to others' opinions about what you are manifesting. Sometimes they are unconsciously setting limits in your mind.

2. Avoid using these statements:

    I am unworthy.

    It's taking too much time. I guess I'm not supposed to have this.

    Maybe I'm not qualified.

    I'm not smart enough to be successful.

Since I've been divorced, I'm not a good partner for marriage.

Everyone in my office is sick. I guess it's my turn.

Everywhere I turn, there are disasters.

Nothing seems to go right anymore.

I guess I'm too old to have fun anymore.

Dramas just seem to follow me.

I always pick the wrong person.

I keep repeating the same mistakes.

Avoiding these statements and thought patterns will help to assure you the successes that you desire. Sometimes, as we speak something negative, we have an immediate reaction or recognition of what we just said. Use the word "cancel" to negate that statement. Then, restate what you said using a positive statement.

Share this information with your family, friends, coworkers, and all new connections. Knowledge is powerful, and sharing this information will not only expand your abundance, but assist others on their journey, as well. I am still amazed at how the Universe gifts us with the magic. It is humbling to watch people and events come into your life just at the right time, thus completing what you had manifested.

Every morning as I am walking, I say out loud **"I expect the unexpected magnificent abundance of all that is and it feels and looks terrific. Thank you. Thank you. Thank you."** Then I allow myself to receive what I have manifested, giving thanks daily, and knowing it is in divine perfect timing.

Begin to see the magic of manifesting and how it changes and shifts your life. As you continue on your journey, the successes begin to build into a life of magnificent abundance…Isn't life grand? Many blessings!!

About the Author

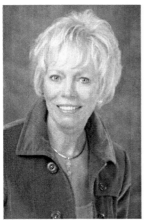

Doreen Lavender Ping has used her spiritual gifts to guide others to unveil the mysteries that are within them for over 30 years. She knows that with spiritual guidance, you can gain the resources to create your reality and realize your higher spiritual self.

Doreen states that "Guidance is a gift. Acceptance is our responsibility, and often reminds us, "That today is the tomorrow you created yesterday."

Doreen is a published author of Stretching Beyond Life's Boundaries and producer of multiple education and meditation CD's.

Currently she is presenting a four part series of seminar Events entitled "Circle of Light – Discovering the Knowings," channeling specific guidance for each participant. Her intention is to share the secrets that Ancient Masters have always known for further ascension with global impact.

Doreen Lavender Ping can be contacted at:
www.lavender4you.com.
(702) 260-4261

Numerology

Carole Grissett

Numerology is a science that considers each number and each letter (with its assigned numeric value) to be alive. The number values and resulting sums we see arranged in names and dates give off various energies that result in your personal characteristics, your strengths, your challenges, and can even forecast what you can expect to experience in this lifetime. As important as what is represented, is the *lack* of a number and its accompanying vibration. Too much or too little of a numeric value, particularly when looking at the combination of our name and our birth date can create challenges in the way we perceive and react to life. In numerology, as with all things, the goal is *moderation and balance.*

Numbers were mankind's first written language, originating from symbols found in nature. Born about the year 590 BC, Pythagoras, a mathematician and a philosopher, is considered the father of modern geometry and was also the first person to realize that numbers form the very foundation of the universe. Throughout the ages, numbers have continued to provide the common ground of communication for all people in every culture. They are considered such a basic information form that now our deep space probes contain numeric formulas as messages in an attempt to communicate with other beings that may exist in our universe.

The idea behind numerology is that the vibration of the universe reflected in your birth date, as well as the name you are called, have an influence over both your character and your destiny in life. However, letters and numbers are only symbols. They do not of themselves make things happen. It is the specific vibration *behind* each letter and number that gives the individual energy to which we react.

Like music, letters, words, and names create widely differing vibrations. Some music makes us feel romantic, some makes us feel patriotic. Music can be restful and soothing. Certain music is an actual assault on the physical body. Likewise, every spoken word has energy. This energy has a constructive or destructive power, according to its formation. The name you are called constantly sets up vibrations and the repeating of it, over a period of years, has the effect of molding you to that vibration. The ancient Romans said, "Nome nest Omen." The name is the destiny. The name you are known by makes an impression in every phase of your life.

Two examples of how numbers reflect their influence are the presence of an "H" and a concentration of vowels. An "H" (which numerically is an 8), adds strength, power and authority wherever it is placed. This letter is common in German names like Heinz, Heinrich, Hedwig, Hedda, and Hildegard. The vowels (A, E, I, O, U, and Y) are considered 'heart' sounds. An example of a concentration is in Hawaiian names like Kauai, Maui, Oahu, Honolulu, Waipahu, Waimanalo, Kailuku, Kapaa, and Kaunakakai . The Hawaiian and Germanic cultures are perceived very differently. The Germans are known for system and order and are considered shrewd business people, always watchful and alert for opportunities. Being strong on self-control and self-discipline, they strive to keep a firm check on their emotions. Stereotypically, Hawaiian culture is noted for its friendliness and warmth to family and strangers alike, with a more easy-going approach to life.

Our present-day Latin alphabet, which we use when reading and speaking English, contains 26 letters. Spiritually, this symbolizes the level of our modern day thoughts and ideas. Ancient teachings suggest that as mankind moves forward and evolves spiritually, our alphabet will eventually contain 27 letters, although at present we do not know what that letter will be. Numeric values are assigned to our current alphabet as follows:

1	A, J, S
2	B, K, T
3	C, L, U
4	D, M, V
5	E, N, W
6	F, O, X
7	G, P, Y
8	H, Q, Z
9	I, R

Using myself as an example, my birth name , Carole Marie Pole, calculates to a 4, (3+1+9+6+3+5+4+1+9+9+5+7+6+3+5 = 76 = 7+6 = 13 = 1+3 = 4) ushering me into this lifetime on a vibration of balance, organization and practicality. When I married and took my husband's surname in daily usage, Carole Grissett, I began vibrating to its total of 9, (3+1+9+6+3+5+7+9+9+1+1+5+2+2 = 63 = 6+3 = 9) the humanitarian. Although the steadiness of my birth name (4) has remained my foundation, taking on the 9 marked not only the full flowering of my interest and involvement in metaphysics, but also began what was a three decades long career in corporate Human Resources, a profession which involved mediation, counseling and guiding others in reaching their highest potential. Both my spiritual and professional development reflected the blending of the practicality of the 4 with the added humanitarian inclinations of the 9. I continue to practice practical spirituality and humanitarian-based business activities today.

Briefly, basic numerological energies range from:

1 (individual self)
2 (cooperation)
3 (self-expression)
4 (stability)
5 (freedom and independence)
6 (service)
7 (introspection)
8 (strength)
9(humanity)

For our purposes, all numbers are reduced to a single digit except 11 (wisdom, inspiration) and 22 (mastership in handling human affairs). The 11 and 22 are difficult to live up to on a daily basis, so for practical purposes, we reduce them to 2 and 4, respectively.

The odd numbers/letters (1, 3, 5, 7 9) are introverts. Folks with this concentration want to accomplish something all on their own and often want to retire from the public eye.

The even numbers/letters (2, 4, 6, 8) are extroverts. The extrovert truly likes people, needs others to be happy, and seeks to give of himself to loved ones.

The mind numbers are 1, 5, and 7. If you have a lot of these numbers you keep things moving; you're one of the movers and shakers.

The builders are 2, 4, and 8. They take care of business. They're direct, make good managers, and earn their money.

The creative numbers are 3, 6, and 9. These folks like the best in life and allow others to help them. They may need the help of others of reach their greatest success.

In numerological analysis, the six major numerical influences are the Birth Path, as well as the numbers of the Personality, Soul, Power Name, Attitude and Destiny. We calculate each of these using the following formulas:

Your Birth Path Number is the numerical sum of digits in your full birth date. Your Personality Number is the numeric sum of all the consonants in the name you go by. Your Soul Number is the numeric sum of all the vowels in the name you go by. Your Power Name Number is the sum of your Personality Number and your Soul Number (represented your whole name). Your Attitude Number (how people first perceive you, correlating to the Ascendant in your astrological birth horoscope) is the sum of the month and day of your birth. And, finally, your Destiny Number is the sum of your Power Name and your Birth Path. Your Destiny Number is the overlying directional compass your soul strives to follow throughout your life.

What is missing from your numbers is as important as what is present. When you look at your name, missing numbers point out areas of weakness in the character which needs to be addressed.

For example, if you are lacking 1's (A, S, J) you may lack ambition and decisiveness.

An absence of 2's (B, T, K) can indicate that you are not adaptable and have difficulties working with others.

No 3's (C, L, U) might indicate you have an inferiority complex and are uncomfortable in social situations.

If you are lacking 4's (D, M, V), it indicates that you may be lazy, dislike routine or find it difficult to discipline yourself.

An absence of 5's (E, N, W) might indicate being unable to make changes and a lack of interest or curiosity about life.

Missing 6's (F, O, X) might indicate a reluctance to marry, have children, or take on domestic responsibilities of any kind.

A lack of 7's (G, P, Y) can make it difficult for you to think along abstract lines and perhaps accept things because they look O.K. on the surface.

If you are missing 8's (H, Q, Z) you may tend to never be content with how much money, power or material goods that you have. You'll need to work on developing ambition and discipline and work to develop sound judgment and organizational talents in personal and business matters.

Lacking 9's (I, R) is rare, but when this is the case, it can limit the extent of intuition and create situations where you must learn to appreciate others' difficulties.

A belief in reincarnation is not required to get meaning from numerology, but most practitioners do believe we have lived before and will again. Following this line of thought, your birth date represents the general road you chose to travel in this lifetime while your name given at birth is a balance sheet showing the strengths (the numerical values represented) and the weaknesses (the numerical values missing) you bring with you from your past life experiences. Any name changes you make, including the name you use in daily interaction (if different) either strengthens or weakens this basic foundation. It's also important to see if there are repetitions of numbers across both the birth date and name. A concentration of a certain number makes its vibration much stronger.

Although the strengths and weaknesses represented in your full birth name are always present, the name you are currently called is the one which has the most impact on your daily life. For example, if you were born John Stephen Smith (9), but are called Jack Smith(8), then the numbers of Jack Smith (8) are the ones to which you vibrate and people around you respond. As an 8, Jack Smith would come across as a better businessman than the humanitarian 9 John Stephen Smith.

In the case of a woman adopting her husband's surname after marriage, Mary Susan Harris (6), who marries Jack Smith (8), might now be called

Mary Smith (4). Although the domestically inclined 6 would have an underlying influence, as a 4, she would come across as very practical and unflappable in her domestic activities.

Timing is always of interest and it is possible to forecast through numbers. The Christian Bible states in Ecclesiastes 3:1 "To everything there is a season, and a time for every purpose under heaven." When we apply numerology to future events, we are able to prepare for the road ahead and, thus, exert control over not only our reaction to what may be in our future, but also as to the outcome.

In forecasting, four major calculations are made: the Cycles, the Pinnacles with accompanying Challenges, and the Personal Years. These break down your lifetime into various broad periods, the combination of which gives you the picture of what's going on in your life at any point in time and what to expect on the road ahead. The Cycles describe in a broad brush stroke the overall environment. The Pinnacles and accompanying Challenges indicate your potential for achievement and potential difficulties or weaknesses,

Every universal calendar year has its unique theme and lesson. For example, the year 2008 (1) marked a time of firsts. One way this manifested was, as a result of the 2008 U.S. presidential election, there was either going to be an African-American President or a female Vice President. Either possibility represented a tremendous break with tradition.

Your Personal Year vibration is calculated annually. Your Personal Year vibration number describes what's happening specifically for you, during the 12 months of that particular year. You find this by adding your Birth Month and Day of Birth to the sum of the current universal year. For example, if your birth date is August 26, for you the year 2008 would be an 8 Personal Year (8 + 8 +1 = 17 = 1 + 7 = 8), meaning this would be an excellent time for you to forge ahead in business and financial affairs.

Since all letters and their accompanying numerical values have their unique vibration, other ways we can use numerology include, but are not limited to, reducing to a single digit and analyzing our house or apartment number, our building or office number at work, hotel rooms, our car's license number, our telephone number, and our pet's name.

Using the house or apartment number as an example:

In a 1 house, you will want to exercise your independence. There will be a lot of coming and going.

A 2 house is conducive to a loving partnership; if you live here you'll want peace and love.

A 3 house attracts communication, parties, laughter. People who live in a 4 home are solid and steady and look to their home as a place of sanctuary.

A 5 house is good for drama with lots of individual activities going on by all the inhabitants...everyone constantly on the go.

A 6 house is great for families and children. It's a nurturing environment.

If you want some privacy or are a student, you'll want a 7 house. This home is not compatible to having loud parties.

An 8 house gives off a proud vibration. If you live here you'll want to make a good impression and be thought of as financially successful. This is an excellent house out of which to conduct a home business.

The 9 house is home to the humanitarian, the extrovert. Everyone will be made welcome here.

Another entire branch of numerology is the comparison of two people's numbers for compatibility. Some numbers naturally get along, some are relatively neutral to each other, and some are outright challenging when they interact. The two most significant numbers to compare when looking at relationships (whether romantic, friend, or business associate) are the individuals' Birth Path and the calculation of the name they each are commonly called.

Although many factors need to be considered for a thorough compatibility analysis, in general, the extroverts (even numbers) get along well with fellow extroverts, while the introverts (odd numbers) understand other introverts. Also, the 1/5/7's, 2/4/8's and 3/6/9's all harmonize with others in their triad more easily than with those who approach life from a different angle. For example, a 7 would find the 2 too gentle and emotionally needy, while the 2 would find the 7 too aloof and independent. However, although the 5 and 7 have a somewhat different approach to relationship, both would respect and appreciate each other's independence and needing their own 'space.'

The beauty of numerology is that of all the analytical and predictive techniques, it is the most portable and the most unobtrusive. With just an introduction of a first name, you can quickly calculate how that person is presenting themselves at that particular moment in that specific environment. You can glance at a person's business card and get a quick fix on how they carry themselves in that arena. In looking for a new apartment or house, you can quickly size up the overall vibration of each option and choose the one that best fits with what you're seeking at that point in your life. With your annual Personal Year calculation, you can better prepare to "go with the universal flow" as it specifically applies to you.

Numbers are everywhere. If used correctly, they can be powerful data points in every facet of your life wherever your life journey takes you. Bon Voyage and Happy Counting!

About the Author

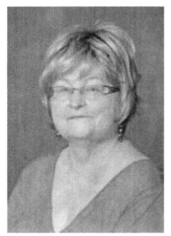

Carole Grissett has utilized Tarot, numerology, and astrology in an intuitive consulting practice serving an international clientele for over 30 years.

In her corporate business career, Carole served in a Human Resources management capacity with several Fortune 500 companies and holds a BA in Journalism, an MBA, and a MA (abt) in Industrial and Organizational Psychology.

She is an ordained minister in both the American Holistic Church and the Universal Church of the Master. Using her practical, positive approach, she continues business and individual consulting practices, as well as continuing to lecture and write.

Carole Grissett can be contacted at:
www.mypsychicpathfinder.com
polestar@netscape.com

Past Lives

Doreen Lavender Ping

Do you believe you have lived another life prior to this one? Are you curious about the concept that you could have multiple lives? Have you ever walked into a room full of people, your eyes can see everyone, yet there is one person that you cannot stop looking at intently? You begin to speak to him or her realizing there is something so familiar. You feel an overwhelming attraction. What is this connection?

Have you ever wondered how a preschool child sits at a piano for the first time and plays a Mozart concerto magnificently without any instruction? How could this happen?
Do you have an intense curiosity about another culture? Is there a time in history that has always fascinated you?

These experiences can be explained by understanding that you have had past lives. In these other lifetimes, you developed associations with other souls, lifestyles, fears, and even life lessons that have contributed to your intense connection with these souls, places, or lifestyles. Knowing you are a composite of lifetimes is an advantage in processing how to interpret what happens in this one.

There are certain cultures and religions that do not accept the concept of past lives, but how do you explain these bizarre strange feelings of intense attractions, fears, or unusual abilities at an early age, or knowing things about a place you've never been to or does not even exist in this lifetime?

Traveling through Europe for the first time, I found the language of one particular country so incredibly easy to speak and understand while other languages just did not flow for me. Even the lifestyle of that particular country seemed to feel like home. As I toured different churches or castles, it felt as though I had been there previously. This happened to me when I first traveled in France. The language was fluid and I just "knew" I had been there at different times, especially when I toured the castle of King Louis XIV of Versailles. I even knew of a secret door before the tour guide told us about it!

Maybe there have been times in your life when you have had off-putting reactions. Maybe when meeting someone for the first time, for some unknown reason, you immediately have a negative feeling. There is no explanation for it other than you both felt as though you were enemies. This could be the result of being in battle with this individual in previous wars in previous lives. Knowledge of your past lifetimes together will assist you in identifying a potential problem in this lifetime.

Extreme fears of a particular animal or insect could be based on frightening experiences in past lifetimes when you had been threatened. What about the first time you spent the day in a zoo? Did you enjoy seeing all the wonderful animals until you came upon one particular animal that immediately made you uncomfortable? Even though these animals were safely caged, did you feel strong feelings of fear, even to the point of nervousness or sweating? Can this be explained by a possible lifetime where you were harmed by a pack of this particular animal?

Do you have a fear of drowning? Is the thought of taking a vacation on a cruise ship upsetting? Perhaps, you experienced a catastrophic sinking of a large naval ship where many of your fellow officers and crew drowned leaving you unable to explain to your family why you won't take a cruise vacation.

Unexplained problems or repeated scenarios can be corrected by viewing your past lives and seeing how these incidents began. Knowing the people in this lifetime that were involved with you can be an added benefit to work on different outcomes now, thus concluding what is referred to as "karma," a person's actions in one reincarnation thought of as determining his fate in the next.

These are just a few of the questions that can be answered with an openness and acceptance that you have had "past lives." Answers to questions about fears, attractions, skills, compulsions, and certain sensitivities can be discovered from knowledge of our many past lives.

Understanding the connection between past lives and your present reality can lead to the most profound and interesting spiritual and practical usages. A past life therapist can regress clients back using hypnosis to discover the journeys of the client's past lives. Generally, there is a theme that runs through the grouping of lives that are discovered.

"The wisdom you carry in yourself is a direct reflection of all the lives you have lived."

It's amazing to know the similarities and tendencies that exist in your previous lifetime experiences. They are in many ways very diverse, and yet, quite similar. Your last few lifetimes could each have had an emphasis on helping others with careers in the medical profession, such as a medic in a war, small town physician, or volunteer in a global organization that helps with disasters. In this lifetime, perhaps you are a fireman or helicopter pilot in rescue missions in the military.

Many years ago, as I was being introduced to a new group of clients for readings, I began channeling and seeing information about their past lives and connections to their family. I had read many books on past lives and knew there was tremendous strength in the understanding of where you were versus who you are now. When a new client comes for his or her reading, they usually refer new clients to me. I began to see a pattern in their past lives, which I found fascinating. Sometimes, this group of people, who had been referred to me, had been in the same country at the same time in history. Perhaps they were not part of the same family, but certainly knew each other in that previous lifetime, maybe as best friends or neighbors.

Here is an example: The first client lived in the area that we now call Australia as the owner of a large shipping company. A friend that was referred by her was the Captain of one of the cargo ships. Weeks later another referral came. It turned out that she was a young boy in the galley of that same ship and was then chosen by the Captain to be his personal liaison on the ship in protection of him from the other seamen.

These three people in this lifetime were friends from the start. They each also play a similar role together in this lifetime. The first is a good business owner. The second is quite adventurous and loves to travel, especially on cruises. The third is somewhat naïve and young at heart, being protected by the two others in making the right relationship decisions. Even though they were men in the previous lifetime, they each incarnated into this lifetime as women.

The repetition of habits became apparent to me as I have done more and more past life readings. I will never forget a past life about hats. A client came for a reading for the very first time. I knew nothing about her at all. She requested that I do a past life reading without first doing a general reading. In one of the lifetimes, I saw her as the creator and owner of a Haberdashery in England. She designed hats with real flowers and bright colors, which were sold to the elite of London for special royal events.

As the reading ended and we were reviewing her past lives, she began to laugh. It turned out she had 33 hats in her closet, each in a special box that was as pretty on the outside as the hat inside the box. She never could understand her fetish for hats. Ironically, in this lifetime she bought very large plain hats and recreated each using large silk flowers and expensive ribbons. Thus, she understood her obsession with hats, flowers, and special hat boxes.

Sometimes, you do the opposite of what you did in previous lifetimes. An example was a client who had experienced leadership roles in major wars in history. Death caused by differences in religious beliefs was common. Not only had my client been killed in battle, but was also responsible for deaths in wars. In this lifetime, she incarnated as a female. She grew up in a family where her father, uncles, and brothers loved hunting and was surrounded by guns and gun cabinets in the family homes. The usage of these weapons was to provide food for their families, yet, she still had a major aversion toward weapons. Not only was she adamantly opposed to guns, but also to violence and wars. She consciously directed her sons against going into the military. After the past life reading, she finally understood her strong sensitivity to guns and wars. It just made sense after hearing her lifetimes of war and destruction.

We tend to travel together as a group in lifetimes. Our roles differ, but the connections are there. Today you and your spouse could have six children. In a previous lifetime in Ireland, you and your spouse could have been brothers, giving your parents a difficult time with your enthusiasm to see the world, and not helping with the family farm. And now, the roles are reversed, you are the parents. Your oldest child in this lifetime was previously your father in Ireland. Now, the challenge is to allow your son his pathway, encouraging him, but not restricting his creativity to travel, and to choose his own lifestyle. There is a saying *"What goes around, comes around."* In other words, we attract back the same people and reverse the life experiences in order to see both sides of any situation.

Gathering different people for a workshop that I present always creates an excitement for me, especially if part of the process is discovering the past life connections of this grouping. In one particular event, I was amazed at the strong past lives during the Roman Empire. Everyone in the workshop had shared a lifetime at the same time. There was no mistaking that each was brought together in this workshop to honor the other souls, getting to know each on a more personal level, and discovering the true integrity and love of all. As the different past lives was announced, you could actually feel the intensity of the group heighten as information was released as to their connections with each other. There were tears, hugs, laughter, and eyes lit up with enthusiasm of their past together. To this day, these bonds continue with a great appreciation of the connections they are experiencing now. Aware of their role from that lifetime gives them an additional advantage on how to approach the others knowing their previous background. Now, they have the choice to shift or change their roles, thus completing the cycle of reversing their pathways together.

With a past lifetime reading, not only do you get to acknowledge others from your past lives, but you experience patterns of living. At the ending of your past life reading, I review with you the theme or repetitious pattern of those lifetimes. With one particular client, she was always in the background. Instead of being a leader, she was an assistant. Even in her marriage, she was not considered an equal. Perhaps the saying *"Always a bridesmaid, never a bride"* would be appropriate here. By understanding her past, she began to realize in this lifetime why she always hesitated to step out into the limelight. She never had a problem speaking up or defending something she believed in, but to stand in front of a crowd giving a formal presentation was way out of her comfort zone. Thus after her reading, she began to take steps to assure her success by manifesting, classes in public speaking, and partnering to present workshops for others. The result was an added elevation in self-esteem and confidence. She is now the leader of her own destiny, having gained strength and understanding from her past.

Your spirit is a composite of all of your lifetimes. At birth, your past is veiled from your ability to see and know, but by acknowledging now that you have had many past lives, it is important for you to recognize that you are "whole." Yes, you have all the information about your many journeys of the past...it is just a matter of discovery.

The wisdom you carry in yourself is a direct reflection of all the lives you have lived.

How do you discover your past lives?

Meditation Practices.

If your intention is to meditate, find a very quiet, secluded room, either lie down or sit in a comfortable chair. With the palm of your hands facing upward, begin by deep breathing through your nostrils. Hold the breath in excess of a count of five. Repeat breathing in and out. Focus your mind on your intention.

Practice meditating several times with the thought of relaxing and enjoying this process. Perhaps you will begin to see the movement of colors and shapes. Eventually, you will visualize different scenarios, i.e. ocean scenes, familiar home, traveling through space, flying with your angels and guides.

When you feel you are ready, ask the Universe to show you a past life where you can see yourself and present family members or friends. If your mind tends to wonder, just mentally say *"cancel"* and come back to your intention.

Now allow yourself to let go and receive the blessings of discovery. It might take several attempts to actually be able to see or participate in this exercise. *Remember, there are no mistakes and whatever you experience is for your highest and best good.*

When you come out of your meditation, write down whatever you remember. As you continue this process, you will begin to see patterns or repetitive scenarios of the past.

The only drawback to an unguided meditation is questioning what you experienced. Our logical left brain sometimes gets in the way of discovery. If so, perhaps you may want to listen to a recorded meditation.

Regression With a Licensed Therapist.

During this process, you can be regressed back to your early childhood as a preface to your past lives. Again, this process may take several attempts throughout this life to begin the unveiling of your past lives. It is important to let go of the control and allow your body, mind, and spirit to travel. This is a controlled session with guidance from a therapist. The advantage is that you are listening to a directed journey to your past. It is recommended that this session be recorded so that you can recall the past scenario.

Channeled Past Life Reading.

When you come to me for a channeled past life reading, I ask you if there is anyone you want to specifically know when and where they were with you previously. We set the intention of the session to include in excess of six past lives.

The first thing shown to me is a world map with a focus on the name of a country as you know it today. You are shown as a male or female and occupation. Everything is verbally described to you.

The next step is seeing your family setting. This is where you begin to know if any of your current family members were with you previously and what role each of you played together in that life. Then a particular experience or more of that lifetime is given. Sometimes, the information is only a single day of time while other lifetimes can be stretched over several years. There is no strict rule here. If the time is only shown as a one day experience, generally it is really powerful in a lesson learned. Examples would be the accomplishment of a major mission or someone who had done harm to you by extorting money or some other negative action.

There is no chronological order in what is shown to me, but in the end it all makes perfect sense. Rarely, do we see the ending of your life unless it is significant in the understanding of that lifetime. I ask you if there are any questions in regards to this lifetime. If not, then we move on to the next lifetime repeating the same scenario of the world map and then focusing on a single part of the world.

When you have completed these lifetimes, there is an evaluation of how many times you were a male vs. a female. Who was in those past lifetimes that you know now is important. There is a review of the themes of each one. It becomes obvious what you learned or did not learn in those lifetimes. There is a grouping theme that becomes evident. That theme can assist you in helping to answer your questions. For example, you might have:

A fear of a particular animal, flying, water, heights, etc.
Immediate dislike or attraction for someone.
Interest and knowledge in an unusual technology.
Strong attraction or aversion to the military.
Unexplained problems that keep repeating.
Addictions.

From these interpretations, you gather strength and information on what is happening now, especially with your family and friends. That's the value of knowing the past. Life has a way of gifting us when we least expect it. You cannot change the past; however, with the information of your past, you definitely can change how you participate in your life today. Remember, today is the tomorrow you created yesterday!

About the Author

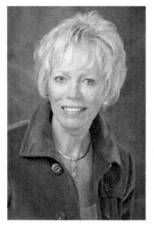

Doreen Lavender Ping has used her spiritual gifts to guide others to unveil the mysteries that are within them for over 30 years. She knows that with spiritual guidance, you can gain the resources to create your reality and realize your higher spiritual self.

Doreen states that "Guidance is a gift. Acceptance is our responsibility, and often reminds us, "That today is the tomorrow you created yesterday."

Doreen is a published author of Stretching Beyond Life's Boundaries and producer of multiple education and meditation CD's.

Currently she is presenting a four part series of seminar Events entitled "Circle of Light – Discovering the Knowings," channeling specific guidance for each participant. Her intention is to share the secrets that Ancient Masters have always known for further ascension with global impact.

Doreen Lavender Ping can be contacted at:
www.lavender4you.com.
(702) 260-4261

The Path of the Wise One

Precious Bautista

"How do I become more spiritual?" There are an infinite number of paths you may choose as you embark on the most mysterious and honored of journeys – that of the spiritual quest.

Whatever path you choose, this journey of spiritual and self-exploration, that is seeking to understand the whole by seeking to understand what lies within, can and should be enormously fulfilling. The rewards of knowledge, connection, healing, expanded world and spiritual perspectives, multi-dimensional philosophies, and much more, are bountiful for the journeyer.

For many, this bounty is more than sufficient. After incorporating select lessons learned into their lives, they can quietly go about their normal day-to-day existence although with increased awareness and joyfulness. Some may become authors or healing, metaphysical, or spiritual practitioner-teachers, or both. Others may decide that this way is not in alignment with their life journey and step off that path altogether. There is much merit to all those mentioned and each is honorable in its own right. However, for a very few, the gentle, but unstoppable, call will come - urging them beyond mere self-exploration onto what I refer to as the *Path of the Wise Ones*.

Hallmarks of the Path of the Wise Ones

The Path of the Wise Ones begs two questions… "What is a Wise One?" and "What is the Path of the Wise Ones?" The definition of the Path of the Wise Ones naturally resolves the first question. The major hallmarks of this sacred path are as ancient as humankind itself.

The Path of the Wise Ones is a path of Truth. One cannot realize wisdom without first having found the Truths within oneself. Every Wise One undergoes a transition period in which inner work is required to become conscious of all that resides within. Some Truths are readily apparent while others are pleasing, but as you may expect, some Truths are still harder to identify, acknowledge and accept. Every person has aspects that operate in darkness or shadows. Only when the Wise One has completed this inner work, which includes "shadow work," accepted his or her Truths, pierced the veil of illusion residing within, and sought to transmute that which must be changed can they progress forward on their path. This process, which unguided, can be long and painful, even torturous, on multiple levels, creates a deep appreciation for Truth and the liberation it offers all who embrace it. Importantly, this process paves the way for compassion and the finely honed (and rare) skill of discernment for both Truth and illusion in others, and the world in general.

While other paths require the acknowledgement of our Truths, the Path of the Wise Ones differs in that Wise Ones accept that this process is a continuous one. A true Wise One accepts that he or she is constantly transforming in accordance with natural laws and, therefore, must acknowledge that inner Truths and aspects are doing the same. It follows logically that the inner work of knowing one's Truth is one that is life-long, continuous, and necessary to continue, walking the path which by its very nature is based on Wisdoms, which are fundamentally rooted in Truth.

Importantly, Wise Ones value and seek Divine Truths. The Wise One understands the delineation between relative truths, which can vary depending on the person, and Divine Truths which are Truths that remain constant throughout time and across all peoples, perspectives, and cultures. It is these Divine Truths that serve as guide posts to all on the spiritual journey. Knowledge of these Divine Truths allows us to transform our lives and the world on the deepest levels.

Many Wise Ones are born with foreknowledge of many Divine Truths that the world at large seems to struggle to grasp. Thus, the young or emerging Wise One often struggles with frustration over the inability to make him or herself understood by others, and feeling out of step with society. Merciless teasing, cruelty, and even physical harm has been experienced by many Wise Ones in their youth as a direct consequence of expressing what they took for granted everyone else knew. For this reason, without the guidance of a conscious parent or an experienced

Wise One, it is common for the young Wise One to submerge these beautiful aspects of their being in order to "fit in" and to learn to fear or despise them. Thankfully, life situations or teacher-guides inevitably present themselves to assist the Wise One in developing the necessary patience, courage, communication skills, recognition, and appreciation for the unique gifts he or she possesses to effectively share this wisdom with others.

Divine Truths serve as guide posts along our spiritual journeys and assist us in realizing deep transformation. Ultimately, *Divine Truths are the basis for true Wisdom and bring us in closer relationship with Divinity itself.* For this reason, one of the most important roles of a Wise One is to continuously seek Divine Truths and Wisdoms and to share them with humanity.

The Path of the Wise Ones is a path of Teaching. Wise Ones are compelled to share their wisdoms and knowledge, whether in the form of seminars or workshops, authoring books and articles, blogs, fine arts, music, one-on-one mentoring, hosting radio shows, informally teaching friends and family, or any combination of the above, Wise Ones inevitably find themselves in the position of being teachers, advisors, counselors, guides, and facilitators. Teaching comes as naturally to them as breathing and, in their inner work, most Wise Ones realize that they have been teaching, even if informally, from a very young age. They also recognize that throughout their lives, they have displayed a talent and adeptness for one or more forms of communication that, in the context of their work as Wise Ones, provides a perfect vehicle for them to share their wisdoms and knowledge with the world.

Wise Ones are *sharers*. They have an innate understanding that wisdom and knowledge are worth nothing if they are not exemplified through actions, thoughts, words, and shared with all those who wish to learn. One of the most unique traits of a Wise One teacher is that they tend to *dispense and share freely* of their wisdoms and knowledge. While many others tend to dispense information in a miserly fashion if no monies are involved, Wise Ones are sharing all the time and in any way possible. This is not to say that they don't charge for their formal offerings and services, but they usually find ways to provide information to everyone in a very accessible way. Some work by donation, which allows everyone, regardless of economic situation, to access their services, while others may charge for workshops, or write a corresponding book sharing the same knowledge at a much reduced price. Whatever the case might be, Wise Ones don't turn it on and off, so to speak. They have a strong belief in their purpose and that the wisdoms they carry is of great importance to humankind. In turn, this makes them truly effective and passionate sharers and teachers, who will ensure that their messages are made available to all.

The Path of the Wise Ones is a path of Healing. It is rare to find a Wise One who is not a healer. One of the tenets of the Path of the Wise Ones is to help alleviate or to ease the suffering, especially unnecessary suffering, that is so prevalent in our world. Thus, Wise Ones are healers of not only the body, but are healers on emotional, mental, and spiritual levels.

As with the teacher role, Wise Ones may use any number or combination of mainstream and alternative healing modalities to affect healing in those they serve. While many engage in formal studies to learn a healing modality, it seems that the majority of Wise Ones are natural healers who from a very early age, without formal training, displayed an inexplicable ability to heal illnesses and alleviate pain. As they age, Wise Ones realize that this is not deemed normal by the world, and healing others often becomes one of their abilities that is suppressed. Fortunately, when they consciously begin to heal again "on purpose," their healing abilities blossom and seem to increase exponentially.

One interesting hallmark of the Wise One healer is the ability to use words and voice to heal on the emotional, spiritual, and mental levels. The voice of the Wise One is usually distinctive and quite mesmerizing. People report feeling lulled to a place of serenity and feel distinctive shifts in energy during verbal sessions with a Wise One.

Wise Ones are strong empaths. I believe it is this empathic ability to acutely feel the suffering of others that make Wise Ones such powerful and compassionate healers. For this reason alone, it is impossible for a Wise One to deny those who are suffering, or in need of healing, or requesting help. It is not uncommon to find Wise Ones proactively working or volunteering in hospitals or healing centers so as to be readily available to any and all who seek healing.

The Path of the Wise Ones is a path of Remembering. One of my favorite admonishments and refrains is, "Remember, Remember, Remember!" Each Remember signifies three *remembrances* that serve all Wise Ones walking the path.

Remember Your Infinite Nature! This first entails remembering and connecting with the Divinity that is within and surrounding us. It involves remembering the Beingness from which we originate and to which we return when we transition from this plane of existence. This is not only a cerebral remembering; Wise Ones must remember on all levels – physical, spiritual, mental, and emotional. The totality of their being must resonate with this knowledge. When this remembering is accomplished, the Wise One's energy matrix is powerfully transformed and what happens thereafter cannot be described in any way that does it justice. Without this transformation, one cannot proceed further on the Path of the Wise Ones.

Remember All That You Know! Wise Ones have either completed or reached near completion of their required cycles on this plane of existence and have returned lovingly and voluntarily to assist the collective during this particular phase of evolution. However, in order to assist, there is often a need for additional resources above what is taught or available through traditional means. For this reason, the second *remembering* is a remembering and re-integrating of wisdom - skills, abilities, talents, and other specialized knowledge - from current and past lifetimes. These remembrances may take the form of long forgotten healing ways, talents that can only be described as extrasensory and defying the laws of science, such as the ability to read others' energy patterns without the use of technology, and the list goes on. This recall of past lifetimes is not intended to be an egotistic exercise in frivolity or vanity, but rather an intensely purposeful recalling and integration of only the gifts, talents, abilities, and skills that best serve all beings inhabiting our planet, and indeed, Gaia (personification of earth) herself.

It seems Wise Ones are able to access wisdom of past lives naturally and quite unconsciously. Upon sharing this wisdom with others, they are frequently asked how they acquired such knowledge. They are often at a loss to explain. They just *know* – they are not sure how, but are so sure of the truth of their statements that, if they were the gambling sort, they would place money on it. This same scenario at an early age can create awkward or painful social situations that are alienating to the point that the young Wise Ones cease offering their wisdoms. However, over time, Wise Ones begin to notice how their seemingly unfounded wisdoms, or *knowingness*, seem to stand true each time, and their confidence increases. This stage of growing confidence paves the way to the acceptance of wisdom nature and is pivotal in the full emergence of the Wise One within. Fully emerged Wise Ones understand that their wisdoms flows from present and past lives, as well as from deep connection to the Divine. The questioning and doubt fall away and in their place resides only a desire to use their wisdoms to serve the highest good of all.

As the connection with past lives deepens, Wise Ones develop a strong affinity with the old ways. There is an intense attraction for ritual, ceremony, and shamanic practices, especially those of native and past peoples, perhaps for the reason that they themselves have conducted and participated in such events in past lives. While they may use technology as a means to an end in terms of gaining and dispersing wisdoms, there is a longing in them to live simply and in a balanced manner, in connection with nature and all its beings. They regard much of modern society's must-haves as somewhat perplexing, and are unmotivated by the common drivers of wealth, fame, power, and the accumulation of material possessions. Without these drivers, Wise Ones experience difficulty working in mainstream careers that offer no higher purpose or little in terms of inner fulfillment. Inevitably, Wise Ones end up creating roles that are extremely unique and allow them to fulfill their life purpose(s).

Remember All Are Equal on this Infinite Path! The third *remembering* is very simple. No matter how powerful the abilities, no matter how much knowledge is carried, and no matter how far along on the spiritual path, Wise Ones must always remain humble knowing there is always more to learn, always room to expand and grow, and since the path stretches ahead infinitely without end, there is no need for competition or haste. Wise Ones view all with compassion, especially toward those who are in the earlier stages of their spiritual journeys. It is a common pitfall for journeyers to forget the challenges and fears they faced, or perhaps certain behaviors they displayed in earlier stages of their own journeys. If this occurs, it becomes very easy to view those who are at these earlier points on the path in a judging or patronizing manner. Wise Ones see no one ahead or behind them on the path. All path walkers are exactly where they are intended to be on the path, all are equal, and, if anyone needs assistance, the Wise Ones offer all the love, support, compassion, and wisdom at their disposal. They bear this responsibility with joy, grace, and dignity. Any other way is inconceivable to the Wise One.

<u>The Path of the Wise Ones Honors Gaia</u>. The Wise Ones have a profound appreciation and connection with Gaia. Rather than viewing nature and its resources as separate entities to be plundered and used for their own means, Wise Ones intuitively understand that we were always intended to live in harmony with Gaia and all beings she sustains. Thus, Wise Ones seek to honor her in all ways. How this honoring is expressed can vary, such as offering gratitude and blessings through ceremonies and rituals, eating and living consciously in day-to-day lives, acting as stewards and guardians for specific aspects of nature and animal friends, raising awareness of issues and concerns that impact our ecosystems, etc.

While Wise Ones may differ in how they honor Gaia, they all share in the need to personally connect with nature on a frequent basis. It is rare to find a Wise One who does not regularly engage in some sort of nature-based activity like walking, hiking, climbing, gardening, or kayaking or canoeing. This time spent communing with nature invigorates and uplifts all, but for the Wise Ones, this time with nature seems to be mandatory. Wise Ones who do not spend a significant amount of time outdoors often are quite depleted in energy and vitality. Once they begin reconnecting with Gaia, the transformations in terms of vitality, energy, and demeanor can only be described as amazing. It seems Gaia and Wise Ones have an ancient bond and symbiotic relationship in which both benefit tremendously when in connection with one another.

Wise Ones frequently integrate Earth-based modalities, such as herbs, crystals, aromatherapy, and dowsing into their healing work and general practice. They are especially drawn to shamanism and display an innate ability to not only easily grasp complex shamanic rituals and concepts, but to also affect powerful healing, communications, and transformation for themselves and on behalf of others. Many Wise Ones have an incredible aptitude for these ancient practices because they are consciously or unconsciously drawing upon past lives' wisdom and experiences.

The Path of the Wise Ones is the path of Love, Honor, Compassion, Humility and Courage. These qualities are the most important hallmarks of one who walks this path. Love, honor, compassion, humility and courage infuse all Wise Ones' actions, words, and thoughts. Wise Ones begin _everything_ from these energies for the purpose of ending with a multiplying of these energies. While it may be easy for most people to overlook Wise Ones, as they tend to shy away from self-promotion and pretensions and to reflect this in their simple speech, dress, and mannerisms, those who spend even a small amount of time in their company can sense these very energies emanating from Wise Ones. It is rare for these interactions to end without the other person(s) feeling a renewed sense of vitality, serenity, and joy... and a sometimes discomfiting sense that something unexplainable just occurred.

Walking the Path of the Wise Ones

If what you have read of the Path of the Wise Ones resonates with you and there is a feeling of "Yes!" then, I encourage you to delve deeper and explore this path as an option along your journey of self-discovery.

Although only a few may hear the call to walk the Path of the Wise Ones, the truth is that this sacred path is available to all. Each one of us has the potential to emerge as a Wise One. However, one must be _present, conscious, and prepared_ in order to hear this call and know it for what it is... which is why so few hear the call when it occurs.

Presence, consciousness, and preparation are only realized when inner work is undertaken. And this inner work required of you at the onset can be among the hardest things that you will ever have to do. However, if you prevail and complete this work, *it will also be one of the most liberating and transformative experiences of your life.*

As a transformational mentor, I work with all, not just Wise Ones, who are beginning or in the midst of the awakening process. This inner work is powerful and transformative. Importantly, it is only after this inner work is completed that each person is able to fully step into the role(s) of her or his life mission.

So, I urge you to begin this inner work as it will only serve your highest good. My period of inner work was unguided and took many years... years that can accurately be described as, amongst other things, agonizing. I realize now that this was by divine design, as this solitary experience aided me in becoming a better teacher and created a deep compassion for all who have chosen to engage in this courageous work. However, with the help of a guide, this inner work is greatly accelerated and wise guidance will assist with the challenges everyone encounters in this work; and I encourage you to seek the wisdom and guidance of a teacher or mentor.

You may be conflicted in regards to walking this path because you are already engaged in formal work or have already committed to a particular path. The beauty of the Path of the Wise Ones is that it can be overlaid across all traditional and non-traditional roles and paths. There are Wise Ones in every imaginable field and profession – doctors, spiritual leaders, clergy men and women, energy workers, entrepreneurs, convenience store clerks... the list is endless. Unlike other modalities or paths that require you be this or that, the role and Path of the Wise Ones do not require formal designations or titles. Nor does it confine you to one path only. It allows you to be in perfect expression of *you* and will exponentially multiply, not interfere with or detract from your ability to experience full realization of your unique life purpose and mission.

If you choose to walk the Path of the Wise Ones, know that once you have connected to the inner and outer Divine and have full access to the infinite wisdom available to you, you are obliged to have the courage to share this wisdom, knowledge, and teachings with all. Along with the Wise One hallmarks, you do this with grace and dignity, with the purpose of *serving the highest good of all beings.* And ultimately you, the Wise One, will perform this service to all beings by raising consciousness in a world that must awaken, by bringing healing and hope to the many who weep in needless suffering, by recognizing and honoring the Divine in each being you encounter, and uplifting all through the highest energies of love, compassion, and joy.

I hope that this chapter offers some useful insight into one of the many paths leading to the Divine. In terms of how to live the spiritual life, I simply offer you – be Spirit*full*. Do your inner or soul work, know your Truth, connect to inner and outer Divine, be discerning as to what energies you allow into your life, and without any additional effort, you will become rich in Spirit or Spirit*full*. All actions, words, and thoughts that flow from the energy of Spirit will be a natural reflection of its wondrous nature. And, *that* is as spiritual as it gets.

Blessings to you, dear reader, on your journey of self-discovery and awakening.

About the Author

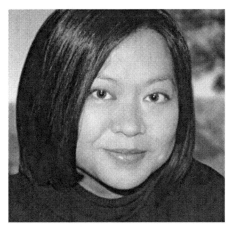

Precious Bautista is a herbalist, transformational mentor, healer, and writer.

She resides with her husband and young son in Henderson, Nevada.

Precious Bautista can be contacted at:
precious@PathOfTheWiseOne.com
(702) 608-5483

Power Animals

Leeza Robertson

When I first set out to write this chapter on power animals, I was unsure how the format of this would work. I didn't want just another power animal guide that gave endless accounts of what the animals mean, as I think both Ted Andrews and Dr. Steven Farmer have already done a wonderful job with animal meanings. I highly recommend that if you chose the path of working with power animals or animal guides that you keep all of their books in your library.

I, however, want to show people how to see past the animal itself and teach them how to engage with the energy of the animal, and to align with its energetic vibration. This is how my power animal soul meditations came to be.

Regardless of whether you are working with animals, angels, faeries or some other guide, you are at a source level, always working with energy. It is the energy that we want to focus on, not the form of the guide. How they are in form is not important. It is how they make you feel, react, interact and process that is. You do not need to get into the theatrics of imitating your animal in order to feel. All you need is to get into the feeling energy of your animal.

Let me give you an example. I have a very strong, female wolf spirit guide. I know when she is most present as she pushes me to be more social and mingle with like-minded people. She wants me to be part of my pack. This is not limited to biological family. It also includes spiritual family or all like-minded people in form and out. When I start to feel myself becoming a little too isolated and withdrawn, as I have a habit of being a hermit, I call on my wolf and allow myself to get into her

254

vibration. This does not mean becoming a wolf or howling at the moon, but harnessing the energy of the wolf to assist me when it comes to being more social and active in my community.

Sometimes, the message, lesson, or skill the animal is giving us is not always in the definition of the animal, but more in its energy. This is why it is so important to be awake, alert, and aware. Do not have preconceived ideas about your animal (s). Allow your relationship with them to unfold and evolve on its own with its own flow and set of communications. Be open to your guides and allow them to assist you, share with you and love you. Acknowledge them when they are around and thank them when they have finished working with you. Treat them the same as any other loved mentor. And in return, you will have the most fulfilled experience you can possibly have in this time space reality.

Random Animal Sightings

I am asked all the time about the significance of random animal sightings. The short answer would be that not all animal sightings have meaning. For instance, if it is common to find blue jays in your garden, seeing them in your garden does not necessarily mean they have a message for you. However, if one were to fly up to your face and hover for a second, then that would warrant some further investigation. This used to happen to me with humming birds.

A few years ago, I took to the craft market road selling my goods. Over the summer, I would set up along with other crafters and sell my crafts. One of the places where I sold my crafts is inundated with humming birds during the summer months, so seeing humming birds was not out of the ordinary. On one particular day, I was starting to become a little discouraged, as it was late in the day and I was yet to make any sales. I was sitting there panicking about the fact that I had failed to even make booth money and would have to write the day off as a loss.

While brooding to myself, a humming bird swooped down over my head and stopped a couple of inches from my face. It just hovered for a few seconds then off it went. This was not ordinary behavior from these birds. This made me pay attention! Hummers are the bird of joy and happiness. They also have the ability to move backwards, forwards and hover, fluid motions between past, present and future. Hummers don't get stuck and don't spend time dwelling on things past or yet to come. In other words, my humming bird was telling me to lighten up!

Still in shock about what had just happened, I was surprised to see that I had a group of eager buyers at my table. I was able to realign myself with my true reason for being there: the joy of offering my wonderful creations. I also ended up making more money than I had planned.

So keep in mind that not all sightings are messages from the spirit realm, but be alert enough to notice when the message comes through loud and clear.

Animals & the Elements

When we are looking at our power animals and wanting a deeper understanding of our animal spirit guides, something to consider is the element of the animal. Some animals are associated with more than one element like the frog, which is connected to both water and earth. And then there are some that start with one element and through metamorphosis change to another element like the butterfly, shifting from earth to air. This is important as it further assists us in understanding not only the animal and its energy, but the lesson or message it has for us humans.

Animals associated with fire tend to show us ambition and enthusiasm. They deal with rebirth and regeneration, creativity, illumination and passion. This is evident with myths and legends surrounding the Phoenix. They also deal with death, destruction, anger, chaos, or out of control energy.

Animals associated with water deal with our emotional side. Water can be used to heal, purify, cleanse and to move blockages, but it can also become stagnant, polluted, blocked, or even dry up all together.

Animals associated with the element of air connect us to our higher self through our thoughts, meditations, dreamtime, and subconscious mind. These animals are the gate keepers to other realms and can act as messengers of divine inspiration. They can also be flighty, scattered, and allow themselves to be dictated to by the direction of the winds.

Animals of the earth not only ground us, but show us the way to our earthly resources. They are our foundation in this physical plane. These animals show a more practical side to our problems or questions. They can also become stuck, still, and unmovable.

So next time an animal comes your way, or your animal guides want to get your attention, pay close attention to which element or elements are associated with them. Their element will connect you to the energy of the animal and how it relates to people, places, and things around you. By understanding your animal's elemental energy, you will be more equipped to align with its vibration and get the answers you're seeking.

Animals we Fear

Like most people, I have a fear of snakes. In fact, I cannot even talk about them without having my feet raised up off the floor, which is more than amusing for my participants when I am teaching classes on power animals. But here is the interesting thing, the animal you fear the most is the one with the most vital life lesson for you. In fact, it will be your most fierce protector and your most active guide. Snake is about fluidity, transformation, shedding outgrown ideas or situations, knowing when it is time to let go, and busting out of the old.

Depending on the particular type of snake, its message does change somewhat; however, my fear is of all snakes, hence the generalization here.

Having grown up in the Australian bush, it was not uncommon for us to have encounters with brown snakes, which are highly poisonous and can grow up to 7-8 feet in length. The summer times in particular, we would all be on high alert as they would on the roads sunning themselves and would even come closer to the farm houses in search of food. As a teenager, I rode my push bike everywhere. It was my form of escape. I could get on my bike and ride for hours in the bush and not come across another person, just the sound of magpies and flocks of local galahs talking nonstop in the trees.

Once in a blue moon, however, I would come upon a brown snake curled up in the middle of the road basking in the sun. I would say, "I am sorry Mr. Snake, I will just stay way over on this side of the road and not bother you"... sounds silly I know, but snakes have always ignored me. They act as if I don't even exist, which is more than fine with me!

I had a similar experience while hiking through forests in upstate New York a couple of years ago where I came across a blue snake coiled up on the moss warming itself from the heat of the forest floor. Again, I said my little line, and around him I went, and again the snake totally ignored my presence.

One thing I have noticed though, when I do come across a snake, be it in the wild or in my animal cards or even on television or something someone has posted on face book (yes animals pop up online all the time), it does mean my life is about to go through some big changes. I truly have outgrown where I am. It is almost like snake says to me, I know you are resisting because you're so comfortable here, but it is time to move on, shake it up and get some new energy flowing. I have yet to figure out if I actually enjoy getting these messages. But like them or not, they always prepare me for what is coming and for that I am thankful.

So look more closely at the animal that terrifies you, as it has some important messages for you. See how and when it has appeared in your life, and what has happened before and after each encounter. Look for the lessons and blessings from this encounter and learn through your animal how to feel fear yet walk through it anyway.

Helpful Definitions
These definitions are ones that I personally have developed in my work with animal energy as a way of not only keeping it simple, but to assist in identifying the message and meaning associated with my animal encounters.

Power Animals
A power animal is an animal that shows up at a certain time to give us a healing, to energize us, or to deliver us a particular message. It may show up in the form of oracle cards or physically in your environment. It will not, however, stay after you have received its gift.

Animal Guides / Totems
An animal guide or totem is an animal that stays with you. It is an animal that you continue to work with and align yourself to. It takes on the role of teacher, master, mentor, companion, partner, protector, and friend.

Animal Archetypes
These are our inner animals. They represent our fears, doubts, triumphs and strengths. They connect us to the locked parts of our psyche. They become symbols for our inner self. These animal archetypes will connect with us during our dreamtime and meditation to assist us in our inner spiritual growth.

Animal Soul Connection Meditation Script

This meditation was designed for you to connect with your animal guide or totem. You may also wish to read the script into a voice recorder and play it back with head phone. Or go to my website and purchase the meditation. Find a comfortable place to sit, get comfortable and begin.

Close your eyes and concentrate on your breathing, in through your nose and out through your mouth, in through your nose and out through your mouth. Focus on extending the exhale as you relax your body. Breathing in through your nose and out through your mouth. Just relax and feel your shoulders drop, feel the base of your spine as it slowly relaxes and settles into your hips. Feel your knee joints, the heels of your feet, your feet and your toes all relaxed now.

Place yourself on a beautiful beach with powdery white sand, feel the sun as it dances across your skin, notice the wind as it rustles your hair as if almost speaking to you as it passes by. Hear the rhythmic motion of the waves as they come in and out, the beautiful turquoise sea. So relax now. Know that in this place there are no worries, no concerns, no one who needs anything from you or your time. In this peace and tranquility you notice a flicker of light to your left hand side, it just catches the corner of your eye and you turn your head to see what it is. As you turn your head to the left, you notice a huge rocky outcrop that you had not noticed before. You get up and walk towards this rock formation as it glistens in the sun. As you get closer, you see that it is not a rock formation at all, but a beautiful amethyst cave.

As you approach the cave, you can see the amethyst growing from the ceiling and the walls, and up from the base of the floor of the cave. On entering the cave, you can feel the amazing vibrating energy of the crystals; you feel it coming up through your feet, through your legs, up through your hips as it travels all the way up your body. A little further into the cave now, you see a clearing in the middle and there in this clearing is a beautiful amethyst bench that looks like it has been carved out of the cave floor. You walk over to this bench and sit down. You feel that the bench is not cold at all but warm and inviting and it almost moves to comfort to the curves of your body.

As you sit there and feel the energy of the crystals, you relax even more. All of this divine energy that surrounds you starts to slowly open the crown chakra at the top of your head. You can feel the tingling around the top of your skull as this chakra begins to open. You feel the energy of the amethyst as it starts to pour in through the top of your head and down connecting to the third eye, down connecting to the throat, down connecting to the heart, down connecting to the solar plexus, down connecting to the sacral, down connecting to the root chakra, and through the root chakra, through the bench and into the floor of the cave, anchoring you into the earth. The energy can now travel through the crown chakra right through to the root chakra and send earth energy back up the root chakra and out the crown.

You sit in silence as this wonderful energy runs through your body, filling you up, making you even more aware, more alert, more sensitive than before. You once again allow yourself to relax just a little deeper and just for a minute allow yourself the feeling of this amethyst energy pumping through your body.

Now that you are both grounded and connected to the divine you are aware of the fact that you are not alone in the cave. You see movement out of the corner of your eye, but cannot make out what it is. Turning now to face the inside of the cave, you notice that there behind one of the crystals formations shooting out from the floor is one of your power animals. You call it to you, and tell it that it is ok and safe at this time to present itself. Thank your animal for coming to you today. As you both stand in this cave, ask your power animal if it has a message for you at this time. If the message is just a word or a sentence or a sound take note of it. Now ask your power animal to shrink down and fit into the palm of your hand and gently hold it.

Feel the energy of your animal, notice its vibration. Ask your animal to forgo its physical form and become an amethyst carving of its self. See it now as a beautiful crystal being full of amethyst energy, sparkling in the light radiating with the energy of the cave. Take this amethyst carving of your power animal and place it to your heart. Allow the animal carving to become one with your chest as it merges into your heart chakra. Feel the animal's energy as it unites with yours. Feel it as it vibrates through your chest cavity uniting its heart beat to your heart beat. Feel your energies merge into one and know that now you are not separate, know that now you can call on the power of this animal at any time. its ability to see, its ability to hear, its ability to camouflage, its ability to hunt, its ability to flee, its rituals and mating habits are now yours to call on at any time you feel you need assistance. Feel your whole body filling up with this combined energy, as you merge into one.

Sit back down on the amethyst bench now, as we will ask the crown chakra to close and go back to its normal size. We shall also ask the root chakra to disconnect from the cave floor and go back to normal size also. Just take a deep breath and relax. Now you will make your way out the cave and back to your spot on the beach.

Once again you feel the sand beneath you, feel the sun on your skin, the breeze in your hair and the sound of the waves. Breathe in through your nose and out through your mouth bringing your focus back to your body. Feel your toes, your feet, your ankles, your calves, your knees, your thighs and your hips as you become more aware of your body. Now, feel your stomach, your chest, your shoulders, your arms your hands, your neck and your head. When you are ready you may open your eyes.

There are many ways in which one can connect with their animal guides. You can find an animal energy master or shaman who sees animal guides and have them tell you the energy that surrounds you. You can do an animal vision quest again with a shaman or animal energy master and have them guide you through the underground to bring the energy into your being. You can pay attention to the animals that present themselves to you on a daily basis, be it in magazines, television, and internet. But ultimately the best way I have found to connect people to their animal guides is through guided meditation. This allows you the power to make your own journey and make your own connection. Although it is fine to have some one assist you, there is nothing like walking the path yourself, for at the end of the day it is your path and your journey. In this chapter you have just completed reading a meditation script that is one of many I use to connect people with their awaiting animal energies. Use it as often as you need, as not everyone makes this connection the first time. It is, however, worth the wait and worth the work. Your life will forever change because of your connection to your animal guides.

About the Author

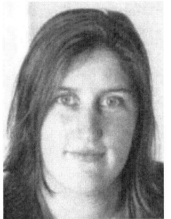

Leeza Robertson is gifted and has helped hundreds of people to make enormous positive changes in their lives as a result of working with her. She is well known as an internationally respected holistic teacher. With her considerable knowledge and training as a Reiki Master, ordained Spiritual Minister, Certified Holistic Stress Management Coach, Intuitive Healer and Meditation Teacher, she is able to choose the exact combination of skills and techniques to maximize each client's experience.

As a master teacher, Leeza also provides various tools for her clients and students to connect with their non-physical guides. Leeza says "We all have guides and they come in many forms with various energies." One of her favorite energies to work with is animal guides. She enjoys teaching her clients and students to connect, align and form spiritual and energetic relationships with their animal guides and pets. Leeza is also a Conscious Trance Channel who works alongside Archangel Uriel.

Leeza Robertson can be contacted at:
www.energyxchange.info

Quantum Biofeedback

Helping the Mind-Body Help Itself

Mary Jo Clark

During these days of ever expanding information dispersed at top speeds, we have available a variety of healing modalities, some of which are fairly new comparatively. Some of the modalities include tapping, meditation, acupuncture, hypnosis, herbal baths, warm stone application, rituals, prayers, and many more. Depending on the person, the malady or the philosophy of the person, when a discomfort strikes, there is always something for you to choose to help the situation and make you feel better.

Energy work in various forms is gaining popularity and effectiveness. Some practitioners do their energy work over bodies with their hands, some use machines and some use computers with straps attached to their client. This chapter discusses the last and the program is called "biofeedback." The straps read the galvanic skin response which is a reflection of your stress to your body and mind. The goal is relaxation because once you are in deep relaxation your body's meridians allow more electrical flow to the physical body, helping it to maintain itself. You know how much better you feel when you can state: "I have great energy today and feel wonderful!" Then, there are times when you have so much to do you begin to feel less energetic or even become ill. That's when you might want to choose biofeedback for energetic support.

What is biofeedback and how can it help me? In lay terms, stress causes most illnesses. In contrast, deep relaxation allows the body to do its job in helping to repair issues – physically, mentally, emotionally and spiritually. A biofeedback program helps with deep relaxation. The program, through the straps, talks to the body and the body tells the program its stress points. Once identified, cellular needs can be addressed. That is, energy can be given to cells at a Quantum level.

What are examples of Quantum energies? They are very tiny vibrations which are abstract senses, such as the sense of expectation or intention, consciousness, or attitude or creativity. Many more energy frequencies causing outcomes can be called Quantum. Results of these Quantum energies can be felt on the four levels mentioned above, causing certain outcomes both positively and negatively. Examples of positive outcomes would be a sense of well-being, energy to face the day, motivation to complete a project, feeling compassion for others, and loving yourself and others. Examples of negative outcomes might be exhaustion, depression, fatigue, hopelessness, boredom and lack of initiative-not wanting to set goals, feeling weak. These "tired" energies can be addressed by biofeedback and by the help of your intentions to help yourself. It might take a while and some changes in your lifestyle and your attitude, but there is help. It is at a depth that you don't normally think about. Energies can be balanced which many of us can't do alone. Thank goodness technology is evolving along with the recognition that we all are personally responsible for our own health and well-being.

Biofeedback (bio=body-feedback=to give back) in this chapter is a huge computer software program and a system using 5 straps that are attached to the client and connected to the computer. Then, through the straps, Quantum energy is fed back promoting relaxation. Many techniques, such as electro-acupuncture and electro-hypnosis, use approximately 80 panels on certain programs and are available to help the body. There are many biofeedback programs of different sizes and abilities. More are being developed as time passes. In my opinion, we are living in a magical age and I am grateful to be studying this in these times.

According to the testing board, biofeedback is a technique grounded in the awareness that matter, time and space are relative and this technique is activated by physical and mental intent. Since the discovery of sub-atomic particles that could be seen only when observed, science has been coming to terms with the fact that matter and thought are influenced by the participants. Philosophers have known for centuries that thought can be controlled and that actions are produced from thought.

The Board also states that Quantum biofeedback is a non-invasive technology based on Quantum Physics. Every thought and feeling is accompanied by electrical activity in the nervous system and can be measured. The more we live these thoughts and feelings, the more electrical activity we generate. The higher the electrical activity, the higher the stress and pain experienced by the person.

The Board continues that Quantum biofeedback helps clients learn to reduce this electrical activity and thus reduce their levels of stress and pain. This is done through a process of relaxing deep within and letting go of the attachments to these thoughts and feelings that are at the root of their stress and pain. Simply stated, quantum biofeedback helps people deeply relax so they can reduce their level of stress and pain.

Deepak Chopra, M.D. states in the preface of his new edition book, "Quantum Healing" his beliefs that "consciousness creates reality...that expectation decisively influences outcomes...and that awareness, attention and intention should be as much a part of health care as drugs, radiation and surgery." He also states "There are heartening signs that Western medicine, after years of resistance, is beginning to accept and incorporate these ideas. In my view, this change is coming about because many people are no longer comfortable with purely materialist interpretation of health and illness. Patients are influencing their physicians to become more familiar with mind-body concepts, and physicians, in turn, are seeing the benefits that these approaches can bring to their patients." And other doctors agree with Deepak Chopra.

According to Carol R. Keppler, M.El chronic pain and disease are the result of cells running out of voltage before repairs are completed. Amazingly, once the voltage is corrected, the system returns to a normal and healthy pH of 7.35. Much more information on nutrition, water, meridians and voltage can be found in the four hundred pages of the book, "Healing is Voltage: The Physiology of Cellular Self-Repair" addressed in layman language by Jerry Tennant, M.D. The point of biofeedback is to help the system by checking voltage and finding ways to return voltage so the body can use it. The paper entitled "In Light Times," has an article in October, 2010 that explains more about this statement.

Years ago, as a teacher of Personal Power, I taught students about learned attitudes causing Feelings which caused certain Actions. The idea is this: Attitudes you learned from home, school and society cause Feelings. Feelings are expressed in Actions. Then, those Actions give more information for a change of Attitudes which change Feelings and new, more mature Actions result. And so you grow. In your life, you can find the times when you reacted from already learned attitudes compared to when you responded after having time to think.

Here's an example: Two students are walking down the hall and each one was bumped by another. The first student turned quickly, ready to hit someone. The other student glanced around wondering if they could help the situation. The question presented was "What made one student react defensively while one reacted proactively? The response was that the learned Attitude in the minds of the students caused the Feelings and the Feelings caused the Actions taken. Therefore, the first student had learned defensiveness as a first response, while the second student learned to investigate before acting.

What does this have to do with biofeedback? Sometimes, we cannot remember the reason for our reactions, positive or negative emotions/energies. Maybe it is subconscious, inherited or even genetic. Whatever the reason, the "hidden" anger frequencies may be sabotaging relationships we have in our daily lives. We still need our own Quantum energies to be balanced for that sense of well-being. This is the time to turn to energy balancing techniques, one of them being biofeedback. It reaches the cellular level and balances the smallest imbalances and even the smallest inner change can result in some of the greatest differences. Have you ever made a bad decision when you were in a bad mood? Have you been either ecstatic or depressed and still made a big decision which didn't turn out as you would have liked? Was the decision different than the one you would have made had you felt a sense of well-being?

We all have made decisions that we wished we hadn't. You need to be energetically balanced on these four levels...physically, mentally, emotionally and spiritually for the best health and self-control to move your life forward. Research shows that stress causes 90% of our illnesses on some level and that it is important to remember that you can get help through biofeedback programs.

Most people find biofeedback techniques relaxing, soothing and beneficial. It can give you the ability to relax quickly; improve your sleep; reduce your stress, tenseness and nervousness; reduce your anger, fear and gloominess; heighten your muscle mobility and flexibility; enhance your mental clarity, memory and attention; and decrease pain and headaches. The biofeedback system helps manage and retrain stress patterns, educates clients on crucial information about stress and empowers them to make lifestyle changes to support overall health and well-being.

The sophisticated wave-form generator also works to re-train harmony to the physical and emotional bodies by addressing aberrant stressful reactions, thus helping the client to create more cohesive and coherent patterns.

So we understand, improvement for the individual will depend on the type of issue, the length of time the issue has been a problem and the willingness of the individual to change his or her lifestyle and thinking. Re-training takes time. However, remember, even a small change in balancing the frequencies and re-training can make a big difference in an outcome. Everything depends on you, the individual, and your ability to self-heal. You are in charge of you. That is your personal power.

Congratulations! You understand how biofeedback can help you!

About the Author

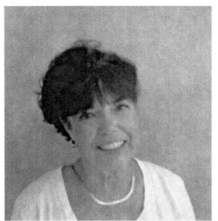

Mary Jo H. Clark, M.S. Sp.Ed, CH at a very young age, discovered there were unseen friends repeating her name and instructing her to help people. Since then, now and again, she hears her name being called and remembers that there still are people to help and things to learn.

Mary Jo, as a teenager, was a babysitter for some challenging children and discovered that it was lots of fun working with them. As time went on, her education became focused on teaching elementary, then K-12 working with the emotionally challenged and mildly learning disabled. She realized that each student was unique in all ways and delved deeper into learning about I.Q.'s, which naturally led to the idea of energy work on all levels, Physically, Mentally, Emotionally and Spiritually. Because she had been told by one of her unseen friends, "You will learn about energy in very different ways," Mary Jo was naturally drawn to the Biofeedback work which she finds intriguing, and helpful to people and animals. Mary Jo is a biofeedback practitioner, and lives in Las Vegas, Nevada.

Mary Jo H. Clark can be contacted at:
buphie@aol.com
(702) 533-0843

268

Reiki

Garry Douglas

Reiki means "Universal Life Energy." The source of this energy, therefore, is the universe itself. As you can imagine, this energy is quite powerful. Its source is endless and its power, limitless! When the trained Reiki practitioner connects with this infinite energy, he or she, as a channel of this Reiki energy, enables this energy to be transmitted directly to you.

Stress and worry have been with humans for millennia, but perhaps no more so than at this time. With the personal concerns we have for family and relationships, work and careers, health and our overall peace of mind, it is no wonder that in today's world we are likely to feel these pressures so deeply and so often. When the mere survival of our homes, communities and nations are threatened, whole new levels of concern seem to grip and threaten our very being.

Reiki helps to alleviate stress. It helps you to step back from the edge of fear and worry, allowing you to see situations far more realistically and with less threat. You can approach these situations with more confidence and focus, and be more in control than you would otherwise have thought possible. Reiki opens you up to the possibilities that already exist, but which you have somehow managed to block from your consciousness. Answers and solutions can be attained more easily because the pathways to them are clearer than they were before the blockages were removed. Simplicity and practicality come to the fore, with actions and results achieved more quickly and appropriately. Your thought process is uncluttered, realistic and positive.

Reiki energy encourages your body's natural healing ability to return it to its healthy state: homeostasis. It helps increase the flow of blood, and the assimilation of your body's oxygen needs. It energizes and revitalizes the lymph system which improves your body's natural ability to remove the toxins and wastes that can clog the blood stream, musculature and vital organs.

Because the essence of Reiki is healing, the results achieved are all for your better good. The situations in which you find yourself – health, relationships, career – may not be part of the plan that was originally planned for you or by you for this lifetime. Time and circumstances have brought you to this place in which you now find yourself. But is this where you really want to be?

We are beings of change who are often nervous or worried about the natural and inevitable changes that are part of our lives. Reiki can help you reach a place where the natural cycles of change and opportunity are welcomed and acted upon with confidence and certainty. Your own physical, emotional, mental and spiritual self, individually and in combination, play such pivotal roles in your life journey that you need to be tuned in continually to the opportunities and choices that are constantly being presented to you. These opportunities can be important and life changing. The process of Reiki can significantly improve your preparedness and awareness of these opportunities when they come your way.

<u>Origins of Reiki</u>

Reiki's beginnings may, in fact, be the rebirth of ancient healing techniques similar to those practiced by earlier Buddhists and Christians. The spirituality and sensitivity of Reiki is a complement to the higher beliefs and ideals of those practices and the followers who embrace them.

Dr. Makao Usui is the founder of the Reiki System of Healing. He was born in Taniai village, in the Yamagata district of Gifu prefecture, near present day Nagoya, Japan. Most likely from a wealthy family, he is thought to have entered a Tendai Buddhist school on or near Mt. Kurama. He also studied a Japanese version of qi-gong. With this ancient practice, based on the development and use of life energy for the purposes of healing and health, Usui found difficult the buildup and eventual depletion of his own life energy during the healing process. He wondered if there could be an alternative method by which the healer's own energy would not be drained.

The young Makao Usui travelled to China and Europe to further his studies, which included medicine, psychology and religion. After his return to Japan, he was employed in an important position at a government health and welfare department. His standings in the community helped him become a successful and prosperous businessman.

When his personal and business life began to fail, he decided to enter a retreat. He returned to the place of his earlier Buddhist training, Mt. Kurama. He enrolled in a twenty-one day training course at the Tendai Buddhist Temple. Usui would probably have followed a routine of meditation, fasting and chanting - traditional in such retreats. Standing under a nearby waterfall, retreat participants would meditate as the waters would flow about the head in an effort to open and activate the crown chakra. Japanese Reiki Masters believe Usui may have followed this waterfall meditation as part of his practice. Whether this is the case or not, it is certain that during his twenty-one day retreat, the Reiki energy entered his crown chakra, greatly increasing his healing abilities, and without draining his own energy.

Following his retreat, Makao Usui practiced his newly found healing abilities on the poor of Kyoto. In 1922, he moved to Tokyo where he formed the Usui Reiki Ryoho Gakkai (Usui Reiki Healing Society). He also opened a clinic where he gave treatments and taught classes. In modern day Reiki, an attunement is essential in the process of passing Reiki from a Master to student, but early on in Reiki's development and teaching, it seems there was no formal attunement process. The mere act of studying alongside Usui and the mutual intention of the teacher to pass the ability on to the student through his presence and example was sufficient for it to take place.

One of the sixteen teachers initiated by Usui was the respected Master, Dr. Chujiro Hayashi. He had a Reiki school and clinic in Tokyo where he recorded his treatments and provided manuals to his students. It was in this clinic that Mrs. Hawayo Takata came in 1935. Hawaiian born Hawayo Takata had returned to Japan for her sister's funeral and to visit her parents. While there she was diagnosed with certain health problems. Rather than undertake an operation, she decided instead to follow a course of treatment with Dr. Hayashi. After four months of continual treatment and with her condition improved and her health restored, she decided she wanted to learn the Reiki process in order to pass on its benefits to others in Hawaii. She studied alongside Dr Hayashi, eventually returning to Hawaii in 1937. Dr. Hayashi soon after went to Hawaii where, in 1938, he initiated Mrs.Takata as a Master.

Mrs.Takata established several clinics in Hawaii, including one in Hilo, on the Big Island. She also taught and gave treatments on the United States mainland, as well as in other countries. At the time of her passing she had initiated twenty-two Masters who continued her methods of teaching. When Mrs. Takata initiated a Master, she charged $10,000. Thankfully, this practice has ended and becoming a Reiki practitioner and teacher is now more affordable. Also changed is the drawn out process of training that prevailed in the early days of Reiki's rediscovery.

Reiki classes are now taught in a more concise and efficient way, but in a way that still passes on the skills and knowledge required. The lineage of Masters can be traced from those currently teaching and practicing, directly back to the founder, Dr. Makao Usui. The energy of this unbroken connection with Reiki's foundation, which has increased immeasurably over time, adds to the effectiveness of the energy that is passed on, whether during a healing treatment or an attunement.

With the increase in the Reiki energy and the variations of life experience practitioners and Masters have brought to that energy, Reiki continues to evolve and develop in a world that itself changes by the second. The founders of Reiki sought to encourage those who would follow them, to develop and enhance the techniques already learned to meet the needs of an ever changing world.

Reiki Classes

As a result of our self-imposed time structures and restraints, the study and training process in the teaching of Reiki has attained a simpler, perhaps more straightforward approach. Extensive study and long internships are no longer believed necessary to pass on the knowledge required to perform Reiki or attain an attunement. As a result, classes and workshops can be completed within a very short time, typically in a day or weekend.

There are three degrees that are taught in Reiki:

Reiki I

Reiki I is all that is actually needed in passing on the ability to self-heal and heal others, and once this level is completed, and the attunement attained, you will be able to apply the techniques taught in the class for the benefit of yourself and others. Undertaking Reiki II and Reiki III/Master builds upon this initial training and expands your options and possibilities greatly.

You will learn the history and basics of Reiki, and the hand positions that facilitate self-healing and the healing of others. You will receive an attunement from the instructor that will open the channels to the Reiki source. Your energy channels will be opened and your chakras cleansed and balanced. You will also benefit from the strong physical healing that will occur as a part of this attunement. You will be on a path of self-discovery and development that will greatly improve every aspect of your life.

Reiki II

This class attunes you to healing treatments with an emphasis on the mental and emotional levels of clients. You learn three symbols that enhance the healing abilities attained in the previous class, adding strength and focus to your treatments. You also learn how to perform long distance treatments. The Reiki II class is perhaps the most powerful of the classes undertaken in that you will have embarked on a process of self-healing that affects your physical, emotional and mental self.

The process begun in Reiki II can help change your life most profoundly. This is a step that is extremely rewarding and enlightening, but should not be undertaken lightly or without expectation. It is as a result of this class that relationships, careers and surroundings can change significantly. The possibilities are limitless for the improvement of your circumstances, and may lead you to find your direction and, ultimately, your life's purpose.

Reiki III – Master

You learn additional symbols and further deepen your understanding and experience as a Reiki practitioner. A spiritual aspect is heightened in this class that further strengthens your experience. Upon completion of this level, you will become a certified Reiki Master and teacher. You will learn how to pass attunements onto others and, as a Master, be qualified to do so.

Attunement

Reiki is not a part of any religious belief. Anyone can learn and practice Reiki. It differs from all other healing modalities in that the ability to heal is attained through an attunement. This attunement is passed on to you by a trained Reiki Master/Teacher. Though some ritual may be included in the process, the actual passing on of the ability to heal is very simple. Typically, the attunement itself takes a few minutes.

During the attunement, the Reiki energy, or Chi (universal life energy) unblocks the recipient's energy channels, clearing them of the many blockages that may have built up over time. The connection to the Source of all energy is opened and that connection, strengthened. It is the energy that breathes life into all living things: humankind and the animal kingdom. It is the vital energy of the trees, the earth beneath our feet, the water, and the air we breathe. It is the energy that first formed, and still enlivens the stars and planets.

Once the attunement is complete, you have the ability to administer Reiki to yourself and others, and this ability stays with you for life: it cannot be lost. The mere action of touch at the commencement of a Reiki healing treatment is all that is necessary for the Reiki to begin flowing through you and into the recipient, and for the healing to begin.
Reiki can be seen as a twofold blessing... you will have this newly attained ability to heal and improve the lives of others, but just as importantly, Reiki will benefit you in so many ways.

Once a Reiki attunement has been received, the "little things" take on a whole new dimension. Instincts are heightened and are observed more easily. You may start to notice certain little incidents or anecdotes that you would probably have dismissed or ignored previously. These happenings may be opportunities or chances worthy of further consideration.

Reiki and the Laying on of Hands

The natural instinct to heal and bring comfort is as old as life itself. When you bump your elbow or suffer the excruciating pain of an ear ache or toothache, your natural instinct is to ease the hurt with a warm hand, lightly pressed, to bring some comfort to the pain.

The laying on of hands is an automatic reaction we have all experienced. It is a natural act that is often shared between individuals to bring comfort and relief. Whether it is a crying child, a distraught friend or family member, or a sick or injured animal, you want to help end their pain and suffering. Your energy has a natural way of blending and soothing the pain through the positive intention behind the simple act of touch. The healing warmth of your touch can ease the pain of an injury and calm the troubled mind.

The laying on of hands - this natural instinct that we all possess- can be further developed and enhanced. You can find various methods of training undertaken in some church and religious groups, and in many metaphysical disciplines. Classes can vary greatly, depending on the teaching group, and can consist of widely differing courses of study, practice and examinations or tests. When a healing session is to take place, you may find certain methods of preparation are often followed, sometimes requiring specific meditations and rituals.

Reiki treatments

If you become a new Reiki practitioner, you may choose to focus on yourself, your family and friends, while others may see this as an opportunity to go out into their larger community and work on a grander scale. Either way, everyone can benefit.

Typically, Reiki treatments are most effectively given on a massage table, although clients may sometimes be seated in a comfortable chair, especially if only a short treatment time is possible, or if the treatment does not require the client to be fully reclined, e.g., neck and shoulder work, or basic stress treatments. A full body treatment is usually an hour to an hour and one half. Sessions of a lesser duration can also be beneficial if the treatment is specific or the client's schedule does not permit more time.

Chakra cleansing and balancing is also possible with Reiki. If you wish to develop your psychic and mediumship abilities, Reiki can help clear those channels and assist you in that development. Reiki clients who are in search of answers to specific questions or concerns can also benefit from a focused Reiki session.

Reiki helps relieve stress, tension and strain. It empowers and enhances the healing process and can aid in the relief and healing of many illnesses and diseases including arthritis, diabetes, high blood pressure, cancers and tumors, kidney stones, fibroids, insomnia, headaches and migraines, flu and colds, wounds and skin ailments, broken bones, digestive disorders and cardiovascular disease.

The Reiki Session

The Reiki treatment session starts with a consultation between you and the client. During this interview, you will provide an explanation of the Reiki process and how the session will proceed. You will also discuss any health issues or concerns that the client wishes to address during the treatment or any problem or questions that the client wants addressed and answered.

The client will then lie on a massage table, fully clothed, except for his or her shoes. You, the Reiki practitioner, then follow a routine of hand positions that will bring energy focus to those specific areas of your client's body. The Reiki energy emitted through the hands is so strong and effective that the hand can either make contact with the client's skin or clothing, or hover just a few inches above the client. When in the proximity of the more intimate areas of your client's body, you will not make contact directly, but continue the treatment at a respectful distance above.

During this full body treatment, the body's circulatory systems are revitalized and strengthened. The client's body will relax and the stress and tension levels will be greatly relieved .You will also focus directly on specific areas of the body that have suffered recent or past injuries where the causes and symptoms associated with chronic pain can also be relieved.

How I came to Reiki.

I came to Reiki in a very roundabout way. Following my education, my earlier working life in Australia saw me in a corporate background of supermarkets, then shipping. Fulfilling my childhood dream I moved to London at the age of twenty-one where, though not my intention when moving there, I became entranced with the dance. Almost immediately, I began my training in ballet, jazz and tap, with a view to an eventual career in theatre. Upon my return to Australia I eventually joined the company of *Irene,* the national touring production, and managed to have a rewarding and satisfying career for several years that included a number of regional tours, and finally, another national tour that took me throughout Australia and New Zealand. I returned to London where I toured England and Wales performing in a production that toured for almost a year and included a memorable summer production in Eastbourne.

There followed an unexpected move to Los Angeles, New York, back to Los Angeles and, eventually, Las Vegas. The years in Las Vegas that followed brought more employment and personal changes when, in 2002, my long-time friend and mentor, the late Australian medium, Margaret Dent, moved to Las Vegas. I took on the role of personal manager to Margaret and her business partner. Over the course of the following year I produced Margaret's psychic presentations in the Madrid Theatre at Sunset Casino, as well as her many seminars and workshops.

Having known Margaret for almost thirty years, I had myself studied under her and participated in many workshops and classes. Margaret had encouraged me to develop my own abilities to heal as she recognized this as a calling that I could develop. On occasion, she would refer her clients to me for a specific healing concern. Positive results seemed to follow my short sessions with people, although I was very unclear as to what I was doing, or how I was affecting the healing. Because of this uncertainty and my lack of understanding, I was most hesitant in developing this seemingly natural ability. I backed away from continuing any further efforts; I felt I needed some kind of formal training that would show me what I was doing on a more tangible level before I could feel comfortable in offering such a service.

My desire to heal eventually saw me enrolled at the Cayce/Reilly School of Massotherapy in Virginia Beach, Virginia. A division of Edgar Cayce's Association for Research and Enlightenment, the school's curriculum and methods are strongly based on the Edgar Cayce readings and research. As well as the extensive massage therapy course at the school, they offered additional classes in Reiki, reflexology, cranio-sacral therapy and other healing and energy modalities. I was drawn immediately to the Reiki classes. Through Reiki, I felt I could develop the healing abilities I had long wanted to make available to those in need of healing. I undertook training in the three Reiki levels and became a Usui Reiki Master. Upon graduation from the massage therapy course I returned to Las Vegas, Nevada.

Further Reiki study

I undertook further training in Reiki at the International Center for Reiki Training (ICRT) in Maui, Hawaii, under the tutelage of William Lee Rand. I completed all levels of Reiki, including the Advanced/Master training, becoming a Usui/Tibetan Reiki Master.
I subsequently flew to England where I trained once again with Mr. Rand to become a Karuna Reiki®_Master at Glastonbury. A memorable attunement within the stone circle at Stonehenge highlighted an incredible journey that has brought me to where I am today.

Following my certification in massage with the National Certification Board for Therapeutic Massage and Bodywork, and after obtaining the state and local licenses, I set up practice in Southern Nevada, where I continue to offer my services in massage, reflexology and, with a major focus, Reiki. As well as offering Reiki healing treatments, I teach all levels of Reiki and Karuna Reiki®. I also teach a course in reflexology.

Karuna Reiki ® and Rhythmyo Reiki®

Variations in methods of Reiki healing have evolved and developed over time, some with remarkable results. As well as the original Usui style of training and development, methods drawing on Tibetan and Buddhist foundations have found acceptance. Another development, Karuna Reiki ®reaches into the recipient's deeper cellular structure and addresses issues on a karmic level.

The observations and insights I have experienced through my own Reiki, massage, reflexology and other training and practice, have added a dimension whereby my own Reiki work has been further developed and enhanced. This development, Rhythmyo Reiki®, heals at a deep and extremely sensitive physical level. Troubling experiences and traumas can find a permanent foothold in the recipient's muscular memory, and are often the cause of chronic symptoms and maladies. I have found that this form of Reiki energy heals at a deeper level. Rhythmyo Reiki® also enables me to tune into the body's extremely sensitive natural rhythms in order to return calmness and balance to the body.

<u>Reiki complements other Alternative Therapies and Traditional Healthcare.</u>

Reiki also adds to the effectiveness of other alternative therapies such as reflexology, massage and nutritional therapy.

For those receiving traditional medical or psychological healthcare, Reiki can improve the results of any treatment and reduce the side-effects of chemotherapy, surgery and other invasive procedures. It shortens healing time, reduces or eliminates pain, relieves post-operative stress and helps create optimism. It has regularly been shown that patients receiving Reiki leave the hospital earlier than those who don't. There are many controlled studies now that support the effectiveness of Reiki treatments. However, patients should continue to consult with their doctors, physicians and other medical professionals.

<u>The Possibilities</u>

The twenty-first century has seen humankind bring upon itself untold benefits and concerns. Families and communities alike are faced with options that a short time ago would have seemed quite unimaginable. It is little wonder that stress and worry seem to be at an all-time high, in individuals and nations.

Reiki heals and calms. It helps you to live a more relaxed and focused life. It can help relieve pain and illness, as well as remove or lessen the negative symptoms and effects of stress. Imagine living the life you were truly meant to live and enjoy!

Reiki attunements bring balance and harmony to the body's natural cycles. It revitalizes and energizes the circulatory systems of the body: cardiovascular, nervous and lymph. This results in better flood flow and oxygen assimilation, stronger more efficient muscular coordination and reaction, and an increase in removal of body's toxins and waste.

A healthier body, a rosier outlook, increased energy and a more productive and joyous life can be expected when Reiki becomes a constant part of your life.

About the Author

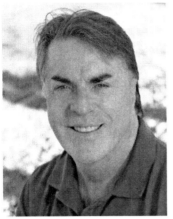

Garry L. Douglas has travelled the world to become knowledgeable about Reiki, training at several locations to earn even more credentials. Garry has set up his own successful practice in Southern Nevada, where he continues to offer his services in massage, reflexology and, with a major focus, Reiki. As well as offering Reiki healing treatments, he teaches all levels of Reiki and Karuna Reiki®.

Garry often visits his family in Australia, but resides in Las Vegas, Nevada.

Garry L. Douglas can be contacted at:
www.garryldouglas.com
www.bodydominion.com
garryldouglas@hotmail.com
(702) 812-6304

Seasons

In each and every one of us
There lives a magic place ~
A secret meant to share with all
To wear upon our face.

The reason I know of what I write,
I'll tell you since you ask ~
It's in my soul, a part of me
I brought it from the past.

It's flutes and bagpipes-Shamrocks too ~
The forty shades of green
Awakening to the Seagull's cry
An evening by the sea.

My wings they glimmer as they lift
To depart from a time now gone~
Soaring on a virgin path
To live with purpose and song.

~Barbara Botch, 2011

About the Author

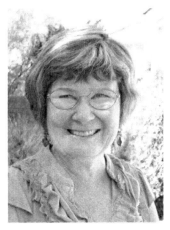

Barbara Botch is a poet and the author of Poet's Crossing. Her strong Irish roots and love for the Emerald Isle inspire much of her writing. She retired after 30 years in the nursing profession, but her compassion for people did not.

Coupled with her love for the written word, she developed a workshop called Healing Through Poetry and is working on a book by the same title. Barbara reads her poetry and holds workshops at the Ganesha Center in Las Vegas, NV.

Barbara Botch can be contacted at:
www.emeraldjourneys.blogspot.com.
barbbotch@gmail.com
(702) 806-0809.

Sound Therapy

Choosing to Heal: A Courageous Journey

Regina Murphy

No one can take this journey for you. It is a journey each of us must choose for ourselves, and when it is your time, you will know. Studies show that being an active participant in your own healing, even if you just start to exercise, increases the results exponentially. Beginning with a minimum investment of time, and just testing the waters of your own power can be interesting at the very least and miraculous if you are truly ready. Becoming aware of your thoughts and being willing to forgive yourself and others are the only real commitments. The rest is simply a commitment to a process that can take less than eight seconds each time you catch yourself having a thought or feeling that feels bad.

This process is called "Energy Psychology," "Thought Field Therapy," "Emotional Freedom Techniques," "Emotional Self-Management," "Power Tapping," "Be Set Free Fast," and the list of titles goes on and on. It all began with Dr. Roger Callahan over thirty years ago when, after taking a class in Acupressure, he tested it on a patient named Mary. Dr. Callahan had been treating her severe phobia of water for eighteen months with no progress. He asked her to tap under her eye (a point on the stomach meridian) while near his pool. Within seconds her phobia was gone. This was the birth of this entire field that has grown into the most effective treatment for PTSD for our troops. It is so simple that children as young as three can do this. Children are much more willing to do this because they are happy to give up the bad feelings they brought with them. As we become older, we become addicted to feeling sad or blaming someone else for our lot in life. Frustration, disappointment, fear and self-loathing become our constant silent companions without even realizing it. Then, we stuff these emotions deep into our body and eventually become depressed or sick.

When we have suffered enough we start to look for answers. Blood work and brain mapping prove the effectiveness of these techniques, but the real proof is the millions of people that participate in free "LIVE" Tapping Summits on the web several times a year. Free manuals for tapping are some of the most popular on the Internet. Any of these modalities, once Googled or searched in YouTube, will start a free and miraculous journey into emotional and physical health. The energy of negative emotions or thought or feelings that feel bad eventually causes the body to become diseased. The Buddha says "What you resist persists" and the key phrase in many of these techniques is "I accept myself EVEN with this problem".

Again intention, awareness and acceptance of self and others are the foundation of change, but combined with tapping or cueing the body in some way, these techniques become very powerful.

The second piece of the puzzle involves deleting an unwanted belief and replacing it with a new one. A belief is something that your conscious and subconscious mind holds as true. Although it may not be true to anyone else, it is true to you. You are very much like your computer. Unless you delete the old belief or program before you install the new one, you only create confusion and conflict for your computer. You are very much the same. According to Dr. Bruce Lipton Ph.D. respected cell biologist and Hay House author of "Biology of Belief," we "must" delete the old program before installing the new. This is a four minute process and well worth the daily commitment if you are interested in altering the course of your life. At the end of this chapter, I have included the protocols, websites and YouTube's that explain in detail everything I refer to.

Once you have reviewed the Energy Psychology protocols on the websites or YouTube's and decide which protocol to try, make a list or inventory of the things you dislike about yourself. Then, add things you are most frustrated about, fear the most and regret. Hurt feelings are also important to include. Then, make an effort to prioritize the list with absolute honesty. Keep in mind that we "lie" the loudest to ourselves. Being honest with yourself and creating your list is no easy task. Make sure you put effort into this list. When you feel you have really become OK with something on the list by using the tools listed above, cross it off but keep the list. By OK, I mean that the "emotional charge" or bad feeling connected to an issue is gone. This will show you how powerful this technique is and how far you have come.

I suggest that you allocate five minutes a day for raising your vibration. Everything is vibrating at a certain frequency and our vibration changes every time we choose to heal. When this list is complete, you should create a new one. We are never finished and continue to evolve. These techniques actually work best if used when you are deeply experiencing negative emotions in your life. Usually, it takes a long time before you have the discipline to use the techniques when you are upset. This is because we actually like the adrenalin and other chemicals released when we feel justified in having a negative emotion. Most people say that they don't want to tap when they are angry.

These tapping points are based in Traditional Chinese Medicine and are key meridian points that correspond with the energy channels in the body. Although tapping works just fine, the Chinese use needles to stimulate these points. They even do open heart surgery with no anesthesia, just needles. Because I am a sound therapist, I use the OHM tuning fork which carries the actual vibration of the fundamental tone of the earth; a very healing vibration. It is also effective to use laser or led light to stimulate meridian points. Laser and needles can require advanced education or in some cases - certification; however, the OHM tuning fork is harmless. My grandchildren have been treating themselves since they were about five.

Officially, according to Fred Gallo Ph.D., Energy Psychology addresses the relationship of energy systems to emotion, cognition, behavior and health. These systems include electrical activity of the nervous system and heart, meridians, biofields and bio photons. Dr. Deepak Chopra says that EFT offers great healing benefits.

My personal experience with tapping procedures occurred in 2001 just days after 9/11. I was in the World Trade Center on the Friday before the planes hit. Although I was suffering from having my period for a year without any relief, as soon as I walked into the WTC, I began hemorrhaging. Upon my return from New York, I went to the Nevada Clinic and was treated with tapping by Dr. Fuller Royal M.D., Las Vegas' only Homeopathic M.D. My tests showed I was very ill. After my tapping session Dr. Royal said I would be fine. Not only did I not believe him, I thought he was crazy! Of course, the following day when I was no longer bleeding, I began to change my opinion. After about a week, I was so amazed, I took a class in Thought Field Therapy. At the time, I was a volunteer massage therapist for the Dioceses of Las Vegas working at an HIV outreach center. The Saint Therese Center for HIV and AIDS provided me a wide range of subjects to test my new tapping skills and I have been working in this field ever since.

I also used this on my son who had a terrible behavior problem in school. In 7th grade, he had had 67 parent teacher conferences within a six month period when I tried tapping with him. After only one treatment and from that time forward, he always got an A in conduct. For a single mom, this was nothing short of a miracle. Tapping also worked miraculously on his fear of flying. To date, I have treated and taught thousands of people how to tap and continue to use this as a part of my own life.

My personal favorite protocol is "Be Set Free Fast" developed by Dr. Larry Nimms. He is an icon in the field of tapping and is probably the kindest man I have ever met. I use his technique along with healing frequencies in a very inexpensive iPod case daily as part of my daily routine. What is so special about "Be Set Free Fast" is that it begins with a (one time) ten minute conversation with your subconscious mind that Dr. Nimms perfected. I include this in my free workbook and on my YouTube's.

After the so called "program" is installed, using a "Cue" when you notice a bad feeling, pain or emotion, the subconscious automatically deletes the root cause of the discomfort you intended to treat. A "cue" is a simple word or gesture. This technique makes use of the power of the subconscious mind in a way most modalities have not yet tapped into, even in the field of Energy Psychology. You can think of this as having a new "app" from iTunes on your phone only it is installed into your consciousness. It is my highest hope that you too find the desire to heal and have the courage to begin or continue this path. It not only heals you, but everyone you are connected to because of an energetic ripple effect.

The spiritual aspect of yourself is activated automatically when you acknowledge the true power within yourself to heal. If you cannot deny that you have the power to make yourself sick with worry, then the opposite must be true. Clearing away the emotional debris opens the path for a greater connection to your spiritual self. Often, as children, we are taught to stuff our emotions. Nowhere along the way to adulthood are we taught how to process or clear them. Energy Psychology is not the only way, but it is very fast and more effective than anything else we can measure.

Another gigantic stride in the field of Energy Psychology has been the use of sound to stimulate the meridian points instead of the tapping. This can be done with tuning forks placed directly on the meridian points and other devises explained in the section on sound.

Before I introduce the power of sound and how it can be incorporated into your life and Energy Psychology, I have two basic protocols for you to try and become familiar with at the end of the chapter. I strongly suggest you practice these even before you read the balance of the chapter. After you try this on yourself and experience the results, see if someone you love is willing to let you try this with them. To find the YouTube on the Four Minute Reprogram and "Be Set Free Fast" just search those phrases along with my name and they will come up. There are qualified practitioners in every major city with contact information easily found online.

Sound Alters Matter and Changes Consciousness

"In the beginning was the word". And the Lord said,"Let there be light". The act of speaking the "light" created the light.

Jonathan Goldman

Every senior scientist in the first congress to study Quantum Physics in 1938 in Copenhagen was a master musician. Here are some astounding facts about the power of sound:

Sound brought down the Tacoma Narrows Bridge in 1940 due to a vibrational disaster believed to have been caused from the frequencies from the wind. Video of this can be viewed on YouTube.

Sound can grow plants twice the size in half the time with no need for pesticides.

Chanting healed 91 of 98 monks of an unknown disorder within a week after a team of scientists from all over the world could not diagnose or treat the illness. Chanting is considered "self-created intentional sound." Any sound created with LOVE is a healing sound.

In UCLA with an atomic microscope, scientists can hear the frequency of a single yeast cell.

In a Petri dish, the sound from a tuning fork can kill a cancer cell.

Sound is being used to alter severe depression and treat addiction with dramatic results at the NIH.

Recently, research into binaural beats and brain entrainment has resulted in amazing success in the areas of stress relief, pain management and peak performance both mentally and physically. In Germany, doctors prescribe CD's for common ailments and are promptly reimbursed by their insurance carriers; a fact dreaded by the pharmaceutical companies because sound cannot be patented.

NASA has long been researching the uses of sound for civilian, military and space applications. Radar became functional in 1934 using the principles of sound reflection off objects. NASA uses sound generators and vibroacustics delivery systems to keep our astronauts healthy in space. Vibroacoustics is the science of delivering low frequency sound directly into the body by a system that actually touches the body. These vibrations trick the body and end the problem of bone loss in space.

Changing the molecular structure of the water we drink and the liquid in our bodies is how sound can have immediate results on the body's cells. Sound travels five times faster in water than in air, and humans are approximately 70 - 80% water. Even the beloved planet we live on is largely composed of and operates on water. Many sound programs are available free on the internet as well as the information of the effect of each frequency on water and biology. The list of companies that make healing music, tuning forks and vibroacoustic devises are endless and easily accessible to anyone with internet access.

Many of these vibroacustic delivery systems allow a person to recline on a sound bed or sit on a sound chair in which special transducers have been placed which convert the music into sound vibrations in the unit. I personally have never experienced anything that feels so good and is actually good for you. This is medicine at its best!

In 1992, NIH Clinical Center began using vibroacustics. The results are astounding and are available at www.musicandlearning.com. These studies include 750,000 people with positive results for autism, pain, anxiety, chemotherapy symptoms, cerebral palsy and invasive medical procedures on infants. In one study done with autism spectrum disorder, the results were as high as 80%.

Dr. Jeffery Thompson, D.C., B.F.A., the most respected man in the field of research with Vibroacoustics says "The obvious stress reduction benefits of listening to relaxing music have been proven through numerous research projects in hospitals, universities and private clinical practices over the course of many years. Normally, hearing involves sound waves pushing air pulses against the ear drum, moving the mechanical joints of the middle ear bones which amplify these vibrations to the inner ear, which pushes fluids into wave pulses, which move tiny nerve endings, which fire signals through the 8th cranial directly into the Temporal lobe of the brain, which interprets the impulses as "sound."

By delivering these sound frequencies through the body directly, an entirely different system of the body – spinal cord and areas of the brainstem and brain – are brought into play, with the possibility of direct cellular stimulation. Direct stimulation of living cellular tissue using sound frequency vibration has shown marked cellular organelle response with a corresponding measurable increase of cellular metabolism and therefore a possible mobilization of a cellular healing response. Since the human body is over 70% water and since sound travels 5 times more efficiently through water than through air, sound frequency stimulation directly into the body is a highly efficient means for total body stimulation, especially at the cellular level.

Sound frequency pulse waves played directly into the body has a profound effect on the nervous system. The entire posterior 1/3 of the spinal cord consists of nerve tract bundles whose sole purpose is the transmission of vibration sense data to the Brain Stem, Cerebellum,

Pons, Medulla, Hippocampus/Limbic System (emotional processing areas) and various areas of the Cerebral Cortex.

Far-reaching possibilities are inherent in using this type of vibrational technology in the areas of massage, energy work, physical healing, emotional release work, hypnosis, stress reduction, relaxation and meditation."

The vibroacustic delivery systems that have now been developed certainly are able to deliver sound frequencies directly into the body. Each company that manufactures the vibroacustic delivery systems has their own variety of chairs, beds, pads and musical CD programs. Each of the systems can be used with all forms of healing music available; medical music CDs, medication CDs, and an enormous array of free healing programs online. IPods can be used to hold the frequencies if the input setting is on "lossless", and then put into an ipod case with metal speakers for less than $15 creating a personal portable vibroacoustic devise by holding the metal speaker directly on the body.

Working with tuning forks at an average cost of $40 on the meridian system is another way of targeting specific emotional, physical and spiritual illnesses. If you have no interest in learning how to do this yourself, vibroacustic delivery systems are the most effective way to influence your health with sound. Finally, the one thing we all have available at no cost and is the most healing instrument on the planet is the human voice. Each charka becomes a speaker as we sing, tone or OM sacred sounds. Wayne Perry wrote the masterpiece in this field, **Sound Medicine**. We all know the power of kind words delivered with love. This is an undeniable force and costs nothing. You may not be aware of just how powerful your kind words are when you use them to greet one another.

Just as with all variations of healing methods, there must be an intention to receive the healing and a vibrational match of the person receiving the healing for sound therapy to reach its full potential. What makes sound unique in the healing arts is its ability to reach the masses with various delivery systems on every level and within each family's budget. The most economical delivery system is putting your own speakers up against your own bath tub or foot bath using water as the carrier of the sound waves into the body. For about $100 waterproof speakers can be acquired and the healing frequencies in water can be used in crystal bowl footbaths, handbaths or directly in the bathtub. Clearly, sound therapy applications are available to everyone. Using a tuning fork instead of tapping or an ipod case with the four minute reprogram or "Be Set Free Fast" is a magical and easy way to combine two powerful modalities. As Jonathan Goldman, the most respected Sound Therapist in the world said "Sound plus intention equals results."

If you visit www.templeofsacredsound.org you can begin to learn about the toning of sacred sounds in the interactive toning chambers. This website is free.

We are being blessed at this special time on planet earth with tools available for self-healing and self-awareness never before available to us. The time has come to share these blessings with those we love.

The hardest part of the journey is taking the first step. Once you do that, the journey has begun. We all have these tools available to take with us on our "Courageous Journey." *Let the Journey begin*!

"THERE IS NOTHING MORE POWERFUL THAN AN IDEA WHOSE TIME HAS COME"

Victor Hugo

POWERFUL TAPPING TECHNIQUE

While rubbing on the chest spot

(repeat <u>EVERYTHING</u> 3 times)

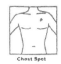

Chest Spot

I deeply and completely accept myself – even with my_____

While Tapping on the Brow Spot

I am healing all the sadness in all the roots and the deepest cause of this problem.

While Tapping Under the Eye

I am healing all the fear in all the roots and the deepest cause of this problem.

While Tapping on the Little Finger Inside of Nail

I am healing all the anger in all the roots and the deepest cause of this problem.

While Tapping on the Brow Spot Again

I have healed all the emotional traumas in all the roots and the deepest cause of this problem.

<u>When you feel the problem is gone, you can do optimizer protocol.</u>

Envision the perfect outcome to the problem you have just worked on and create a positive affirmation. Say the affirmation while Tapping 3 times on each spot: **brow, under nose, under lip, and inside nail of middle finger.**

<u>Repeat until you believe your statement 100%!</u>

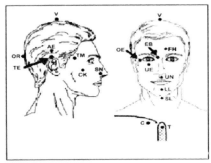
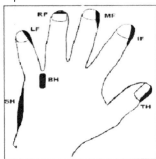

Four Minute Reprogramming

Step by Step Reprogramming Procedure

The picture below depicts the woman performing this reprogramming procedure. Have the person sit on a comfortable chair.

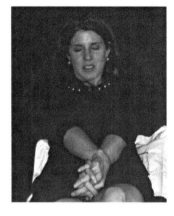

Cross your right ankle over your left ankle.

1. **Put your right hand on your left knee. Put your left hand on your right knee.**

2. **Now clasp the palms of your hands together and intertwine your fingers.**

3. **Create your positive affirmation such as "I am wisdom, truth and grace" or "I am love incarnate" or "I am INFINITE love and gratitude" or "I am feeling a little bit better."**

4. **Begin to feel this as truth in both your physical and emotional body.**

5. **Inhale through your nose a deep breath and as you exhale, whisper your affirmation. Repeat this breathing exercise for two minutes.**

6. **Reverse your ankles and hand positions and repeat the breathing exercise for another two minutes.**

The science behind this is ancient and the power it has to intentionally create your day is astounding. If this is all you do once a day, preferably in the morning, you will gradually change your experience of life. If you do this before you fall asleep, you will expand your consciousness and this will aid you in having a good night's sleep. It is an easy habit to form and your dreams will be much more peaceful. And isn't that what we all want?

Her Recommended websites are:

www.TheSecretsOfSoundTherapy.com

www.erergypsych.org

www.emofree.com

www.nexneuro.com

www.MusicalMedicine.net

www.musicandlearning.org

www.sound-remedies.com

www.neuroacoustics.com

About the Author

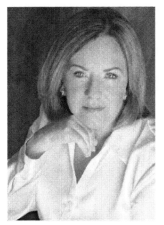

Regina Murphy is a Licensed Massage Therapist since 1996 and an Approved Provider by the NCBTMB of CE hours for Massage Therapists. She is the Founder of "Emotional Sound Techniques" an emotion/meridian based therapy that has the added benefit of Sound Therapy; more specifically, Vibroacoustics. Much of Regina's work includes research into these fields.

She is the President and founder of Excelsis LLC which has partnered with Dr. Susanne Jonas of MusicalMedicine.net and together they created special Musical compositions for health enhancement.

She is an author, guest speaker, teacher and practitioner in the healing arts. Regina is passionate in her belief that self-healing is the greatest responsibility we have to ourselves and others. She teaches the techniques and use of the tools to do this.

Regina is one of the cast members in a movie called "The Keeper of The Keys" along with Jack Canfield and John Gray which features her creation "Project Heartbeat." It presently is scheduled to have the premier *Red Carpet* opening at the Palms Hotel in Las Vegas on December 8, 2011.

Regina Murphy can be contacted at:
www.TheSecretsOfSoundTherapy.com
murphyfour77@hotmail.com
(702) 525-7312

The Tarot

Carole Grissett

"A picture is worth a thousand words" probably says best why we're drawn to the Tarot. We are intrigued by the colors, the images that date back to antiquity and the possibility that these seventy-eight pieces of paper might actually have something to tell us.

There are many worthy books available on the definitions of various Tarot decks, so a detailed description would be much too lengthy for this chapter. Simply, the seventy-eight-card Tarot is actually comprised of three decks: the twenty-two cards of the Major Arcana, the forty-card Minor Arcana; and the sixteen Court cards. The combined Minor and Court cards is actually the ancestor of the familiar fifty-six card deck that we use for entertainment today.

The Tarot can teach you many things. You may consult a reading for specific information, to find direction, to gain a greater understanding of the events, or gain insight to the individuals that make up the daily drama of your life. The Tarot reminds you to pay attention and become more aware of how you choose to direct the course of your life. It can alert you to any upcoming bumps in the road of life, giving you the opportunity to change your actions and arrive at the potential result that is currently indicated. You must always remember that the outcomes of your life dramas are a result of *your* choices and, ultimately, rest in your hands. Forewarned can be forearmed.

How do you find someone to "read" the cards for you? One of the best ways to find a reader is to ask your friends if they have one they like. Or you can take a class and see if you like your teacher. Also, talk to people at your local metaphysical bookstore and ask them about Tarot readers they know and like.

It is a common misconception that all Tarot readers are psychic. Broadly speaking, there are three types of reader. The first is one who strictly interprets the classical meaning of the cards. The second largely ignores the cards and counsels totally from their own psychic input. The third type combines an in-depth knowledge of Tarot (and possibly numerology, astrology, and other modalities) with their intuition. Each of these styles can provide valuable input. The type of reader you select will depend on the style with which you feel most comfortable.

Regardless of your choice, the more your reader knows about you, the more they can help you understand what the cards are indicating and how that fits with your needs and desires. Although discretion and common sense are always advisable, taking a totally skeptical stance and playing the "Impress me by what you can tell me about myself" game is a waste of your money and the reader's time. Also, keep in mind that your own attitude when you approach the cards can make a difference. If you see the reading as a joke or a game, you most likely will receive a shallow reading. If you think deeply about your questions and keep an open mind, a reading of some significance will usually result.

Tarot is a visual medium. However, the best readers understand that no card has any one meaning, but rather is a metaphor for a variety of interpretations. These interpretations will expand as our world changes. For example, The Tower classically means traumatic changes, total upheaval. However, I have seen this card happily represent the "cable guy", a fireman, and an electrical engineer in various relationship readings. The Empress often speaks of pregnancy for those in a relationship, yet many times she has indicated that a business client or their project is "pregnant with promise" and "fertile with prosperity." The Devil generally represents either addictions or a very nasty character, but I have seen him speak to "Better the Devil you know than the Devil you don't know" in business consultations, assuring the client that they would be aware of those people whose agendas did not correlate with their own, and that they would navigate their political landscape successfully.

Why have a Tarot card reading at all? Isn't it scary? There is a not-uncommon fear of looking into the future; however, this should not be so. Forecasting is a much more accepted term than fortune telling or divination, and it is done all the time. Forecasters, after all, are the people who tell us where a hurricane might hit or whether to take our umbrella when we leave the house; what traffic conditions we can expect for our daily commute; predict what stocks will be hot; and suggest what future trends will be in fashion. We look into the future in strategy meetings at work, with guidance counseling at school, and with business planning in corporate offices across the globe. The Tarot may not give us names or dates, but like the weather, investment, and business forecasters, the Tarot alerts us to the patterns in the past that have influenced patterns in the present, and pinpoints patterns which may happen in the future.

Why do the Tarot card readings work? The practice of Tarot comes from the concept that everything is connected, everything has meaning, and that nothing occurs at random. Events or patterns in an area of living correspond to patterns in other areas, explained by the Swiss psychiatrist Carl Jung as "synchronicity." I believe that Tarot cards and other techniques work because there is a great cosmic ordering principle that results in the outer events in our lives mirroring our inner realities.

It is critical to remember that although predictions may speak the truth about your human nature, they only *infer* your future. Any foretelling modality, such as the Tarot, Astrology, the I Ching, Runes, sticks and bones should be used with the understanding that nothing is inscribed in stone. What is *not* shown in a reading is your free will, the human ability to make choices, which gives you the power to write the scripts that you live, to change what you don't like, and to create more of what you do like. *You* determine the course of your life, *not* the Tarot, *not* the reader. The alternative would be to be told by your reader, "The sky will fall in tomorrow, there's nothing you can do about it. Thank you, and have a good day." If that were the case, and if this were the way it worked, there would be no constructive purpose in ever having a reading. Let the Tarot show you what is now, at the moment, so that you can decide whether to exercise your option to change the outcome.

In order to have a Tarot card reading, you don't have to be in the same place as the reader. Many readings today take place over the telephone, online, or even with you merely thinking about the question as the reader deals the cards. It works because we are all connected to the same streams of energy, a consciousness "grid," so to speak. I serve half my clientele by telephone and have found through the years, neither I nor my clients have seen any difference in accuracy between readings in person or readings by other means.

What if you want to know about another person? The Tarot will answer the question through your own energy. Whatever information is revealed will have to do with your own relationship to the person you want to know about. It's *your* energy that influences the cards, and yours that will come through.

There are times when the Tarot seems to have a mind of its own. I have often seen that the cards that are drawn don't seem to apply to the situation the client has asked about. For instance, they ask for advice about love, and get a bunch of cards that relate more to business matters. It's my experience that what they're being told is that they have some other issues that are (or should be) vying for their attention, or are possibly getting in the way of the other things they're asking about. It continues to amaze me that the Tarot always seems to give the information that's *needed* versus necessarily what the client *wants* at that particular moment.

No matter what the reader tells you, it is important to weigh and balance the information you get out of a reading with your own knowledge, experience, and common sense. Tarot card readings can be inaccurate. If a reading turns out to be false, it may be there are external facts or conditions you failed to consider. The other people involved in your situation may have exercised their own free will and, thus, altered the outcome. When predictions don't materialize, it may be that you having been forewarned altered something in your attitude, behavior, or circumstances that, in turn, altered the outcome. In fact, there are times when this was the entire goal of you having a reading in the first place.

The Tarot cards are endlessly interesting and each has multiple levels of meaning. The Major Arcana with its 22 cards, on occasion, represents people or material events, but in general, they are more concerned with psychological or spiritual matters. Almost all the Major Arcana cards show a figure sitting or standing. Only The Fool and The World move. The Major Arcana depict archetypal forces rather than real people. The Fool and The World move, because only they fully embody these principles. The Majors describe your soul's journey from the innocence of The Fool through all the developments and challenges you encounter in this life until, finally, your soul as The World is ready to ascend to the next level on your Spiritual Path.

The Minor Arcana with its 40 cards have to do with material events. All the scenes show something happening, rather like a frame from a video. These cards show aspects of life as you actually live it. In the different combinations these forty-eight cards form when they are spread out, the reader reads the cards you've drawn as a condensed story board of your current situation and you are given insights into potential outcomes as the pictures indicate.

The sixteen Court Cards (kings, queens, knights and pages) represent real people. A heavy weighting of Court Cards in a reading would indicate that your inquiry (and its resolution) has much to do with dealing with friends, relatives, loved ones or business associates rather than specific actions on your part as would be indicated with a larger number of Minor cards.

If your interest is peaked enough to go a step further, the next decision will be what Tarot deck to choose as your own. There are decks to suit every taste. They come in several sizes, most rectangular, a few round. Myths of many societies are represented from Egyptian to Native American to Goddess. Certain images are common to all Tarot decks: male and female; child, adult, aged, for example. The colors and designs have a variety of meanings. There are even blank cards so you can create your own deck. Although each deck is accompanied by what is unofficially called the "Little White Book" of instruction and explains that particular deck's orientation, what you see in a Tarot card is up to you.

If you are beginning your journey into Tarot, I would recommend starting with either one of the Rider-Waite decks or a close clone. These have pictures or scenes on each of the seventy-eight cards which will make it much easier for you to make sense of the reading's message. Other types of decks can be beautiful and interesting, but many have pictures on only the Major Arcana and Court Cards, with simple symbols on the 40 Minors, leaving a novice to struggle with remembering what "the book" said about a certain card.

There are two approaches to learning to read Tarot, the intuitive and the classical. I recommend students begin with the intuitive approach because this frees them up without placing any limits on interpretation. This means ignoring what the "books" say a card means and just "step into" the picture represented. What does the card look like? What are the colors? As you look around the scene from the inside out, how do you feel? Are you happy? Do you feel threatened? What figure or item in the scene catches your attention? How do you think this relates to your question? In considering multiple cards in a reading, how do the people shown look toward one another? Are they facing away from each other? Are figures in several cards all looking in the same direction, possibly toward another card? Which figure are you? Why? Open a dialogue with the other figures, what do they say regarding your question?

The classical approach is one which involves learning the traditional meanings of the card, the astrological assignments of the Major Arcana, the elemental designations of the Minor cards, and astrological and age associations of the Court cards. Although I think your intuition should always be in play with readings, I also believe that a thorough understanding of the classical meanings of the cards, the numbers, the elements, and astrology adds depth and breadth to your reading. The richer the subconscious database of information you have available to access when you do a reading, the more meaningful the message.

It is helpful to recognize if a general pattern is evident with the four Minor elemental suits – Coins (earth/fall), Wands (fire/spring), Cups (water/summer) and Swords (air/winter). Traditionally, the suit of Coins deals mainly with matters of money and material things. Wands are the suit of business, career and creative endeavors. Cups are the suit of the heart. The suit of Swords tells of strife, affliction, or the exercise of intellect. Another key to traditional interpretation is provided by numerology. Each of the root numbers from one to nine appears not only in the Majors, but is repeated four times in the Minor suits.

The question of timing of events indicated is the trickiest element in a reading. Unlike systems like astrology and numerology, the Tarot doesn't lend itself to exact timing. We need to remember that what a reading shows is what is now, at the present time. The future is flexible and open-ended and can be changed in a moment by a change in intent, feelings, or actions by either the client or any one of the supporting cast of characters in the drama in question. One of the most asked questions is "*When* will something happen? *When* will I meet my soul mate? *When* will I be offered the job or get the raise? *When* will I move? *When* will I get married, pregnant, out of debt, buy the house, move, reconcile with my loved one?

There is no one right way to get a potential timeframe. Remembering that each of these methods will yield only a possible answer to the timing question, the more popular approaches include using the seasonal element indicated on a card; using the number shown as being days, weeks or months from the date of the reading; or designing a specific layout to represent a designated period of time. Readers generally develop their own methods to provide dates, but experienced ones preface their answers with an explanation that a timeframe can and often is changed through intent and desire.

The interpretation of reversed cards is somewhat problematic. Tarot readers have not reached consensus about how to interpret reversals and even the various systems vary. Some readers ignore reversals entirely. In my experience, I have found that reversals, generally, represent either the opposite of the card's upright message or a weaker potential of a particular card. This can result in so-called "negative" cards being more "positive," as well as lessening the impact of an originally "positive" card. In any case, reversals should not be taken individually, but only in the context of the overall spread.

Think of the Tarot as a seventy-eight book library of ancient wisdom and intuitive insight, a dear friend, a personal counselor to whom you can turn at any time. The more you study the Tarot, the deeper the meanings you'll unearth, and the more you'll see there is to discover. Although you certainly can read for yourself, I recommend occasionally consulting with other readers to get a different perspective or a sanity check, depending on your emotional involvement in the outcome! We all understand and do it. May your journey into the Tarot be filled with Light, Laughter, and Love!

About the Author

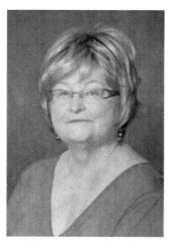

Carole Grissett has utilized numerology, and astrology in an intuitive consulting practice serving an international clientele for over 30 years.

In her corporate business career, Carole served in a Human Resources management capacity with several Fortune 500 companies and holds a BA in Journalism, an MBA, and a MA (abt) in Industrial and Organizational Psychology.

She is an ordained minister in both the American Holistic Church and the Universal Church of the Master. Using her practical, positive approach, she continues business and individual consulting practices, as well as continuing to lecture and write.

Carole Grissett can be contacted at:
www.mypsychicpathfinder.com
polestar@netscape.com
Tarot,

ThetaHealing®

Have faith in yourself –
God was, is, and will be in you forever

Barbara Pasqui

At a young age, I was interested in esoteric theories of all kind. I read about Angels, Spiritual Guides, Tarots, Pendulum, Reiki, energy work, oriental philosophies, and more. One of the most powerful healing techniques I have encountered since then is Thetahealing®.The founder of this technique, Vianna Stibal, says "ThetaHealing is a meditational process that creates physical, psychological, and spiritual healing by focused thought and prayer through the Creator. You must have a pure belief in the Creative Force, in God, in the Creator of All That Is. God, Goddess, Jesus, Buddha, Yahweh, Allah, Shiva are some of the different names for this Creative Force. Anyone who strongly believes in this Source can access and use this incredible healing technique."

Thetahealing is only one branch of the Energy Healing tree. Energy Healing has been used for thousands of years, mostly in the hands of a few and passed on from one healer to the next. Only recently has it become more acknowledged. Thetahealing is a holistic healing technique that directly addresses your subconscious mind, allowing healings and profound life changes, by changing beliefs. Beliefs are strong thoughts, memories and behaviors you accept as true or real, and send as messages to your body. Your mind is like a computer - the conscious mind (approximately 12% of it), sends Programs to the subconscious (approximately 88% of it), in order to perform a task.

With Thetahealing you become aware of negative beliefs and replace them with positive ones. Whether you seek to transform your health, your finances, your relationships or your spirituality, Thetahealing is a surprisingly fast and easy way to make effective changes in your life. There are many positive things that you can learn from Thetahealing that help you grow as a person and recognize that we are all one. You can heal through your thoughts, words and actions.

One of the principals of Thetahealing is recognizing that separation is an illusion. We are all one, and as such, we should love, cooperate with and have compassion for one another. You should not be in competition with anyone knowing that each one of us has an equal connection to Source with the power to bring in information that benefits all of humanity.

A ThetaHealing session can be performed long distance over the phone or in person. The word "Theta" refers to the Theta Brain Wave. This is the brain wave reached when you are daydreaming or in a deep meditative state. As the practitioner, I go into the Theta brain wave state, and command and witness the healing I perform for a client.

At the beginning of a healing session, I ask my clients permission to enter their space. Then I close my eyes, slow my breathing and center my heart. I imagine going down to the very center of Mother Earth to gather some of her energy. I bring this energy up through my feet and legs. I feel this energy opening up all my charkas, coming out of my crown charka in a beautiful ball of light. I imagine going up beyond the Universe, passing many beautiful bright lights until I get to a jelly-like substance that has all the colors of the rainbow. I continue going up heading toward an iridescent white light coming out from a rectangular opening. This is the window to the Seventh plane of existence, to the "Unconditional Love of All That Is." I feel this light passing through me and sense that I am one with this energy. It is from this point that I believe that the "Creator of All that Is" grants me a reading and a healing for my client. I begin by completing a mental body scan on the client. I cannot even begin to describe the joy I experience when I enter another soul's space! Each client is so beautiful inside out especially when seen through the eyes of Creator, through the eyes of love.

Here are the basics for understanding this technique:

The power of words and thoughts
You can find extensive literature about positive thinking and affirmations. Since everything is energy, including words and thoughts, it is important to think positively and to use positive words in your speech. Like the Law of Attraction proclaims, what energy you give out comes back to you, whether it is positive or negative. The universe does not know the difference. For instance, one of the concepts that the subconscious

mind does not understand is the word ' try.' You should never 'try' to do something, you should simply do it. Another example of a negative thought using negative words is "I cannot afford it." By saying that, you are confirming that you will never be able to afford anything or have abundance since you can't afford it. You can find more examples of both positive and negative thoughts and words to use or to avoid in the chapter on Affirmations in this book.

The brain waves
Amplitude and frequency are the primary characteristics of brain waves. Brainwaves may be divided into 5 catego¬ries depending on the fre¬quency:
- Delta waves (0.5-4 Hz) are dominant during coma and deep sleep.
- Theta waves (4-8 Hz) are asso¬cia¬ted with drives, emotions, tran¬ce states, and dream sleep.
- Alpha waves (8-13 Hz) reflect the brain's idle state and are for most people found in the awake condition with closed eyes. Alpha waves are the prime indicators of conscious attention, and they represent the gate between the outer and the inner world and between the conscious and the unconscious.
- Beta wa¬ves (13-30 Hz) indicate an arou¬sed, mentally alert and concen-trated state.
- The fast Gamma frequencies (30-42 Hz) correlate with will, high-energy states and ecstasy.

Thus, both Delta and Theta waves reflect unconscious states, whereas Alpha and Beta waves indicate awake, con¬scious states. Recent research point to Gamma waves as the brain's signature of higher states of conscious¬ness. If a subject relaxes and connects to his or her unconscious, it is been scientifically proven an increase of Alpha and Theta activity.

Alpha is the bridge between Beta and Theta, used by Reiki practitioners. When we imagine going up above our head through our crown charka, our brain is still on an Alpha state on an electroencephalograph. The moment we send our consciousness through the crown with the focused thought of going up to seek "All That Is," the brain automatically shifts to a pure Theta state on the electroencephalograph.

The psychic senses and chakras

The electrical energy of the brain waves is directly connected with the "psychic senses" connected to the Chakras :
- Empathy or Empathic sense (Solar Plexus)
- Clairvoyance or Clairvoyant sense (Third Eye)

- Clairaudience or Clairaudient sense (Ears Chakra)
- Prophecy or Prophetic sense (Crown Chakra)

The importance of learning and knowing the different aspects of your body's seven major energy centers or chakras cannot be overstated. No matter which energy healing technique is practiced, it always relates to the chakras in some way because healing takes place when there is movement of energy. In other words, if healing is required, it is because there is a blockage that needs to be removed to allow the flow of energy. Please refer to the chapter on Chakras in this book for additional information.

Free agency; Co-creation.
The principle of free will has religious, ethical, and scientific implications. In the religious realm, free will implies that an omnipotent divinity does not assert its power over the will and choices of individuals. In ethics, it may hold implications regarding whether individuals can be held morally accountable for their actions. The question of free will has been a central issue since the beginning of philosophical thought. The concept of freedom is very important. Humans have the power to make their own choices. In Thetahealing, we practice that through the gift of co-creation, we can bring the Creator into our reality, heal others and heal ourselves. We believe that as a practitioner, we will unite with the Creator and become witness to readings, healings and manifestations.

The command.
When we perform a healing through Thetahealing, we go up out of our space and connect to the Creator, using in our prayer the word 'command.' Using this word, the mind of a practitioner knows that the statement will be done. The Unconditional Love of the Creator of All that Is is going to do the healing while the practitioner witnesses it.

The power of observation and being the witness.
The act of observation changes our reality. Scientists experimented with the behavior of light in order to prove this theory. When observed, it behaves as particle; in absence of observation it acts like a wave . Based on these experiments, we can come to the conclusion that our mind needs to visualize something in order to accept it as real. It is very important to develop visualization skills when we co-create a healing.

The Creator of All That Is.
As stated at the beginning of this chapter, the founder of this technique says that anyone who believes in God, in the Creator of All that Is, can use this technique. To connect with 'Creator' you should practice a meditation that takes your consciousness to "All that Is" as described previously in this chapter.

Removing negative beliefs is, in my opinion, one of the most useful parts of Thetahealing®. I cannot remember the number of times I have used Thetahealing, but I do remember that it was effective each time! Using a muscle testing technique integrate with kinesiology, you can test yourself for negative beliefs. In an standing position, face north, making sure you are hydrated. Close your eyes and say "yes." Your body should lean forward. Follow the same procedure and say "no," and your body should lean backward. When you have tested yourself for yes or no, then you are ready to test for negative beliefs. For example, you can state out loud "money is the root of all evil!" Your body will tell yes or no, and if it is yes, then you can go into a theta state and command that belief to be removed and replaced with another one. For example, "It is safe to have money." Any negative belief can be removed and replaced with a positive one! Please refer to the chapter on kinesiology in this book for more information on this technique.

I first discovered Thetahealing through a friend of mine who encouraged me to join her for a seminar to become a practitioner of this technique. So on a pleasant evening in October 2008, I found myself headed to Idaho Falls with some close friends. I was curious and excited! I was anticipating the beginning of a remembering process that would lead me to a better understanding of this wonderful experience called life. I believe we all are here to learn by experiencing life, and to heal others and ourselves. Although many tools for healing are available, I searched for years for an effective way to remove the beliefs that were blocking my growth.

The morning after I attended the first of Vianna's classes on Intuitive Anatomy, I received a healing and a reading from one of the students applying this technique. I had recently lost both of my parents and I was unaware of just how afraid and angry I was at the diseases that killed them. The practitioner went in a theta state, and commanded a reading and a healing on me after asking me permission to enter my space. She performed a body scan and then began the reading and healing. In a theta state, she discovered my issue, changed several beliefs that I had and witnessed the healing. I was so ready to receive the healing that is why it so easily and instantly came through the practitioner working with me that day. I also learned right then that the practitioners of Thetahealers® make the command and then just witness the healing process...Creator heals. I realized right away that I had found the very powerful tool and precious technique that would help me to look at and solve my everyday life issues easily and effortlessly. My struggle to find the right modality for me was over!

I started to practice Yoga and became more interested in Reiki, alternative medicine, homeopathy, and Chinese herbal healing. Every day, I found myself experiencing new ways of healing, loving, and living. I gradually improved my relationships with others, and became more open to the wonders of my beautiful journey. I started volunteering at a spiritual center right after its opening and still work there now, teaching and healing others while I learn and heal myself.

I was so amazed by this technique that I arranged to take a course at the Ganesha Center in Las Vegas on both basic and advanced Thetahealing® with a great teacher who deepened me into the Thetahealing® world. She showed me how to keep my ego outside the reading process, how to trust myself, and most of all, how to allow the unconditional love of the Creator of All That Is to do the healing. Now I have the privilege of sharing with others this precious technique while constantly improving my abilities. I was blessed the moment I became aware of the existence of this technique.

I am so amazed at seeing all the improvements in every aspect of my life, and in the life of my loved ones, that I can't stop talking about it! My son is now eleven years old and Thetahealing® helped him to overcome several issues, including my parents' death. He was very close to them as the first and only grandson for nearly seven years. They treated him like their own son, and my son used to tell everybody that he had two moms and two dads. Thetahealing also helped me heal after they died and my son perceives my energy, knowing I am at peace with their departure. We both have accepted their death and have moved on.

Our little dog, Lamby, which we adopted and know almost nothing about, improved his silly behavior after a few sessions and loves both Thetahealing and Reiki. He is communicating with us more and more every day, and even tries to talk to us!

I really appreciate using this technique and I strongly suggest to you to experience it at least once.

Although I prefer to use Thetahealing® for my healings, that does not limit me from channeling precious information during my daily meditations. Recently, my Italian colleague and I together channeled a tool to speed up the manifesting process. It is a plexi-glass pyramid that we designed and had built that I believe helped me to manifest a house, new streams of income, a positive love relationship, and new opportunities. I also created the Seven Day Abundance Meditation where I use a different musical note and color for each of the seven major chakras each day of the week.

Lately, I have begun experimenting with copying and pasting on to myself some characteristics that I appreciate in other people that I know. The results have amazed me!!!
And I know there is more to come.....

Thetahealing Institute of Knowledge is based in Idaho Falls. For more info: www.thetahealing.com

http://www.newbrainnewworld.com/?Brainwaves_and_Brain_Mapping
http://en.wikipedia.org/wiki/Free_will
Vianna Stibal, ThetaHealing .Rolling Thunder Publishing, 2006.pg 40-41
Vianna Stibal, ThetaHealing .Rolling Thunder Publishing, 2006.pg 40-41
Vianna Stibal, ThetaHealing .Rolling Thunder Publishing, 2006. pg.11

About the Author

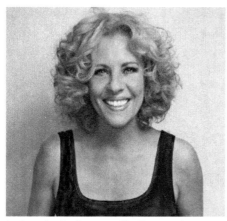

Barbara Pasqui is not only a singer and songwriter native of Milan, Italy, she holds a Masters of Arts in Foreign Languages and an Doctorate in International Law.

Barbara is a born educator with the soul of a songbird. With an accomplished background in many areas, the healer in Barbara has developed fully with an array of modalities to assist with body, mind and soul well-being, including meditation and yoga.

She is a Reiki, ThetaHealing and Intuitive Practitioner. Her natural abilities and connection with Source and Masters guide her intuitively in this process. She works with Young Living Essential Oils and is a practitioner of the Gary Young Raindrop Technique with Essential Oils.

Barbara Pasqui can be contacted at:
papppara@hotmail.com
(702) 994-5356

The Wellness Code

Intentional Code

Sheila Z Sterling

One of the key components of living a spiritual life is the knowledge and wisdom to accept that you are an amazing being…a spiritual being… and an astounding bridge between the spiritual and physical worlds. The fact that you are reading these words verifies that you have already arrived at a place of embracing and welcoming your own evolution.

The key and the "Code" to wellness lay deep within your subconscious intention and your cellular memory. So what exactly does that mean?

Two of our main systems that make up who we are and how we view life are the Conscious and Subconscious systems. Our every thought and action comes from the information we are given from our subconscious and carried out by our conscious system. These systems receive this information from every cell in the body, all 100 trillion of them. From the moment we are born and perhaps before, our cells are recording every moment of life. When we are very young much of what we experience is beyond the scope of what and how we process this information. We are not yet able to understand the information and so our self-preserving subconscious system stores the information for a later date. Yes, this is your cellular memory at work. Your view and your perception of life is a culmination of the cellular memory. If you have ever wondered why some times you react in a certain way and think, "why did I do that? Or say that?" The answer is you are consciously acting out the information given to you that has been stored in the subconscious.

The Wellness Code/Intentional Wellness is an exploration of the cellular memory and a method of communication with your own physical, emotional, mental body for the purpose of attaining communication, and understanding of the original blessing that was meant for you. Embracing and releasing the seed or root of what was stored on the cell allows you to be your authentic self. Feeling harmony and balance in life brings about healing to wellness in all areas of your life.

In 1998, I had my fourth near death experience where I was given information through channeling that would enable us as humans to gain a greater understanding of this process....shift up before the awakening of 2012. The term "shift up" refers to each being taking responsibility for their perspective and their actions, re-actions and pro-actions, creating a life of harmony, balance and joy...being responsible for your own evolution. This information is meant to be shared with all, to be of assistance in the area of Emotional Clarity and moving from healing to wellness. This gave me the platform for creating my own modality, which I named "Opportunity Retrieval" and is part of the Wellness Code/Intentional Wellness.

What is it and why is it a key to our future? What benefits does it hold for you, your family and friends, your community and the whole global village?

It is a shifting of your perception and intention for a greater and more meaningful experience in your lifetime. In fact, the Wellness Code is also called Intentional Wellness and has everything to do with gaining, learning and living from an awakened perspective. You are taken from a perspective of how you view life now to a perspective of life the way it is seen and played out in the universe...a truer and deeper understanding of all that is.

It is like your own personal Alchemy, turning your personal lead (that which may be holding you from your wildest dreams) and turning it to the purest of gold (a state of being where you are able to be in the universal life flow as it was intended for you) to live your highest vision in congruency with your body, mind and spirit.

313

Would you like to be able to unravel the true meaning of events and feelings? Have the benefit of knowing the blessing that was meant only for you?

I had a client that was having a very difficult time emotionally. Her family called me to see if I could help her. During the session, we discovered the seed of the emotional upset; it was something that happened long ago when she was in grade school. She had come to school with a haircut and all the children had made fun of her. It left an emotional trauma on her cells and was now coming to the surface. She believed and viewed what happened to her as a negative event. Through the session and the "Opportunity Retrieval" she was able to realize the event that had occurred so long ago was a blessing. It gave her inside information on how to better understand some similar events that were happening now to her own child, who has Down Syndrome. Through this method, she unraveled the blessing and realized this was a gift "for" her and not something that happened "to" her. By the end of the session all of her symptoms just vanished.

The Wellness Code provides a foundation for emotional clarity. It is the "decoder" and the piece of the puzzle necessary for seeing the whole picture. It then becomes your choice to release and shed feelings and past actions that may not be to your highest good. It is the gateway to your next step in human evolution.

While experiencing the Wellness Code, you will journey towards a deeper understanding of Perception and Intention. Let's look at these marvels knowing your subconscious steers the boat of these two inner mechanisms. These two components are important to know when looking deeper into your own evolution and into understanding the Wellness Code/Intentional Wellness.

1.   Intention:

Through your intention, all things are created. Intention is the link between the realm of possibilities and the reality of creation. Through intention, you have the ability to bring forth information from a unified field, a place that quantum physicists refer to as "outside space and time," the place where cellular memory resides. If you go back and take apart the action of intention, it is like unraveling the fabric of time and space; like taking apart a magic act, giving you a fuller understanding how life itself manifests and flourishes.

Does intention come from universal information or does intention begin within your very own heart and soul? That's the question so many are seeking. It is intention that can move mountains and your intention can take you beyond any limitation...all limitation is perception. When you see your dream within yourself and you feel it, you begin a cellular reaction that puts the wheels of the universe in motion. It is your intention to follow your dream and it is that intention to bring your dream into reality that becomes the driving force. It is something you cannot see or touch, and yet, the reality is that the energy of all of our intentions is what drives all life on this planet.

Without intention, there is no movement. When a child looks at a chair, sizes it up, sees itself grabbing onto the chair and pulling itself up into a standing position, it is the intention that drives the action and the child to stand. It is the same mechanism that allows us to get up from a fall, or to think, believe and have hope for a better future.

Indeed, it may be the power of all of our intentions that will put into motion the reorganization and implementation of a new way of seeing ourselves as the instruments of health and wellness, of peace and prosperity and as stewards of this great and precious earth.

Unconsciously, you are creating intention in every moment. That is why it is so important that you are in touch with your intention, your true intention, and that you look at everything in life with profound gratitude. Coming from that place, your intention can be the driving force for the realization of all of your dreams. Remember, intention is there before the thought. It begins in the spinning fluid space that is within each cell of the body. The place that connects us to spirit is the place where the seed of intentions is born. Therefore, it is the intention that you are learning to work with. As stated in my book "Our intention is the beginning of the outcome" is indeed true.

2.   Perception:

Although perception is defined in the dictionary as: "An act or result of perceiving; awareness of environment through physical sensation", and "ability to perceive," I would add this. Perception is what happens when all your cells and all your views and all your past and present, and perhaps your future, come together in a nanosecond and at that same time, all the input you have had up to that moment defines what your perception will be. It is a wondrous feat of all the systems working together that allows you to have a single thought and a single perspective.

When you feel love or when you feel hurt, it is this mechanism at work. No two people will have the exact same perception of anything. Each one of us has a long history of thoughts, feelings and experiences that define how we perceive.

In the end, your life is your perception of life. Even the perception of "the end" is a perception because the truth is, nothing really ends, it just transforms. Scientifically speaking, that is a fact. When we say, "dust to dust," we mean that literally.

Your atoms have been the same atoms that have been in this time and space since the beginning of this time and space. How you perceive your world and act or react will determine the level of happiness, joy and fulfillment you receive in your life. Your life is your perception of your life.

In your Wellness Code session, you learn and experience a method to communicate with the subconscious, giving it enough information so it allows you to proceed to a cellular level, the place where all healing truly occurs. The subconscious likes status quo (staying in its comfort zone) and you will proceed very carefully with a great amount of respect for the subconscious. You will connect and re-connect with the energy of what some call your inner child, that precious place within you where your truth is stored. We will complete this process together using music that was channeled through me, a gift from the angels and named Sounds of the Soul CD. You are guided to a sacred place that allows you to experience the feeling of being in the quantum field, outside space and time. This experience itself may be very profound as you come face to face with the actuality of your true core feelings regardless of who you are or how long you have been on a path of higher consciousness. We all live in a conscious world. To seek out and synchronize the conscious and subconscious is to discover your own evolution.

In The Wellness Code/Intentional Wellness we explore what I call "pockets of opportunity" that are your stepping-stones to a place of grace. We all have them and now there is a way to embrace and release them. You will gain understanding of the process in which our being protects us and learn the process that can take you into the quantum field beyond space and time, where shift happens. The benefit and purpose for the Wellness Code is to facilitate and assist in this evolutionary shift or change that awaits each and every one of us.

This change is crucial and key for you to be prepared for the energetic and planetary shifts that may occur in 2012. "Everything on the inside is reflected on the outside" and everything which is above is also below. The universe is in perfect balance and harmony. And now it is time for each and every one of us to step into who we were put here to be and to assist all mankind and Mother Earth herself in this great awakening.

Are you in perfect health? Do you experience perfect wellness? Do you have abundance in every area of your life? What is it you truly believe about your health and wellness? What is it you truly desire and how close are you to having it all? Do you believe in your heart that you know with certainty the reason for your being on this earth plane?

What if everything, every event that has happened in your life is happening for you, not to you? In most cases, this viewpoint requires a person to shift their perspective and one of the components of the Wellness Code is to attain this "shift."

We start with a few basics, physics of the form, if you will. Within each of us there are 100 trillion cells, a daunting number to imagine, especially when we know that every single cell communicates with every other single cell in less than a nanosecond. These cells lay down a base code that affects every moment of our life. How we feel, how we act or react, even our perspective on life.

Your cells are like the blue print in which you work from to maintain life. You have automatic systems, such as breathing that you don't think about, yet it is something you can't live without for more than a few minutes.

There are subtle systems that form our thoughts and actions and are directly tied to the "emotional body." Even before you were born, each moment of your life was being recorded and left a trace signature on every cell. When you were happy, that was recorded on the cells; when you were sad or scared, that also left an imprint on the cells and then with every event, those imprints shifted and formed your current thoughts, opinions and actions.

Seated deep within your subconscious lay all the answers. We are such amazing beings that when you were very young and, perhaps, were unable to cope with some of what life was revealing to you, your cells took care of it for you and stored the information for unraveling at a later date. Some of this stored information works it way out on its own. The challenge is we were never taught how to find this information that is in the subconscious or how to unravel the blessing behind it. We did not have a way to decode what was once a helping hand and now may be the hand that unconsciously says stop, do not pass until you are able to decode the past.

I believe this is the answer and the key to why some people heal and some do not; why some experience true joy in their life and some do not; and why some experience success in all areas, including business, relationships, health and wellness, and perhaps Long-Gevity and certainly Young-Gevity, and some do not.

It may sound a bit confusing to say you must go beyond space and time, but that is where all healing takes place. You must journey within to reach that doorway.

In the world of meditation and Yoga, you will hear it said, "It is the moments between the moments." This is another way of saying the quantum field.

Your subconscious must first feel it has enough information to allow you to pass through the door of awakening and awareness…this place where you are in the flow of consciousness.

When you are ready, you will journey to a place where you can call forward "that which is ready, willing and able to be healed." You will know when the time is right because a catalyst will appear in your life and push that button. This is where most people think, "How did that happen to me?" or "Why did that happen to me?" This is the moment you shift to "I am grateful for this catalyst that has let me know that this pocket of opportunity is ready to be embraced, healed and released. Thank you as I know this was for me and not to me."

This method must be experienced in person, as it is a physical phenomenon that occurs when you release from all 100 trillion cells. In psychology it is called "the benevolent witness" and one is needed to complete this method. We take this journey together and the result is that your perception shifts and at that moment your vibratory rate is raised, taking you up a notch on the evolutionary scale as you gain and are gifted a greater understanding of how and why all this was meant for you. You have healed along the time line and as you go about your days, you will notice and see things in a brighter light. It is the ending of unhealthy patterns and the beginning of choices, and choices are always good.

The Wellness Code /Intentional Wellness is a breakthrough modality.

It may not be one way but all ways that woven together in a tapestry of consciousness, awakened consciousness brings about a "shift" that enhances your experience of life.

Taking a universal view of all that is, we can see that our entire universe is a great tapestry, woven into a beautiful universe and life, as we know it. We are all different and unique in a magnificent way, and close in association with all the elements, including the plant world that represents the earth, the air, which we breathe, the water, which is life's flow, and the sun, which is our spark of illumination and transformation. We are not spectators, but interwoven. This is not a dress rehearsal but the moment in time where you have the stage and the seed of truth. All life on this planet is delicately balanced within this beautiful tapestry we call life. Each of us is a unique and beautiful being and creature, one thread of the tapestry. We are all inter-dependent with each other and one cannot thrive without the other. In fact, one cannot exist without the other. It is the acknowledgement and embracing of this symbiotic relationship that brings great joy and gratitude.

May you move forward knowing that you are the bridge; you are the amazing being that is creating and co-creating this universe. Your every thought, your every intention and your every action affects the energy everywhere.

There's no turning back now. You have been touched by the awakening energy of what will be.

I look forward to the day when we can share this experience together and so help to assist in the evolutionary shift that is occurring on this beautiful planet, right here, right now,

In humble awe of all that is…you are the light…shine on…

About the Author

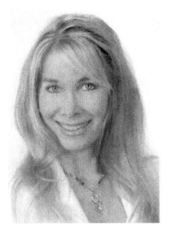

Sheila is an International Inspirational Speaker and catalyst for wellness and success. After a near death experience which changed the course of Sheila's life, she received divinely guided information on raising consciousness, inner clarity, and how to prepare for our future. She is a true visionary of our time and an Award winning Author of books and channeled music.

Sheila works tirelessly with community projects that enrich people's lives. She is the Southern Nevada Coordinator for IONS (Institute of Noetic Science) bridging science and consciousness. She was hand chosen by Al Gore to be part of the Climate Project - promoting sustainability world-wide.

She is a professional intuitive and works with people to understand the underlying causes of challenges in their life, thereby increasing energy, joy and effectiveness in one's life.

Sheila created the Nationally accredited "Intentional Wellness Experience" as a way to share the "missing piece of the puzzle," the key to wellness and success in all areas of your life. A doctor in Natural Health & Philosophy, Dr. Stirling is also a Certified Lymphologist, Acutonics Practitioner, Sound and light therapist, and Reiki Master. She is more than an energy healer, inspirational life and wellness coach; she is a catalyst for your wellness and a lifelong student of human behavior.

Sheila Z. Sterling can be contacted at:
www.Truelife-solutions.com
openwisdom@cox.net
(702) 227-9415

Why Prayer

Janice Marie Wilson

According to statistics, billions of people pray. A high percentage of people "hope" that their prayers are answered, but they are not sure what's really happening. I don't know about you, but when I can't be SURE about something, I don't trust or believe that it will happen. Learning how to pray, so that you can trust and believe in the results is the only reason we should continue to pray. If every time you went to flip a light switch on, and you questioned whether it would work...what would you do? You would stop using that light or you'd fix it.

Prayer works the same way. You should be able to flip the switch (ask) and the light goes on (get your answer). The truth is all prayers are answered, but most of us don't know how to listen for the answer or don't know how to ask believing we will find the answer. Prayer is many things to many people. Some people pray for stuff. "Please, God help me to get an A on this quiz! God, I pray for patience, and I want it now! Please God, help me to pay my bills! God, if you do this for me just this once, I'll never ask for anything again." There are as many ways to pray as there are human beings in this world. We pray when we are scared. We pray when we need help. We pray for answers. We pray that God makes our lives better. We beg, we plead and sometimes, we even barter. Everyone has muttered some kind of prayer at some time. Sometimes, our prayers get answered. Sometimes, we think no one is listening. And sometimes, we are happier for that "unanswered prayer."

What if you were able to harness the energy of a prayer? What if you knew for sure that every time you prayed, your prayers would be answered to your highest good and the good of all those around you? What if you could pray and immediately start seeing the results? What if you prayed and always got what you wanted or something better? What if you could fix your light switch and the light would always go on?

The "WHY PRAYER" is your answer.

The "Why Prayer" is a proven method based on strong spiritual truths and the laws of physics. But don't take my word for it. Prove it to yourself. If it works use it; if it doesn't, keep trying. The "Why Prayer" doesn't ask you to take a leap of blind faith. It is rooted in the laws of physics and the Bible.

The laws of physics state that the total energy in a closed or isolated system is constant, no matter what happens. Another law states that the mass in an isolated system is constant. When Einstein discovered the relationship $E=mc2$ (in other words that mass was a manifestation of energy) the law was said to refer to the conservation of mass-energy. The total of both mass and energy is retained, although some may change forms. The ultimate example of this is a nuclear explosion, where mass transforms into energy.

The Bible states: *"Ask believing it is so.... and allow it to be done for you." It is done unto you as you believe.*

"Ask and it will be yours." Luke 11:9

If the formula to prayer is so simple, why are most of us wandering around lost, unhappy, or angry because our prayers aren't answered. Or worse yet, we are discouraged because most of the answers we hear are "No. Not now. Be patient." Some of us have prayed for so long with little results that we no longer believe anyone is listening. So what are we doing wrong? How can we do it better? What is really going on when we pray?

According to physics and the Bible, everything in life is made up of energy. It is your conscious awareness of this energy that gives it form and substance. The "Why Prayer" is a way to focus your consciousness to unleash the powerful energy of thought to transform substance. Using science to pray isn't a new theory. In fact, the Kabbahlists, a five million year-old religion called prayer a technology and used the Bible to understand this technology. All cultures used nature as their model to pray. We all know about the Indian Rain Dance, offerings to Mother Nature and many of the different gods and goddesses that were named for their energetic influences from nature. Science and nature have natural elements that create substance and mass. The three elements of an answered prayer are:

1. Ask
2. Believe
3. Allow

ASK

In order for the "Why Prayer" to work, you need to ask the question why. When you ask this question, immediately you set into action the energy forces to find answers. The truth is that you only ask why about things you believe to be true. So when you start your prayer with a "why," you are activating your awareness to find true answers. The "why" moves your consciousness beyond what you know in order to find answers. "Why" is the laser beam of energy that lights up these answers.

When you ask "why," you are asking to find the cause, reason, or purpose to your question. "Why" opens your imagination to see things that you have kept hidden from yourself. It implies that there are answers; that there is a purpose; and that you understand what the cause is. These are all reasons why someone wants to pray in the first place. So if you preface your prayer with the word "why," you have already set in motion the energy to find answers. You are asking for the purpose, reason or cause of something in your life. The trick to getting what you want is to ask "why" in conjunction with something that you want.

Why am I so happy?
Why am I so healthy?
Why do I have such great kids?
Why do I love what I do?
Why am I so blessed?

If, on the other hand, you place a "why" in front of something you don't want, you will also find all the reasons, purpose and cause that make this true.

Why does this always happen to me?
Why am I so stupid?
Why don't I have enough money to pay my bills?
Why am I unhappy?

When you use this method to pray, it is tantamount that you focus only on that which you want. If you ask for what you don't want, it will give you that also. The "why" is the light beam that shows you answers. You are the master of that light. Use it to find the answers to questions that will make your life better. Use it to ask for ways that will give you what you want more of...peace, happiness, courage, and an abundance of health, wealth and happiness.

When you use "why" to find more love and happiness in your life, you will find it. If you use "why" to find the reasons for all of your misery, you will also find that. This powerful word when used for good opens your kingdom of heaven. When it is used to find fault, it will take you to the depths of hell.

Note: Always use "why" in your prayers to find what's good, loving, and beautiful in your life. This will show you all the reasons, the causes and the purpose that this is true.

BELIEVE

The only reason we want anything in our life is to feel better. We pray so that we can feel safe. We pray so we can feel in control. We pray so we can feel love and approval. Unfortunately, most of us pray or ask for things that we don't want. Or we pray, and then deep down believe that ultimately it won't make us happy. For your prayers to work, you must ask believing that you can have it. Sounds a little tricky. To believe is to accept something as true or real. So when you pray, you have to accept as true or real that you can have what it is that you want, or something better. But how many of us pray and don't accept that we can have what we want?

When you ask "why" it already implies that you believe it to be true. "Why" automatically triggers responses that prove to you the truth. "Why" activates that you accept the answers you receive as the truth. This is the reason that you must learn to formulate your "Why Prayer" so that you receive the answers that will make you feel good. Stay away from formulating "why" questions that find answers that don't feel so good.

For instance, say a "Why Prayer" that goes like this. "Why am I so happy?" Immediately, you will start seeing all the reasons that you are happy. You will immediately get responses that feel happy. You will be happy because your "why" has beamed a light all around you on everything in your world that makes you happy. It will also bring things to you that you had never imagined would make you happy. "Why" is the magnet that attracts more happiness.

On the other hand, if you ask, "Why me"? You will also attract answers and situations that may not feel so good. You are implying with this question that you believe it to be true that you are a victim of circumstances. You will then find all the answers that show you why this is true.

Formulating your "Why Prayer" to give you what you want instead of what you don't want is the key. You will always get answers when you ask the question "why." You will always find what you believe to be true when you ask "why." You will see how you accept this truth as reality when you ask "why." You shape your world and your experiences with this tool.

Everything you are asking for already exists in some form or another. If you don't see it, it is because you haven't decided to shine your light of awareness that will show it to you. You haven't decided to ask the 'why" question to find what you want. Whatever you want already exists. You don't have to make it, earn it, or struggle for it. You don't have to mint five million dollars to have it. You don't have to create the perfect mate from scratch to have the love of your life. You don't have to build the perfect company to have a great and fulfilling career. The answers are real. Formulating your prayer to ask "why" you have an abundance of health, wealth and happiness is the righteous way to get your answers.

If you want a better job, ask "Why do I have a better job?" Listen for the answers you get. See what starts to unfold. Observe. If you want more love in your life, ask "Why am I so loved?" You'll be surprised at how many ways you can feel loved. If you want more wealth in your life, ask "Why am I so rich?" And as if out of nowhere, good things that make you feel rich will start to appear.

When you ask "why," you show yourself that you *believe* something to be true. The "why" allows you to find the reasons to see the truth. You never ask "why" unless you know that there are answers. So when you pose a "why" in a prayer, immediately it opens your imagination to find the answers that are hidden from your five senses. "Why" by-passes the logical mind and helps you see what you have kept hidden from yourself.

For example, when you ask the question, "Why is the sky blue?" you already *know* the sky is blue. You are only seeking to find the answers that make it so.

When you ask, "Why am I so happy?" you already *believe* that you are happy. "You are only asking to see the reasons for your happiness. "Why do I have such a great job?" You already *know* that you have a great job, the "why" question only opens your mind to show you all the reasons that your job is so great! Asking the question "why?" is how you pray believing that it is so. "Why" also allows the answer to be given to you. All the answers to be happy, rich, and healthy are given to you just by asking, "Why?".

ALLOW

The "why" question allows you to see what is true and real. The definition of allow is to make attainable, open to an opportunity, give permission. When you allow yourself to listen for the answers, you open yourself to new opportunities. You give yourself permission to have what you want. To allow doesn't push the good things away. You are quiet and you are able to see your answered prayer.

Ask and it will be yours. Luke 11:9

The "Why Prayer" is how you can ask and it will be yours.

Below are some examples of how to use the "Why Prayer." Don't take my word for it. Try it and let me know what happens. Write down the answers you begin to see. Watch how your life unfolds in magical and loving ways. See the miracles that come to you with ease, grace and fulfillment of all of your dreams come true.

Why do I believe that I can have what I want!

Why do I know how to le go and allow the universe to give me what is best?

Why do I enjoy so many sources of income?

Why do I have the clarity to get what I want?

Why do I love my life?

Why am I so happy?

Why do I have perfect health?

Why do I feel safe?

Why do I approve of myself?

Why do I have control?

Why do I always get what I want or something better?

> *FAITH – WHEN YOU COME TO THE END OF ALL THE LIGHT YOU KNOW, AND THERE'S NOTHING BUT DARKENSS AROUND YOU, FAITH MEANS YOU KNOW YOU WILL LAND ON STURDY GROUND, OR YOU WILL BE TAUGHT HOW TO FLY!*
>
> *- ANONYMOUS*

You were born to fulfill all the promises of your heart. You were born to have everything you have ever desired that is good and true. The "Why Prayer" is the key to your personal kingdom of heaven on earth. Use it to find all of your answers. Use it to see what you have kept hidden from yourself. Use it to unleash the power of your heart to have fulfillment, riches, health and all the happiness your heart needs to experience. AMEN!

About the Author

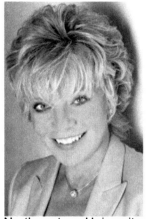

Janice Marie Wilson is the author of four books, The Gift from the Goddess, Athena Leadership Styles for the Millenium, Live Laugh and Love, and THE GOODNESS EXPERIENCE. She is the Life Style and Beauty Editor for Risque Las Vegas Magazine, spa and travel correspondent for Jetsetters Magazine, former columnist for Las Vegas Bride Magazine, keynote speaker, and radio talk show host.

As a former Executive with the IBM Corporation, professional actress, dancer, and artist with a Masters Degree from Northwestern University, she has devoted her life to inspiring, teaching and mentoring women to become self-actualized and live their lives filled with beauty, goodness, love, well-being, success and Divine fulfillment.

She is the mother of two adult children, Kyra and Christopher, and has been married for thirty-two years to an entrepreneur and health care executive. She loves to play tennis, ballroom dance, cook, snow ski, golf, travel, shop and laugh with her friends.

Janice Marie Wilson can be contacted at:
www.janicemariewilson.com
goddesslv@aol.com
(702) 233-8305

Yoga

Christian Kaufman

When most of us think of Yoga, we have an image of a person sitting on the floor with their legs crossed, or turning their body into some type of pretzel. Yoga in the West has established itself as a physical exercise practice much like aerobics. Most of the things written about Yoga go on and on about the great health benefits, even the stress relief one gets from the practice of it. Doctors are starting to take note of it and are recommending it to their patients. The field of Yoga Therapy is starting to grow and many educational establishments are jumping on the band wagon, offering training in Yoga Therapy.

Everywhere you look you can find yoga classes popping up all over with soccer moms running to class all decked out in "Yoga gear," or seniors gathering at community centers for classes. Yoga for kids is being added to some school curriculums and I've even seen classes where dog owners can bring their pets to class and practice with them. Expectant mothers take pre-natal yoga, knowing that they will be able to bring their infants in for "mommy and me" yoga once their child is born.

You can do yoga in the privacy of your own home or you can take a group class.

You can even do it in all kinds of temperature, even110 degree heat for an hour and a half because your practice can be slow and gentle or powerful and fast. It doesn't matter. In a world of stressed out multi-taskers, it's no wonder that Yoga has become a buzz word. But what is Yoga, really? How can one thing be applied so differently for so many different people?

Perception is how we interpret the world around us, and perception is what has given Yoga its numerous meanings. Yoga isn't just an exercise, it is a way of life, a philosophy that was birthed in the Indus Valley where it became the heart of Eastern thought more than 2000 years before Christ. The ancient scientists that developed Yoga found that the major factor of human suffering was the mind. They knew that the mind could create disease as quickly as it could cure it. Through the mind, and its perception, a life of suffering or a life of peace could be created and maintained.

Through their personal experience, the scientists witnessed first-hand that the more they had a certain thought replaying in their minds, the more that thought affected their emotions, bringing that thought to life. Thoughts triggered emotions, which triggered a physical response in the body.

These ancient "mind scientists" quickly saw the connection between control of their thoughts and a life of joy and peace. They understood that the way they viewed the world around them reflected what was going on inside them. Perception was the key. They realized that as well as thoughts, emotions needed to be explored. This brought forth a very important aspect of Yoga that is so often left out in modern Yoga classes. If we want to live a good, happy, healthy life, we must explore the parts of ourselves that have been hidden and wounded.

Yoga's internally directed work of self-examination to heal teaches us the original intention of ancient yogis, self-actualization. They believed the only way to reach that self-actualization is to first tame the wild meanderings of mind in order to witness what is in the mind.

Yoga is a "joining" of the physical body with the mental, emotional and spiritual selves, making the practitioner whole and able to experience the present moment, rather than reacting out of past fears or rushing to the future worries.

Through Yoga, this ancient culture found a way to train the mind, and explore the thoughts and emotions, thereby ending the unnecessary pain caused by their former misguided actions. They understood that everything in life was connected, and through this connection, the actions and thoughts of one could influence the other. They saw that if they were in a state of suffering, their actions would continue like a domino effect out to the community around them. Not only did this ancient science help their individual lives, but it also affected the lives of the people around them, showing that actions affected the chain of life that links everything.

The philosophy of Yoga goes back to a time before people had an alphabet, let alone a written language. The teachings were passed down in an oral tradition from generation to generation. It is interesting that even in a time where it was common for people to travel around in nomadic tribes from place to place searching for land and food, the people of the Indus Valley perceived the importance of the interconnectedness of life. This culture was based on the understanding of creating a life of harmony between the soul and the mind, believing that when those two aspects became joined, it brought the body into balance. They would then become self-fulfilled, no longer needing things from outside themselves to bring them happiness and joy. This brought a deep understanding of spirituality. Without it being a religion, they practiced living a moral and kind life. They knew they had found the key leading them out of the prison of suffering.

When the rest of the world was busy trying to find food and fight off other tribes, this culture was busy implementing a system to correct that damage. They recognized that there was no truth in what other people of the time saw as "things" coming between them and what they wanted. Their strong viewpoint of truth taught them that if they weren't aware of their actions, it would only continue the cycle of suffering.

Shortly after 2000 B.C. a group of nomads arrived in the Indus Valley called the Aryans. Their arrival brought a very important shift to Yoga. They began to develop the written langue of Sanskrit, that later would become the main language of Yoga sutras (texts) that are still used and referenced even today.

Around 200 B.C. Yoga would take another important turn. The great Indian sage, Patanjali, began to take the oral tradition of Yoga and write it down into what are now known as the Yoga Sutras. In the Yoga Sutras, Patanjali collected the best that Yoga had to offer and wrote them down as aphorisms (an idea written in a memorable form). The Yoga Sutras are important because it allowed everyone access to the Yoga texts that had been reserved only for the upper class. The sutras provided a step-by-step guide to attaining mental, physical and spiritual balance. Each aphorism addressed some aspect of self-development leading to spiritual consciousness which later became known as Ashtanga (The Eight Fold or Limb Path).

This Eight Limb Path consisted of eight identifiable social practices that were moral guidelines for living in peace with self and others. Patanjali created another wonderful aphorism helping people better understand the sometimes complex teachings of Yoga into what he called the "Yoga Tree of Life." This symbol shows how connected each limb of the path is and how they influence one another. Just as humans are connected to each other yet maintaining uniqueness and a set of talents with a purpose, each part of the tree is dependent on the other parts to grow and thrive, working as one unit coming from the same original seed.

Patanjali's Yoga aphorisms are the heart of all Yoga practices and serve as a road map for our spiritual journey. Imagine in your mind a tree, see the roots (yama) which contains the five moral and social restraints which keep the outside world in balance just like the roots of a tree brings balance so that it may grow. These limbs are the practice of:

> Ahimsa: non-violence. Non-violence doesn't just take on the idea of not harming others, or ourselves physically. It also applies to nature and animals, as well as not acting violently through thoughts, speech, and action. Through this practice, compassion, empathy and kindness for all of life is born.
>
> Satya: truthfulness. Truthfulness includes not lying to yourself or others, as well as deceiving yourself with the way you view past, present or future issues and actions. With truth one is lead out of illusions, lies and deceit and can view things in an accurate way.
>
> Asteya: non-stealing. Non-stealing teaches us about greed and shows us our selfish desires for money, power, control, status, and attention. When we learn to only take what life has given us, it teaches us to be grateful for those things we have. We become open-hearted and generous the more we understand this connection to life and all the riches its abundance bestows upon

us. We do not need to take more than we have been given so the motivation behind greed disappears.

Brahmachary: control of sensual pleasure. Control of our sensual pleasures teaches about over indulgence and appropriate sexual behavior. Never harming another in the pursuit of fulfilling what we think we need. We also learn that we do have control over our senses. Through learning to control our senses we find what we are truly looking for, self-intimacy; learning to live our lives purely and cleanly.

Aparigraha: non-possessiveness, coveting or grasping. The last of the yamas, non-possessiveness, teaches us to let go of all the identities and images we hold onto. We are no longer addicted to them; we no longer feel we are not enough. Here we find our true nature.

From the roots, we are carried up to the trunk (niyama) and brought to the five personal restraints of the "Tree of Life." The trunk brings us from social ethics of the yamas to the deeper personal actions we take from the guidance of the niyamas. Just as the trunk gives shape and strength to the tree, we find the same with the niyamas of:

Sauca: purity. When our lives are pure and we know all of our actions are clear and clean, we know this is living to our highest potential. We become fulfilled and we move into the next niyama

Santosh: contentment. In each moment, we are reminded to stay content with each thing we do, this includes simple dressing, living, eating, even keeping simple boundaries and principles.

Tapas: burning desire or discipline. We need to develop discipline and are taught that through the third niyama, to continue our practice which fuels our desire becoming a seriousness towards our spiritual practice that gives us the strength we need to lead us into the fourth niyama of self-study.

Svaddhyyaya: self-study. Here we find that we are personally responsible for learning and re-learning the things from our past that are holding us back. All the things that have happened to us now become teaching aids for our growth. We embrace and take ownership of our lives, learning acceptance about our needs and desires, and our life purpose. This self-study brings us to a teaching so deep we understand our connection to something greater than ourselves and the final fifth niyama which is

Ishvara-pranidhana: surrender to a higher power. We surrender our control and move with life rather than against it. By reaching this point, we lose the sense of our ego self and see our true Divinity.

These aren't just "do's" and "don't's" to follow. The wisdom science of Yoga was designed to lead its aspirants out of a life of suffering. Using the yamas and niyamas as a moral and ethical guide to live by teaches us to live in harmony with all of life. Each precept depends on the other and together they form a basis for the "Yoga Tree of Life."

Moving up past the roots and the trunk we come to the branches of the tree, (asana). Asana is the physical practices of yoga that in modern day we see in most classes. Asanas work on the anatomy and physiology of the body. This part of yoga came into being towards the end of the development of the science of Yoga as a way to relax the body in order to sit in meditation (the goal of yoga) for longer periods of time. Yogis of old found that in each part of the body the mind stored memories of tension and past wounds. They also found that moving the body into a balanced yet unusual position, the conscious mind had something to focus on rather than the normal everyday thoughts of fear and worries. They found that the longer they could give the mind a break from its ego thoughts, the more they could witness what was coming from the subconscious.

They knew it was normal for the mind to "think" and that the intense focus that it took to hold the body in the poses they created kept the conscious mind busy. The longer the mind was busy, they found that their memories would bubble up with the events that took place from the past which had created the tension they held in their bodies. They became aware of how their thoughts continued to replay these old wounds in everyday life.

One of the greatest gifts of asana practice is that it gives you a mental break from your life. With a break, it is easier to come back and deal with things with greater understanding of our past and how to help ourselves use the insights received when we move deeply into ourselves.

From the branches of the tree we move out into the leaves (pranayama).

This is the breathing practice that calms the nervous system and brings oxygen to the body as well as prana (energy). Just as the leaves help to nourish the tree, pranyama does the same for the yogi. Through these specialized breathing practices the body is cleansed of toxins and one is able to bring relaxation into the asana or posture. The body relaxes on the out breath, and with relaxation, intuition is able to come forth.

We have moved from the stable roots, felt the strength and shape of the trunk, stretched into the branches of the tree, reaching out into the leaves where we rest with the breath and energy. Now, our journey takes us from the physical to the mental and emotional into where we can work on the deeper spiritual practice of the three remaining parts of the "Yoga Tree of Life."

The bark (pratyahara) is the outer most part of the tree, the barrier between the inside of the tree and the outer world. Just like how our senses (sight, hearing, taste, touch and smell) are the barrier between our inner most being and the world. Our senses are the organs of perception, teaching about the world around us as we experience it.

Without them, we would have no concept or understanding of the outside world. It is here that Yoga teaches us about choice. We can choose to only be aware of the world around us or we can follow our senses inward to the internal world of our infinite wisdom, or ignore our internal "calling" in lieu of the external things that grab our attention.

This action teaches us pratyahara, withdrawal of our senses where we move our attention from the outside world and explore all the happenings going on inside. We no longer hear the clocks ticking around us or people talking. We hear the beat of our own heart. We feel the blood moving through our body, we become aware of the world inside. We must regain our control of the mind and relax its impulse to hold on to the sense of ego where it wants to relate to the outside world - a world that defines who we are. It is here that we start to lose our ego identity and clear consciousness can emerge. With the withdrawal of the senses, we move from the bark of the tree into the sap (dharana).

It takes concentrated focus to remain internally aware for extended periods of time. Through this practice of dharana, we learn the skill of focusing our mind into a one pointed awareness that keeps our attention fixed on our goal. Being so aware of ourselves, we are able to know when our emotions are changing, and our deep attention gets us in tune with our intuition that is guiding us in each moment.

From the concentrated focus of the sap of dharana, we move into the next part of the tree, the flower (dhyana) which is the act of meditation. All of our hard work is starting to pay off as we have moved inward preparing for the deeply spiritual insights that we become aware of. It is here, in meditation, that we observe ourselves, a still quiet, peaceful place where we are able to investigate our beliefs, actions and perceptions. We see both the dark and light parts of ourselves and learn to become comfortable with viewing who we truthfully are. In this place, we experience the whole goal of Yoga, self-actualization. We have a clear picture of what we need, and where we want to go. We see our present situation, insights of our past, and create our future. We learn that we have the power to change our path in life, our attitudes and the way we live.

The act of meditation transforms the beautiful flower on the "Yoga Tree of Life" into the fruit of (samadhi) pure consciousness directed inward. In this last stage of Yoga we are fully present in the moment, aware of ourselves and fully absorbed in the true nature of our Soul. Consciousness is moving through our whole body, and there is no disconnection of body, mind, emotion or soul. In this moment, we are whole and joined with all of life just the way it is. We are united and we can experience harmony in the Universal Spirit.

Through the spiritual wisdom of the "Tree of Yoga," we see how each part of the tree is dependent on one another. It is only natural for humans to try to compartmentalize each part of our lives as being separate in order to understand all. The beauty of Yoga spirituality is through personal experience. When touching spirit, you learn each part slowly flows into the next and the boundaries disappear. Yoga emerged from the human need to find a way out of suffering, a way that can help us help ourselves.

Yoga changed and grew over the years just as everything does when people put their own "spin" and understanding into it. The life philosophy of Yoga wasn't meant to be practiced as a religion; it was more a way of life that anyone could use. It brought the practitioner (yogi/male, yogini/female) in touch with an awareness of something greater than themselves. It had no teaching of what God is or what happened to the soul after death. It was a personal spiritual practice that brought harmony with all life. Many different styles were developed that individuals could better relate to, depending on their unique perceptions. None are better than others. They each offer a different focus that can fit the many different people that make up our world. The eight main branches are still practiced today.

Jhana Yoga (pronounced gyah-nah), known as the Yoga of "knowledge and wisdom." Through Jhana, self-realization and enlightenment are achieved through the teachings of non-dualism, the elimination of illusion and direct knowledge of the Divine. Its focus is on education of self, and understanding nature. Intellectual knowledge of the workings of the microcosmic and macrocosmic universe is also explored.

Bhakti Yoga (pronounced bhuk-tee), is the path that brings union with the divine through love and acts of devotion. It teaches honoring a Higher Power and that commitment to the Higher Power resides within the practitioner.

Karma Yoga (pronounced karh-ma), is dedicated to selfless service and actions. This includes adding those in need, and from that karmic debt is erased.

Mantra Yoga (pronounced mahn-trah), is the Yoga of sacred sounds for self-awakening. This includes uttering scared sounds for healthier energy vibration. Sacred sounds are a focus for concentration to reach a deeper conscious connection.

Kundalini Yoga (pronounced koon-da-leenee). This is the activation of latent spiritual energy stored in the body that is raised along the spine to the top of the head through breath and movement. A vibrational shift occurs to awaken personal and spiritual insight through the movement of life-force energy up along the spinal column.

Tantra Yoga (pronounced tan-trah). This branch of Yoga brings union to all that you are, and that you can achieve by harnessing and utilizing sexual energy for deeper spiritual awaking and awareness. Tantra Yoga has become famous in the West for rituals that spiritualize sexuality, but in its truest form, it is a spiritual discipline of nonsexual rituals and visualizations that activate spiritual energy. It focuses on sacred practices to open spiritual channels, as well as contains rituals to connect the complimentary energies of Yin (female) and Yang (male).

Raja Yoga (pronounced rah-jah) is the Yoga known as the Royal Yoga or Ashtanga Yoga of mental mastery. (There is also a style of athletic yoga known by the same name but they are very different.) Raja Yoga focuses on mental training, emotional equilibrium or control leading to spiritual evolution. ("Yoga Tree of Life" that you read about).

Hatha Yoga (pronounced haht-ha). This branch of Yoga emerged around 1000 A.D. and emphasized only the yamas, niyamas, asana, and pranyama which became a health regime aimed at opening the mind, transforming the body and inspiring spiritual practice. It became much more popular in the twentieth century and we see versions of this form of Yoga all over. Its focus is on physical movement leading to union of mind, body and spirit.

Most Yoga that we see in the West is considered Hatha Yoga. (Iyengar, Ashtanga, Viniyoga, Kundalini, Kripalu, Ananda, Yoga College of India, Integral, Sivananda, Hidden Language, Ishta, Jivamukti, Tri, White Lotus, In-Tu-It, Power, Hot, Anusara, Forrest, Moksha, Restorative, and Yin are all types of Hatha Yoga).

Looking back over the evolution of Yoga, we see how it has changed, grown and found ways to reach out to the lives and hearts of so many different people. It's amazing in itself that the practice of Yoga has grown with people for over 5000 years, and we still aren't tired of it yet. Asking, "What is Yoga?" will give you about as many different answers as there are people in the world because our individual experience of it colors our reality.

In its basic form, Yoga means union...the union of the soul with the Universal Spirit of life. Every definition you hear, or style you practice, is right in its own way. Thich Nhat Hanh expresses it beautifully in *Peace in Every Step*, "Each thought, each action in the sunlight of awareness becomes sacred. In this light, no boundary exists between the sacred and the profane." Yoga's goal is to teach us two things; how to move our attention inward, and how to, then, move into the self-awareness practice of meditation. Classic traditional Yoga emphasizes spiritual health as the pathway to physical, mental, emotional health and, more importantly, happiness.

The ancient yogis of old knew that the mind was the most important energetic force behind every experience we have. They knew that personal growth would be impossible without a way to tame it, so they created Yoga and it has been passed down since, from person to person. The best way to understand it is in simply experiencing it. Namaste

About the Author

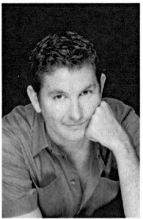 Christian Kaufman has worked in the health, wellness and beauty fields since 1998. He combines his work as a Cosmetologist, Yoga Therapist, Yogatsu Counselor®, and Reiki Master/Teacher into a unique practice that encourages people to learn about themselves and transform their lives from the inside out.

Christian began his studies at the Yogatsu Institute of Conscious Living & Healing Studies in 2002 and has since received numerous certifications. A testament to his dedication to education, Christian is now the Director of Education and Programs at the Yogatsu Institute. There, he strives to consistently improve the Institute's programs for the benefit of the Las Vegas community.

As a cosmetologist, Christian enjoys bringing out the inner beauty of his clients through the varied skin treatments and styling options he provides.

Christian's passion for yoga is put to good use at a Las Vegas area hospital where he instructs a diverse group of students weekly.

Christian Kaufman can be contacted at:
www.christiankaufman.com
Christian@christiankaufman.com
(702) 524-7437

YOGATSU Therapy

Alice Strauss

For those new to the growing field of complementary and alternative medicine, a basic knowledge of the workings of energy, and its creation of physical matter, is necessary in order to alleviate any misunderstandings. Before we begin, let me say that the work I do is a complementary therapy that supports any conventional medicine you may be using, have used, or will be using.

The ancient theory that *energy* is the substance behind the creation of life is now an accepted scientific fact. Studies related to the phenomenon of energy and its future potential to heal the woes of man are so widespread that it has been given a name, *Energy Medicine*. We have entered a new era of medicine that requires a willingness to synergistically blend ancient and modern sciences for the purpose of creating health, prosperity, and harmony for all people throughout the world. In essence, this is the ultimate goal of *YOGATSU* therapy— *healing the world one mind at a time, one spirit at a time.*

Spiritual masters from all traditions and all cultures view the universe as a pulsating vortex of *conscious energy* that is intelligent, intuitive, and intentional. Quantum physicists, who study the possibilities and potential of energy, have known for a number of decades what spiritual masters and mystics have known for centuries, that consciousness is the only reality, and that this reality is inclusive of a creative, intentional energy that cannot, perhaps, be seen by the naked eye yet functions immaculately in its ability to manifest and sustain life on this magnificent planet. The human body is a perfect microcosmic replica of the macrocosmic universe. Similar to the wisdom intentionality of the universe, the human body also vibrates with the intention for life, creativity, joy, and good health.

The human body is made of energy, and so is the human mind. The energies of body and mind are intimately connected, each knowing instinctively what the other is experiencing and in every moment. Here's how it works. From the energy of mind we receive thought, thought creates emotion, emotion dictates energy flow, and energy flow determines health. *YOGATSU* therapy teaches the logic of becoming keenly aware of the mind and its thoughts because thoughts are the catalyst for emotions, which fall into three categories: positive, negative, and neutral. When we are not paying attention and allow negative emotions to inundate the majority of our day, healthy energy flow is impeded, with the body paying the price. With this in mind, *YOGATSU* provides the energy evaluation, spiritual insights, commonsense tools, and practical skills that encourage a new realm of thinking and living that can transform outdated mental patterns, emotional habits, and negative attitudes into healthier ways of perceiving life that will encourage and support greater happiness, and health. The following story describes the work my clients and I do when they are in need of spiritual development, guidance, and healing.

Jonathan is a large real estate developer in another state. A few years ago, he began experiencing difficulty in both his private and work-related relationships. His feeling of being out of control was similar to watching a rock rolling down a steep hill. His fourteen-year old son had begun displaying a belligerent attitude that seemed to have appeared out of nowhere. Jonathan's wife became increasingly frustrated with the growing defiance displayed by their son, and became emotionally and mentally exhausted trying to deal with their son's escalating anger alone. Jonathan's desire to remain at the office more than she believed necessary also caused a great deal of animosity. Jonathan admitted openly that his life was out of balance and that his micro-managing tendencies in the office depleted him so thoroughly that he had no energy, or desire, to assist in the situations at home.

Jonathan's health began deteriorating. He experienced extreme tightness in his chest, lingering headaches, and chronic pain in his middle and lower back. He couldn't sleep most nights, which made him tired during the day. He was desperate. He sought medical assistance from his doctor who prescribed drugs to help him relax and dull the physical pain. However, he didn't like the zombie-like feeling he'd experience every time he took the prescribed medications, so he stopped taking them.

Jonathan also sought the advice of a psychologist, which he soon terminated because he wanted answers to his problems, and he wanted them *now*. He became weary of talking without receiving step-by-step instruction as to how he could change the nightmarish life he had been living. He was impatient for change.

When he felt the most frustrated and to the point of near collapse, he shared his dilemma with a family friend. Jonathan had great affection and respect for Mark and always felt comfortable sharing his work concerns with him when they were together. Mark was a decade or so older than Jonathan and always appeared confident without being arrogant. He moved through unexpected events and circumstances with a tranquil ease, and he enjoyed a successful business. Mark was creative and his life seemed to move effortlessly. When Mark had difficult decisions to make, he made them in a logical, composed manner, which garnered great respect from his employees and clients. Jonathan wanted to know how to live like Mark.

Mark shared with Jonathan that for years he had suffered from several physical conditions himself that his doctors couldn't completely remedy either, and that he began feeling better after starting *YOGATSU* therapy. Mark went on to explain that prior to his *YOGATSU* sessions, he too felt restless, agitated, hurried, out of sync, and not at all well. Despite his initial doubts, Jonathan decided he had nothing to lose by making an appointment for a session with me. In fact, he thought, he might enjoy talking to someone who was not interested in, or working with, bottom line projections, oppressive reports, and mind stifling organizational charts.

After our initial introductory chatter, I had Jonathan fill out the regular client information sheet. As he filled out the form, I began taking notes on the intuitive information I was receiving from his *aura* (electromagnetic energy field that surrounds the body). From his aura, I was able to gather significant information regarding Jonathan's childhood and upbringing. I also saw symbols that represented Jonathan's perceptions and beliefs that hindered his ability to fully appreciate who he was, and thus live happily in his own skin. From his *meridian* evaluation, I was able to identify the emotional habits he relied on when stressed, and how he allowed those emotions to exacerbate his mounting mental agitation, and how often he acted on those exaggerated emotions, which rarely served his life and purpose. From his *chakras*, I was able to determine the life-challenges, life-lessons, and childhood misperceptions that kept playing themselves out in his life, both publicly and privately. I will discuss these three energy systems later in this text.

The body holds a tremendous amount of information. Each cell acts like a file cabinet that holds within it everything and anything we will ever want to know about our past circumstances, present situations, and future events. Candace Pert, Ph.D., neuroscientist and author of the best-selling book *Molecules of Emotion,* says that our state of mind, thoughts, and emotions, all of which are usually ignored by conventional medicine, does, in fact, play a major role in recovery from illnesses that range from a cold to cancer, from diabetes to heart disease. The more Jonathan's world opened up, the better he felt and the faster his body healed.

With all Jonathan was learning, it wasn't difficult for him to see the extremely intimate and influential connection that exists between mind and body, body and mind. Gradually, he understood that the more he ignored his negative thoughts and resulting reactive emotions, which he almost always acted on without considering the consequences first, the more he affected his body's healthy energy flow that, in turn, created excessive stress and tension throughout his body. Naturally, the more physical tension and discomfort he felt, the more negative his mind, emotions, and reactions became. Jonathan realized that until he was 100% willing to do the *work* of facing, and then transforming, his unhealthy mental patterns, he would not enjoy the good health, happy relationships, and respect at work that he so desperately wanted.

The result of the information that I was able to gather from Jonathan's aura, meridians, and chakras showed him how his hyperactive, undisciplined mind—filled with superfluous, fear-based thoughts—created the drive that fed his emotional over reactivity, which then resulted in depletion of his energy, mental exhaustion, physical pain, and the hopeless and depressed feelings associated with spiritual malnutrition.

The following is a concise synopsis of the information inherent in each of the three major energy systems that were mentioned above:

Aura: biography (childhood background and history)
Meridians: behavior (emotional reactions and habits)
Chakras: biology (illnesses, pathology)

As our therapy sessions together continued, Jonathan began to feel a great deal more *self-aware*. The combination of the spiritual modalities I work with: *Yoga Psychology*, *Buddhist Philosophy*, *Energy Psychology*, and *Meditation*, enabled Jonathan to identify and transform the self-sabotaging perceptions and beliefs he'd grown up with that shadowed him personally and publicly. Here is a quick rundown of what the above modalities provide in the way of spiritual guidance and healing:

- **Yoga Psychology**: *mind/body awareness*
- **Buddhist Philosophy**: *sincere and honest reality check*
- **Energy Psychology**: *wisdom inherent in energy*
- **Meditation practice**: *mental training and transformation*

Jonathan learned more about the importance of *self-trust*. He did the homework I gave him wherein he was to practice, in small steps, trusting that he would be okay not controlling others as a result of *his fear* that they would not, or could not, do their work properly without him micromanaging.

Jonathan concluded that while he had been raised in an environment that readily displayed certain emotions like anger, disappointment, guilt, and depression, he seldom observed patience, trust, courage, and authentic compassion. It became increasingly apparent to him that what he was not taught in childhood, he was responsible for providing for himself as an adult, even if it meant seeking out and paying for guidance from experienced professionals. I explained to Jonathan that not taking responsibility for his own emotional education was equal to an adult who blames his parents for not teaching him how to ride a bike when young. At some point, as adults, we have to undertake our own emotional education and healing. Jonathan accepted that while he could not change his history, he could become *greater* than his history.

It was hard for Jonathan to admit that he needed to pay more attention to his own healing, and that he needed to stop making others responsible for not triggering his emotional tirades, and then blaming them for his resulting feelings of guilt. Actually, a lot of what he was learning about himself was rather shocking because he believed that since he was the boss, he obviously was the most well-rounded and capable person in the company. What he found most difficult to swallow was a statement that I, gently, continued repeating throughout our work together: *"Children blame, adults take responsibility."*

Within a few weeks, Jonathan's work relationships began to improve, as did his personal life. His wife responded to his newly attained transformation with gratitude, and told him how proud she was of his willingness to become accountable for his life. She also praised him for no longer letting his vulnerabilities overpower him when expressing his feelings.

For the first time in his life, Jonathan's haunting need to "prove" himself diminished as he realized he didn't have to seek anyone's attention, approval, or respect other than his own. Jonathan was more honest with others than he had ever known himself to be, which greatly bolstered his sense of courage, confidence, and self-esteem.

Make no mistake, after our work together, Jonathan's life was not free of challenges, disappointments, crisis, or stress. The difference was that he knew how to self-manage—quickly analyze his thoughts to see if they were exaggerations and illusions brought on by imagined fear, or if they were real, useful, and valuable. As a result of his new and efficient self-analytical work, Jonathan learned a lot about his need to be seen a certain way. He also learned to forgive himself for believing he had to be *perfect* if he wanted respect and love. Jonathan realized that loving himself meant accepting his humanity—with all its frailties and strengths.

As Jonathan became more aware of his true nature, and how to apply it into all areas of his life, the physical problems that had plagued him for so long slowly disappeared, and he began sleeping through the night. With greater self-awareness his spirit began healing, and so did his body.

WHAT IS YOGATSU?

YOGATSU is a fusion of the energy practices and spiritual teachings of several Eastern healing traditions, with emphasis on *yoga* and *shiatsu*, hence the name *YOGATSU*. After three decades of studying and working with yoga and shiatsu, I feel confident that *YOGATSU* can serve the public in ways that go beyond taking a yoga class or having a shiatsu treatment. The aim of *YOGATSU* is to help each unique individual *heal from the inside out*; healing the nonphysical mental mindsets, emotional reactivity, and attitudinal misperceptions that chip away at our spirit, sense of purpose, happiness, and health.

YOGATSU therapists collect information from the aura, meridians, and chakras, which I refer to as the Triune Energy Systems (TES) to evaluate the state of health in those systems, and to glean data from each that tells the clients energetic and spiritual stories. To understand the TES, a short, yet concise, explanation of each and what they do is necessary.

Aura

The aura is a color infused, electromagnetic, multi-layered realm of intelligent energy that surrounds the body. The aura is the outer most extension of TES, and works closely with the other two energy systems. The aura is responsible for analyzing everything that happens in our external environment in order to keep us safe. It is also responsible for everything we think and feel so that we are conscious of those thoughts and feelings. Auric energy can become torn and injured by the intentions of others, and most importantly, by the self-inflicted wounds caused by our own habitual negative thoughts and automatic nonproductive actions.

Though the aura is normally depicted as extending out from the body to about six feet, it really does extend out into infinity, picking up nonlocal information about people and upcoming events thousands of miles away. The aura is filled with historical background, and can be labeled as the body's energetic depiction of each person's *biography*.

Meridians

The meridians are channels of energy that run up and down the body, just under the skin. The 14 meridians transport life-giving energy and emotional information to related organs or glands. Example, the heart meridian is responsible for maintaining good energy flow to the physical heart while inspiring the emotions of joy and gratitude, lessening the chances of having to experience emotions of unhappiness and ingratitude. The kidney meridian is responsible for sending energy to the physical kidneys, and helps to keep emotions like trust and courage active, diminishing the opposite emotions of distrust and fear. The trick is to make sure healthy emotions outnumber unhealthy emotions, because healthy emotions maintain good energy flow, and unhealthy emotions do the opposite.

The meridians are very sensitive to emotions. Our emotions influence the ability of each meridian to maintain good energy flow. Each meridian receives energy data from the aura, and then delivers that data to the appropriate meridian. When the aura announces that there is some kind of external or internal danger, the meridians immediately transport that message to the related organ or gland wherein that area of the body is notified and can then determine if that emotion is appropriate, useful, and beneficial, or not. When a meridian has to transport a negative emotion too often, its life-giving energy supply is decreased, rendering the meridian much less capable of maintaining balanced energy distribution to that area of the body, ultimately rendering that body part unable to sustain its normal work, which then produces a *symptom*.

Symptom observation is vital in *YOGATSU* therapy. Every symptom announces which meridian is energetically out of balance, and the emotion that is out of balance.

The following list shows the relationship between each meridian and their related emotional states:

1. **Lung meridian**: *grief*
2. **Large Intestine meridian**: *clinging*
3. **Stomach meridian**: *nervousness*
4. **Spleen/Pancreas meridian**: *control*
5. **Heart meridian**: *joylessness, depression*
6. **Small Intestine meridian**: *obsessive thinking*
7. **Bladder meridian**: *guilt, humiliation, blame*
8. **Kidney meridian**: *fear (of repeating past wounds)*
9. **Pericardium meridian**: *defensiveness*
10. **Triple Warmer meridian**: *stubbornness, stoicism*
11. **Gall Bladder meridian**: *resentment, bitterness*
12. **Liver meridian**: *anger, rage*
13. **Governing Vessel meridian**: *"monkey mind" (chaotic mind state)*

14. **Conception Vessel meridian**: *indecision, confusion*

In *Energy Psychology* symptoms are considered "messengers." The 14 meridians are deeply aware of our emotional history and emotional habits. The meridians are the body's energetic depictions of our emotional *behaviors*.

Chakras

The chakras are seven wheels of spiraling colored energy, each related to one of the seven endocrine glands. The chakras are located deep within the body, close to the spine. Each vortex of spinning energy radiates with universal, soul-level wisdom that moves energy upward from the tailbone to the crown of the head. The chakras exude a strong and definitive relationship with the many life-lessons that are part of the human condition. Each chakra receives inspired wisdom from the depths of our divine intelligence, the *soul,* and inspires us in the best way to apply this wisdom in our everyday lives.

The soul does not have an auditory voice. It cannot be heard as we hear sounds outside our window. Without an auditory voice, the soul uses other forms of communication that are not normally perceived as coming from the soul: intuition, dreams, difficult challenges, crisis, accidents, loss, chronic physical discomfort, and debilitating illness. As expected, illness is the soul's strongest voice, and the evidence of ignoring chakra wisdom.

When we are following chakra guidance, trusting our capabilities, and flowing easily with life, things go smoothly. We feel good, uplifted, excited, creative, and healthy. When we are off track and not listening we feel disappointed, irritated, dull, depressed, creatively unresponsive, and often seriously ill. The following list describes the wisdom and intuitive teachings that the chakras share with us so freely:

1. **Root**: *survival issues, clan, family of origin issues, financial stability*
2. **Sacral**: *one-to-one relationships, individuation, creativity, access to money*
3. **Solar Plexus**: *self-awareness, intellect, confidence, accountability, motivation, courage, tenacity*
4. **Heart**: *authentic love, conscious forgiveness, gratitude, compassion, kindness*

5. **Throat**: *communication, self-honesty, choice, willpower, criticism*
6. **Third Eye**: *commonsense, intuition, wisdom, imagination, ideas*
7. **Crown**: *inspiration, altruism, service, oneness, pure consciousness*

In short, the chakras are the body's energetic depictions of our *biology*.

HOW DOES YOGATSU WORK?

Throughout life we learn survival techniques that help us get through the tough spots. We practice being or doing what we think others want so that they will "see" who we are, and love us. We work diligently, though often unconsciously, to become: the good girl, the tough kid, the caretaker, the funny one, the smartest, the most responsible, the leader, the kindest, the most beautiful, the most reliable, the best communicator, the most articulate, the best mediator, the most caring, etc. etc. As helpful as these survival persona may have been when we were young and needed them to gain notice and affection, the problem is that all too often we become reliant on them, and after decades they become our major means of identification—having only a vague sense of who we were originally. These survival personas, and make no mistake we all have them, served us well when we didn't know any other way to get what we needed. After a while our survival personality becomes the glasses from which we see out into the world. Also, we end up showing the world more of our trained personality than our authentic personage. We lose pieces of ourselves that are true representations of whom we truly are, and who we are meant to be.

My survival personality was created by my mother's need to have me be, and act out, the "big sister." While I did not mind this role when younger, as it did indeed provide extra approval-driven "pats on the head" from my mother, I resented the responsibility of it all as I grew into my teen years. Though I loved my siblings, being the big sister to all of them was a weighty responsibility. I grew up wanting a big sister of my own, which led me to trust many strong women, who entered my life at crucial times, who were unable to fulfill that role for me for any length of time. And why should they? It was a heavy burden for them to carry, and was not fair to them. When I finally understood the reason for my unconscious, constant search for my own big sister, I was able to change my perceptions, and neediness, associated with recreating what I didn't have as a child. I realized I didn't need a strong woman to lean on. I needed to be strong for myself. I needed to be the big sister for the little, frightened girl inside who was still waiting. That was the turning point in my life, and the beginning of my self-realization. Now, I was able to understand what my yoga mentors tried to convey long ago when I was studying to become a yoga teacher. They often said: *"Self-realization is the fastest way to contentment and happiness, health and wellbeing."* With *YOGATSU* therapy, we learn to recognize and claim our authentic selves.

BENEFITS OF YOGATSU THERAPY

With *YOGATSU* therapy, we begin to understand the stupendous workings of the miraculous, energy-filled universe within. We see the TES as ready and able to instruct us in spiritual development, psychological maturation, and physical wellbeing. Fear of change lessens, and the necessity for allowing change into our lives becomes clearer and stronger and, in fact, becomes a gift we give to ourselves.

Our view of suffering changes too, as the result of working with Yoga Psychology, the mainstay of *YOGATSU*. We begin to see suffering as a choice. We accept that while we cannot avoid the pain of life, we can decide if we want to prolong it, moving it into suffering. And there's more. The people we once viewed as enemies become our teachers. Failure becomes insight, and crisis becomes the conduit for growth—and meditation, a staple of YOGATSU therapy, becomes our friend.

MEDITATION

Becoming comfortable with *aloneness* is meditation's greatest gift. Meditation is the quiet inner space where *stillness* and *introspection* can happen. Modern life allows very little time for *solitude*—the process of quieting down without distractions. Solitude invites and encourages the will to change parts of our lives that are no longer working. It creates the inner environment conducive to identifying the patterns of our thoughts, the intentions behind those thoughts, and every choice we make as a result. In the silence of meditation, we become intimate with Self, the most profound and loving relationship we will ever have. Meditation practice brings us back to our natural selves, to that place deep inside where self-confidence overrides self-doubt, and divinity meets potential.

Vast amounts of research show the efficacy of meditation to quell the usual fight-flight-freeze responses associated with stress. With regular meditation practice, we create a place of safeness that allows us to see things as they are, without judgment, and we learn to see life as it is without our misguided illusions. Meditation is a safe place to go where we can quietly and privately look at who we are, both the good and not-so-good, without feeling vulnerable or embarrassed. Meditation is also a "soft place to fall" when the world around seems to be collapsing.

Meditation requires focused attention on breathing, with special emphasis on exhalations as they trigger the relaxation response, in both mind and body. The relaxation response relaxes tight muscles, lowers blood pressure, lessens pain sensitivity, calms the nervous system, strengthens immune function, and creates endorphins, the body's natural anti-depressants. Meditation is an enormously self-healing practice. It teaches us to slow down, breathe, focus, and pay attention. Paying attention in meditation, teaches us to pay attention in life.

For most people, learning to meditate, and to pay attention, starts with the physical body...that's why focusing our attention on the breath is so important. It teaches us to feel what is going on physically, making it easier, and less threatening, to experience and identify what is going on mentally and emotionally.

There are many ways to prepare for meditation. Some people find it easier to sit upright in a chair with hands resting easily on their laps, and others prefer the more traditional practice of sitting on a cushion with legs crossed. Explore both ways and see which one suits your body best. Other than when you are unable to sit up or are ill, it is best not to lie down for meditation as it's too easy to fall asleep.

Meditation requires no equipment, financial outlay, physical training, or special venue. In fact, it requires nothing more than a willingness to sit comfortably, undisturbed, for 10-20 minutes every day, while focusing on the breath. Meditation can be practiced by anyone. All you need is a quiet room without the distraction of the television, radio, or phones. The object of meditation is to become better acquainted with your authentic self. For this, you need to have a serene environment, even if that environment is just a tiny little corner of a room that has been set up in a very sacred and inviting way. I have known people who have set up a little altar space in a closet, as they had no other place in which to create a sacred space. The important thing is to have a place of your own that is conducive to quiet, private contemplation. Keep in mind there is no right or wrong way to meditate.

Meditation forces us to become comfortable with our uncomfortable emotions, because there is nowhere to hide. Meditation is our private psycho-spiritual session. As we become unattached observers of our thoughts, we identify the defensive stances we take when we are not feeling confident and self-assured. We see how ferociously we cling to the exaggerations of a false self that makes real our unhealthy attitudes, and orchestrates our defensive actions toward others. We become privy to the hidden material stored at the level of our subconscious. Through the vehicle of meditation, we see how strongly our egoic mind, which is an element of the subconscious, abhors uncomfortable emotions, truth, change, intuition, accountability, responsibility, hard work, and commonsense.

Peace of mind calls for maintaining awareness of body, mind, thought, emotions—and not just when practicing meditation. Peace of mind requires that we focus on whatever it is we are doing: eating, drinking, chewing, walking, cleaning, gardening, standing, falling asleep, waking up, talking, resting, cooking. We take our meditative mind and brain into whatever is occurring in order to know the best way to approach every situation—without second guessing or beating ourselves up later. Here's a parable that the Buddha shared with his monks relating the value and necessity of paying attention.

There was a group of people gathered around a famous beauty queen, watching her sing and dance. A man came along, and was handed a bowl filled to the brim with oil and told he must carry the bowl on his head between the crowd and the beauty queen without spilling a drop, or a man following along behind with a sword will cut off his head. "What do you think monks?" the Buddha asked. "Will that man allow himself to be distracted from the bowl of oil?" Naturally, the monks said no.

Life is just one situation after another in which we have to choose between staying mindful or losing our heads. Meditation establishes and enhances resiliency and psychological hardiness. It helps us practice self-efficacy for management of disturbing moods and painful memories, and empowers us with a skill set that develops our ability to respond objectively to strong emotional experiences, using conscious choice rather than habit-driven, unconscious, and automatic reactivity.

STAGES OF MEDITATION

1. *Breath awareness*—following the breath focuses and calms the mind
2. *Relaxation*—with a calm mind, body begins to soften into a restful state
3. *"Monkey mind"*—overactive mind, restless
4. *Dark night of the soul*—personal truths, illusions, spiritual purification
5. *Surrender*—letting go, humility
6. *Insight*—intuition, wisdom
7. *Pure joy*—bliss from not fighting what is

Every time you meditate, it will be different for no two meditations are alike. Sometimes, you will experience all seven stages, and other times only the first three. The point is practice. The more you practice, the calmer you become, and the more calm, the greater health. Go gently into meditation without expectation. With regular meditation practice, you will receive such stunning benefits that you may no longer dread it, but long for it. Namaste.

About the Author

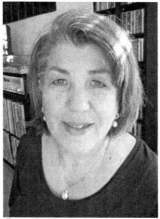

Alice Percy Strauss is the founder and director of the **Yogatsu Institute for Conscious Living and Healing Studies.** She is member of the *International Association of Yoga Therapists*, both as a practicing yoga therapist, and registered yoga therapy school.

Alice is also a member of *Yoga Alliance* as an E-RYT-500 (highest teacher category) and a 200 hour registered yoga therapy school. She is a Certified Master Instructor in Acupressure, Shiatsu, and Reflexology with the *National Therapies Certification Board*, and holds a seat on their Accreditation Council.

Alice has authored two books, several textbooks, and writes a monthly newsletter. In addition, Alice has lectured and taught internationally: Australia, Germany, Korea, and Japan. She is available for private sessions or educational offerings at the Yogatsu Institute.

Alice Percy Strauss can be contacted at:
www.yogatsuinstitute.com

BELIEF

In the dark of the night
in the light of the day
through troubled times
and peaceful ways

In a flower-filled meadow
or hot asphalt road
when you fear "all is lost"
but you know there's still hope

Brains mired in thoughts
hearts flowing with love
A shadow is lurking
feather floats from above

Hands busily working
sweet scents fill the air
Quick! Turn around
but no one is there

You think it's all over
yet it's only begun
petals fall from the vine
seasons turning around

Chest pounding wildly
tears fall to the ground
for Miracles witnessed -
Heavenly Angels Abound!

~Beatrice Hagen April 12, 2011

About the Author

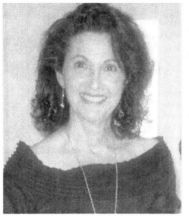

Beatrice Hagen has always found faith and inspiration in her spirituality and an unwavering belief in the angelic realm with their divine power to love, comfort, protect and inspire.

She considers her creativity and writings to be a divine gift, and is blessed with inspiration through meditation and her love of nature and music.

Beatrice spent most her adult life as an executive assistant to a corporate vice president and has an educational background in art and interior design. She currently resides in Southern Nevada with her husband, their dog Oreo, and is the proud mother of three wonderful grown children and two amazing grandsons.

Beatrice Hagan can be contacted at:
www.enchantedbeequilts.com
enchantedbeequilts@yahoo.com
(702) 292-7384

Final Thoughts

It is always amazing to me to see how each one of us who shares our method(s) of connecting to our higher power can say much the same thing as the others, yet, have it be unique. This allows for us to make available to you the reader various techniques to make your own connection. As you have journeyed through this book, you will find the right modalities for you, the ones that resonate with you and make you feel the most comfortable.

For some, to live a spiritual life means doing all the "right" things expected of them by society or what they have been taught in any of the religions that they have practiced.

In reality, to live a spiritual life means to connect with your inner knowings of the ways to live in harmony with your higher power and the spirit of unconditional love where we all are one. We are a people who live with feelings and emotions of which there are two overriding ones – love and fear.

When we live our lives with love, there are no judgments or ego that creates fear.

When we live our lives with trust in the Universe or Source, there is peace and joy, knowing that what happens in our lifetime is either because that is what we contracted for this lifetime or is for our highest purpose.

We have been given "free will" to allow us the opportunity to make choices and to experience what our choices bring about. Sometimes, those choices can be painful and that is when some of us want to blame God for not stepping in to prevent us from any suffering. It must be clearly understood that the Universe wants all the best things for us and it is we with our human ways that get in the way. Part of the journey for each one of us is to learn to take responsibility for what is ours and own it. If it does not belong to you, let it go! Live your life with love!

There is so much wasted energy spent on emotions and worries that have nothing to do with us. Wonder if this same energy was spent on praying for or sending love to those living on the streets, or children without parents or homes, or animals that are beaten and left behind, or those suffering with abuse, or anyone less fortunate that we are? There is power in prayer and if we would take just one minute a day to send out love for those who need it, the vibration of our entire world would change. Remember that the love energy is infinite...

Because the Universe wants the best for each one of us, we are given clues and different messages giving guidance and comfort. We just need to be open to receiving those messages. We create our own life, day by day, minute by minute, second by second. We have that power!

We also have the tools through the modalities presented in this book to create the best energy flow for good health, to receive guidance for the possibilities in our life, to understand the positive spirit energies that surround us, and to appreciate the opportunity to journey on our spiritual path for our own spiritual growth. There are other modalities that aren't a part of this book, such as some of the different types of yoga. I encourage you to seek out any of the other ones to see if they fit into your comfort zone and try them out! Every way that brings love, joy and peace in your life that is to your highest good and the highest good of others, I encourage you to look into and do.

You have heard this expression, I'm sure: "Life is for the Living." There is a lot to be said regarding that expression. It is important to live your life with zest. Albert Einstein said, "There are two ways to live your life. One is as though nothing is a miracle. The other as though everything is a miracle."

Mother Teresa, a magnificent woman and healer, a woman who lived unconditional love of all, and voted "Woman of the Century" had this to say about life:

"Life is an opportunity – benefit from it
 Life is beauty – admire it
 Life is bliss – taste it
 Life is a dream – realize it
 Life is a challenge – meet it
 Life is a duty – complete it
 Life is a game – play it
 Life is a promise – fulfill it
 Life is sorrow – overcome it
 Life is a song – sing it
 Life is a struggle – accept it
 Life is a tragedy – confront it
 Life is an adventure – dare it
 Life is luck – make it
 Life is too precious – don't destroy it
 Life is life – fight for it"

I honor the place in you
In which the entire universe abides.
I honor the place in you
Which is of love, truth, light and peace.
When you are in that place in you
And I am in that place in me
We are one...

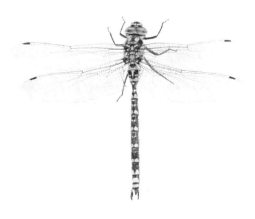

Namaste

CPSIA information can be obtained at www.ICGtesting.com
Printed in the USA
BVOW041619211011

274082BV00004BA/1/P

9 780982 460726